Mountain Medicine

Mountain Medicine

A clinical study of cold and high altitude

Michael Ward, M.A., M.D., F.R.C.S.

Crosby Lockwood Staples   London

Granada Publishing Limited
First published in Great Britain 1975 by Crosby Lockwood Staples Limited
Frogmore St Albans Herts AL2 2NF and
3 Upper James Street London W1R 4BP

ISBN 0 258 96989 X

Printed in Great Britain by
William Clowes & Sons, Limited, London, Beccles and Colchester

Acknowledgements

Thanks are due for permission to reproduce illustrations from the following sources:
Figures 2, 3, 15, 16, 17, 19 and Table 10
   High altitude by L. G. C. E. Pugh, in *Physiology of human survival*, ed. O. Edholm and A. L. Bacharach. Academic Press: New York and London, 1965.
Figures 5, 8, 13 and 14
   Textbook of medical physiology by A. C. Guyton. W. B. Saunders: Philadelphia, 1971.
Figure 9
   Everest. The unfinished adventure by H. Ruttledge. Hodder and Stoughton: London, 1937.
Figure 20
   L. G. C. E. Pugh in *Nature* **209,** 1966, 1281-1285. Macmillan Journals Ltd: London.
Figure 21
   J. D. Nelms in *Journal of the Royal Naval Medical Service* **58,** 1972, 192. Institute of Naval Medicine: Alverstoke, Hants.

Preface

Mountaineering and mountain exploration have always presented two faces—the romantic and the scientific. The physical and mental disciplines imposed by the mountain environment are exacting and the penalty for failure to observe these disciplines is usually severe. Everyone who goes into the mountains is exposed to the stress of cold; the stress of high altitude is an additional factor in the Andes and Himalayas and the topography of mountain country carries its own inherent dangers.

The origins of mountaineering and of respiratory physiology are interwoven and many important observations have been made by laymen as well as scientists and especially by those who have been to Mt Everest.

This book has been written for all who are interested in the effects that the stresses of the mountain environment impose—it is for doctors, physiologists, human and medical geographers, mountaineers and skiers. It explains how adaptations are made, how the failure of these mechanisms leads to illness. It describes the treatment of these illnesses. It also includes a section on accidents and another on the biology of mountain populations, as well as an historical survey.

Because of the differing interests and knowledge of those who may wish to use this book I have included a certain amount of basic physiological information. With this background the more complex adaptations to and the clinical features of cold and high altitude can be more easily understood by those who are non-specialists.

Much of the work has been carried out in the field and my interest in the subject dates from the time when I was working for the Primary Fellowship of the Royal College of Surgeons of England and concurrently taking part in the first successful ascent of Everest in 1953.

So many people over the years have contributed both directly and indirectly to this book that it would be impossible to name them all. I would however like to mention four. Dr O. G. Edholm, Head of the Division of Human Physiology of the Medical Research Council to whom I, and many others, owe a great debt over many years for the constructive influence he has had on expeditions to the Himalaya and Polar regions, has looked through my manuscript and advised me on its final form.

Dr Griffith Pugh of the MRC's Laboratory of Field Physiology has been responsible for much original field work on cold and high altitude and it has been a privilege as well as a pleasure to work with him in the field, particularly on Everest in 1953 and during the Winter of 1960 and 1961 in the Silver Hut in the Everest region.

Dr James Milledge of the MRC's Clinical Research Centre, Northwick Park Hospital, has commented on the section on respiration and high-altitude disease; while Professor Edward Williams, Director of the Institute of Nuclear Medicine, Middlesex Hospital Medical College, has advised me on the endocrine section.

For the omissions that may be found I must apologise and take refuge in the words of the Chinese historian Tai T'Ung— 'Were I to await perfection my books would never be written'.

Lastly I would like to thank my family for maintaining their equanimity in the face of my absences in the operating theatre, in the Library, and in the field.

Michael Ward
November 1974

Contents

Photographs between pages 138 and 139

Large goitre
Frostbite of feet
Feet of a pilgrim able to walk barefoot in snow
Silver Hut in the Everest region
Bicycle ergometer
Exhaustion and frostbite
Protective clothing

CHAPTER ONE

History

The following short historical account traces the development of interest in high altitudes from the level of a traveller's tale to the establishment of permanent research stations.

Inevitably it is also concerned with the exploration of the world's mountain ranges and with the ascents of the highest peaks, particularly Mt Everest.

Many of the earliest and very accurate descriptions of clinical conditions were made by laymen, who have made important contributions to this subject.

Possibly the first communication on illness in mountains is contained in Plutarch's account of the crossing into India by Alexander in 326 BC. He comments: 'Many then were the dangers he (Alexander) underwent in those encounters and serious the wounds he received; but the greatest harm to his expedition came from their lack of necessary supplies and from the unsteadiness of the atmosphere' (alternative translation, 'severity of weather') (Plutarch 1912).

A Chinese official, Tu-Chhin, in about 100 AD, advised the Prime Minister, Wang Feng, not to send ambassadors to Chi-Pin (probably an area including Afghanistan, Gandhara, Kashmir, and the Upper Indus Basin). He argued that 'after passing the Phi-Shan Mountains...one must cross the Greater and Lesser Headache Mountains, chains of naked and burning rocks so named because they cause headache, dizziness and vomiting. Then comes the San-Chhih-Phan Gorge, thirty li long where the path is only 16 or 17 inches wide, on the edge of a precipice and where travellers have to be tied together with ropes. From here to Hsientu it is 3000 li and more, on a road full of dangers.'

The Phi-Shan mountains have been identified with the Kara-kach pass between Khotan in the Tarim Basin and the Head-ache Mountains (the Tibetan plateau), and the San-Chhih-Phan as the Karakorum Pass.

It has been suggested too that mountain sickness may have been taken as a sign for the Chinese not to transgress their natural geographical boundaries (Needham 1954).

In 1519, Cortes sent Diego Ordaz with nine Spaniards and some Indians to attempt the ascent of Mt Popacatepetl 17,500 ft (5334 m). The Indians fled at a height of 13,000 ft (3962 m)—but the Spaniards persisted above the snow line. They remarked 'to increase their distress respiration became so difficult that every effort was attended with sharp pains in the head and limbs'. Two years later, Francisco Montano and four Spaniards reached the summit and obtained sulphur from the crater for the manufacture of gun powder (Prescott 1891).

Reports in 1557 on the Government of the Incas indicate that they were aware of some of the affects of altitude. 'It was an order of the Inca that the upland Indians, those of the cold country, were not to go down to these coastal plains, since they were lowlands and hot lands ten leagues wide and they would die, and likewise that the lowland Indians should not go up to the cold highlands' (Urteago–Romero 1920).

Father Joseph de Acosta gave one of the first and probably the most detailed descriptions of 'mountain' sickness, when cros-sing a pass 14,000 ft (4267 m) in the Andes in 1570.

'I have wanted to say all this in order to describe a strange effect which the air or the wind which blows has in certain lands of the Indies namely that men get seasick with it no less, yea even more than at sea. . .' (De Acosta 1608).

The Spanish Conquistadors noted the infertility of their livestock at high altitudes and this may have been a factor in the transfer of their capital from Jauja 10,900 ft (3300 m) to Lima 500 ft (150 m). In the Act for the founding of Lima, it was pointed out concerning the city of Jauja, that the 'great disadvantage and lack felt by the citizens who peopled this said city in that neither there nor in its surroundings nor anywhere in the Upland could pigs be raised nor mares nor fowls because of the great cold and sterility of the land and because we have seen by experience among the many mares that have dropped colts their offspring usually die'.

Fertility in man could also be affected. When the Imperial City of Potosi 13,000 ft (4002 m) was founded there were 100,000 native Indians and 20,000 Spaniards. The Indians reproduced with customary fertility whilst the Spaniards either remained infertile or their babies did not survive. The mothers used to leave Potosi and stay at lower altitudes in order to give birth. They remained until the child was more than a year old.

The birth of the first Spaniard did not take place until 53 years after the founding of the city, and this occasion on Christmas Eve 1598 was attributed to a miracle by St Nicholas of Tolentino (Calancha 1639). Later the Spaniards did reproduce intensively and crossed their race with the local inhabitants.

In 1661 a Jesuit, Father Grüber remarked of travel in Tibet: 'Man cannot breathe in the Langur mountains because the air is so subtle'. He adds, 'In summer certain poisonous weeds grow there which exhale such a bad smelling dangerous odour that one cannot stay up there without risk of losing one's life, nay, not even cross the mountains without danger to life'.

In 1716, Father Desideri, another Jesuit, comments

> Many people believe that the discomfort one experiences arises from the reek from certain materials that occur in the interior of the Langur mountains: but as no unmistakeable traces of such minerals have been found hitherto, I rather believe that the unpleasant symptoms are due to the thin sharp air. I am more inclined to this view because my pain became still more unendurable when the wind rose, and I suffered from excruciating headache just on the tops of the Langur mountains.

Father Beligatti in 1739 alludes to the 'Singular influence which the mountains exercise over both men and animals whether this arises from the rarefaction of the atmosphere or from deleterious exhalations' (Hedin 1913).

Table 1.   Altitude–pressure table based on the United States Standard atmosphere-feet-millimetres of mercury.

| Altitude | | Pressure | Altitude | | Pressure |
Feet	Metres	mmHg	Feet	Metres	mmHg
0	0	760·0	21,000	6,401	334·8
1,000	305	733·0	22,000	6,706	320·8
2,000	610	706·6	23,000	7,010	307·4
3,000	914	681·0	24,000	7,315	294·4
4,000	1,219	656·4	25,000	7,620	282·0
5,000	1,524	632·4	26,000	7,925	269·8
6,000	1,829	609·0	27,000	8,230	258·2
7,000	2,134	586·4	28,000	8,534	246·8
8,000	2,438	564·4	29,000	8,839	236·0
9,000	2,743	543·2	30,000	9,144	225·6
10,000	3,048	522·6	31,000	9,449	215·4
11,000	3,353	502·6	32,000	9,754	205·8
12,000	3,658	483·2	33,000	10,058	196·4
13,000	3,962	464·6	34,000	10,363	187·4
14,000	4,267	446·4	35,000	10,668	178·7
15,000	4,572	428·8	36,000	10,973	170·4
16,000	4,877	411·8	37,000	11,278	162·4
17,000	5,182	395·4	38,000	11,582	154·9
18,000	5,486	379·4	39,000	11,887	147·6
19,000	5,791	364·0	40,000	12,192	140·7
20,000	6,096	349·2			

In Europe, the physiologist Borelli described the phenomenon of mountain sickness during his ascent of Mt Etna in 1671 and endeavoured to explain this by theories of 'blood effervescence and force' (Mosso 1898). Prior to 1760 it was considered dangerous even to climb above the Montanvert, about 3000 ft (900 m) above Chamonix in the French Alps and now a small station, and in the latter half of the eighteenth century, fear of mountain sickness was very great.

De Saussure in 1760 describes symptoms occurring between 10,000 ft (3048 m) and 14,000 ft (4267 m) as 'faintness accompanied generally by vomiting, indescribable uneasiness, anxiety, thirst, no appetite, and tendency to sleep' (Mathews 1898).

Balmat complained of a severe headache at about 13,000 ft (3962 m) the night before his successful attempt on the summit of Mt Blanc in 1786 with Dr Paccard, who suffered considerably from breathlessness.

Humboldt in 1802 climbed to 18,500 ft (5637 m) on Mt Chimborazo in the Andes of Ecuador. During the latter part of his ascent he complained of malaise, nausea, and giddiness. He and his companions also suffered from bleeding from the lips and gums (Bruhns 1872). He explained the fatigue of mountain climbing as a simple physical effect of diminished barometric pressure. 'The thigh bone tends to slip out of its socket in the pelvis, because the pressure of the air does not suffice to keep it in its place. On this account we must first perform a greater muscular effort, and afterwards can no longer move the legs with ease' (Mosso 1898).

J. Tschudi relates how after a year in Peru, he rode up to a height of 15,000 ft (4500 m) on a mule. As the mule was tired he dismounted and proceeded on foot. 'An indisposition such as I had never felt before caused me increasing discomfort at every step...My heart beat so violently that I could hear its palpitations. My breathing was short and broken...My senses became inert, a mist spread before my sight, I trembled and had to stretch myself on the ground' (Mosso 1898).

In 1804 Gay Lussac and Biot ascended to 13,000 ft (3960 m) by balloon. About three weeks later Gay Lussac reached an altitude of 23,000 ft (7020 m). He reported difficulty in breathing, increased pulse and respiration, and difficulty in swallowing due to dryness of the mouth and throat resulting from breathing the 'dry attenuated air' (Wise 1873).

In 1808 the Italians, Andreoli and Brioschi reached a height of about 30,000 ft (9000 m). At 23,000 ft (7077 m) Brioschi was overcome by a 'gentle sleep'; at 30,000 ft (9060 m) Andreoli observed that he could not move his left hand. The lowest barometric reading was 216 mmHg (c. 31,000 ft (9450 m))—however the balloon burst and the ruptured balloon acting like a parachute, they landed unharmed (Bert 1878). Glaisher later pointed out that Andreoli had made many balloon flights and was tolerant to the effects of lowered barometric pressure.

The Gerards explored the Spiti–Tibet frontier of Central Asia in 1818 and 1821. In addition to the usual symptoms of mountain sickness they noted that headache was almost constant above 17,000 ft (5182 m).

The Schlagintweit brothers and eight natives slept for ten consecutive nights on Mt Ibi Gamin in the Garwhal Himal in 1855 at heights ranging from 16,642 ft (5060 m) to 19,326 ft (5800 m). The two brothers reached a height of 22,259 ft (6900 m). This record stood for 30 years. They were experienced mountaineers and they considered that complaints due to low barometric pressures were, 'Headache, difficulty of respiration even to occasional blood spitting; bleeding at the nose rare; bleeding at ears and lips never experienced; want of appetite, muscular weakness, and general depression of spirits. All symptoms disappeared on return to lower levels'. They noted that symptoms varied greatly in different individuals; and in general humans began to feel low barometric pressure at 16,500 ft (5030 m) whilst horses and camels suffered above 17,500 ft (5334 m) (Schlagintweit 1862).

During the ascent of Mt Demavend 18,500 ft (5670 m) in 1862 Michele Lessona and Filippo de Filippi commented, 'The rarefaction of the air occasioned me more distress than the cold: at an altitude of 12,500 ft (3600 m) I suffered from a severe attack of nocturnal asthma...My symptoms were nausea, dizziness, oppressed breathing, and an invincible desire to sleep as soon as I stopped to rest a little' (De Filippi 1865).

Glaisher with Coxwell between 1862 and 1866 made a series of balloon flights and obtained much valuable meteorological information. In 1862 they ascended to over 29,000 ft (8839 m) where Glaisher became unconscious. He was aroused by Coxwell—who having lost the use of his hands opened the escape valve with his teeth. Neither seems to have suffered any serious cerebral damage and Glaisher lived to be 94 years old. He summarised the effects of low barometric pressure thus

> The number of pulsations usually increased with the elevation, as also (did) the number of respirations: the number of my pulsations was generally 76 per minute before starting, about 90 at 10,000 ft (3048 m), 100 at 20,000 ft (6096 m) and 110 at higher

elevations; but the increase in height was not the only element for the number of pulsations depended also on the health of the individual. They also, of course, varied in different persons, depending much on their temperament. This was the case too in respect to colour; at 10,000 ft (3048 m) the face of some would be of a glowing purple whilst others would scarcely be affected. At 17,000 ft (5182 m) my lips were blue; at 19,000 ft (5791 m) both my hands and lips were dark blue; at four miles high the pulsations of my heart were audible, and my breathing was very much affected; at 29,000 ft (8839 m) I became insensible.

Glaisher believed that repeated balloon flights led to acclimatisation to high altitude. He stated 'that the diminished pressure of the air...acts with far greater force upon an individual who ascends for the first time than ever afterwards'. He goes on, 'at length I became so acclimatised to the effects of the rarefied atmosphere that I could breathe at an elevation of four miles at least above the earth without inconvenience. At six and seven miles high I experienced the limit of our power of breathing in the attenuated atmosphere' (Glaisher *et al.* 1871).

Mt Elbruz in the Caucasus 18,470 ft (5637 m) was climbed in 1868. The actual ascent of 6500 ft (1882 m) was made in $7\frac{1}{2}$ hours, and none of the party was affected by illness (Freshfield 1869). Between 1860 and 1865 W. H. Johnson climbed peaks of 21,000 ft (6400 m) in the Kuen Lun in Northern Tibet and ascended to 22,000 ft (6706 m) whilst crossing a ridge in Ladakh. He mentions no symptoms of mountain sickness and experienced less discomfort than in a decompression chamber.

Paul Bert was able in 1869 to build a decompression chamber large enough to hold a human being and his experiments led him to conclude that the effects of altitude could be avoided by breathing oxygen.

In 1874 Croce-Spinelli and Sivel ascended by balloon to over 20,000 ft (6000 m). The lowest barometric reading recorded was 300 mmHg (23,000 ft (7000 m)). At an altitude of 12,000 ft (3600 m) they breathed a mixture 40 per cent oxygen and above 20,000 ft (6000 m) a 70 per cent mixture of oxygen. They experienced less discomfort than in a decompression chamber.

The next year Croce-Spinelli, Sivel and Tissandier, despite a warning from Paul Bert that their oxygen supply was inadequate, started a balloon ascent. They decided to use oxygen only when they considered it necessary. The results are well known. At an altitude of 26,000 ft (8000 m) Croce-Spinelli and Sivel died. Tissandier only survived. In his account Tissandier states that the last record of height he wrote in a book was a barometric pressure of 300 mmHg at an altitude of 24,000 ft (7450 m). He wanted to use the oxygen tube but could not raise his arm. He noted that the pressure fell to 280 mmHg c. 25,000 ft (7620 m) and he then became unconscious at 1.30 pm. He regained consciousness about 40 minutes later when the balloon was descending. Croce then threw out more ballast and the balloon ascended—Tissandier fainted again to open his eyes at 3.30 pm and found both his companions dead.

In 1878 Paul Bert published his book *La Pression Barométrique*. In this he showed that oxygen deficiency was the main feature in all the biological effects of decreased barometric pressure.

Edward Whymper—best known for his successful and tragic first ascent of the Matterhorn in 1865—gave one of the best accounts of mountain sickness during an expedition to the Andes of Central America. At his second camp at 16,664 ft (5000 m) on Mt Chimborazo 20,545 ft (6250 m) Whymper and his two guides were incapacitated although they had ridden up by mule. Intense headache, laboured respiration, increased pulse and a temperature of 38°C, were the symptoms which lasted for 24 to 36 hours. Two days later they moved to a camp at 17,285 ft (5250 m). They seemed to have grown weaker though their headaches had gone. They reached the summit a few days later.

In the following month they stayed for 26 consecutive days at or around 19,000 ft (5791 m) without serious inconvenience. They ascended Mt Antisana 17,623 ft (5350 m) and Mt Cayambe 19,186 ft (5800 m) without headache or unpleasant symptoms beyond some shortness of breath that was also noted on the second ascent of Mt Chimborazo 20,545 ft (6250 m).

Whymper divided the clinical effects of low barometric pressure into two categories, transitory and permanent. The first included an increase in heart rate, rise in temperature, and in-

creased pressure in blood vessels. The second consisted of increased rate and manner of respiration, indisposition to take
food, and lessening of muscular power. At no time did they or
any of the natives they employed show any sign of haemorrhage
or nausea (Whymper 1892).

In 1883 Graham ascended Mt Kabru 24,000 ft (7315 m) in
the Sikkim Himal. He camped at 18,500 ft (5637 m) and reached
the summit in $9\frac{1}{2}$ hours without suffering any symptoms.

Viault made the first careful red cell counts during his journey
through the Andes of Peru and Bolivia in 1890. He found that
his red cell count had risen from 5×10^6 at sea-level to $7\cdot5-$
$8\cdot0 \times 10^6$ at Morococha 15,000 ft (4540 m) and that this increase had occurred during a short time (Viault 1891). By
contrast, Paul Bert had thought that this change could only take
place gradually through adaptation over generations staying at
high altitude.

In 1891 Egli-Sinclair and two companions spent ten days at
the Bosses hut on Mt Blanc at 14,500 ft (4420 m) suffering
considerable loss of appetite, loss of weight, and an increase in
pulse and respiration (Mosso 1898).

Egli-Sinclair also commented in a book that he wrote about
mountain-sickness, that the respiration 'had the Stokes character' (Egli-Sinclair 1893). In fact a disorder of respiration at
high altitude had been noted by Hirst when he made an ascent
of Mt Blanc in 1857 with Prof. Tyndall. Tyndall fell asleep
near the summit and Hirst roused him saying, 'You quite
frightened me. I have listened for some minutes and have not
heard you breathe once' (Tyndall 1906).

In 1891, after ascending Mt Blanc 15,800 ft (4800 m) Dr
Jacottet became increasingly breathless, cyanosed, and coughed
a great deal. After a few hours in a hut at 14,300 ft (4360 m)
he died. The initial diagnosis was pneumonia, 'confirmed' at
post-mortem. There seems little doubt, however, that this was a
case of pulmonary oedema, and probably the first so recorded
(Mosso 1898).

In 1892, W. M. Conway ascended Pioneer Peak 22,600 ft
(6850 m) in the Karakoram Himal. From the last camp at
20,000 ft (6096 m) to the top took $6\frac{3}{4}$ hours, whilst the descent

took an hour only. As a general observation he commented: 'We seemed to become less able to hold out against altitude the longer we remained at a higher level'. He also mentions 'that in the Himalaya he experienced discomfort when his arms hung down by his sides and relief when he supported them on the hip' (Conway 1894). This was an example of using the accessory muscles of respiration to aid breathing by fixing the arms, clavicle and scapula.

In 1894 a group of men with seven scientists and two guides climbed up to the Théodule Pass 11,800 ft (3500 m) above Zermatt in the Swiss Alps. One of the first physiological expeditions to enquire into the effects of high altitude, it was led by Hugo Kronecker, Professor of Physiology at Berne. He was studying the effects of passive transport on human beings because plans were being discussed for the building of a railroad to the top of the Jungfrau 13,800 ft (4158 m) (Kronecker 1903).

In the same year, 1894, Angelo Mosso climbed the Italian side of Monte Rosa with a group of twelve scientists and a large number of soldiers. At the Cabanna Regina Margarita, constructed by the Italian Alpine Club on the Punta Gniffeti 14,900 ft (4560 m) one of the summits of Monte Rosa, he carried out a number of physiological experiments.

Later, Mosso exposed himself for 25 minutes to a pressure of 13·4 inches Hg (23,000 ft (c. 7010 m)) in a decompression chamber. He felt dull and apathetic. Recovering, he lowered the pressure to 11·5 inches Hg (27,000 ft (c. 8230 m)). Oxygen was then let into the chamber and the pressure further lowered to 7·5 inches Hg. Oxygen then formed 8·14 per cent of the atmosphere. At this point he became too apathetic to pick up a pencil that he had dropped.

In 1895, Collie, Hastings and Mummery attempted Mt Nanga Parbat 26,658 ft (8130 m). Beyond some minor symptoms when first ascending to 18,000 ft (5486 m) they felt extremely well up to 21,000 ft (6400 m).

In 1895 the Russian Central Asian traveller, Roborowsky, whilst crossing the Mangu Pass 14,000 ft (4267 m) suffered a transient stroke which lasted eight days, before he recovered enough to move (Roborowsky 1896).

In 1901, the Cabanna Margarita on Monte Rosa was created an International Laboratory for high altitude research with financial support from Ernest Solvay. This was the first permanent site to be set up for such a purpose.

During the British Expedition to Lhasa, 1903–4, L. A. Waddel of the Indian Medical Service noted how people gradually became acclimatised. The Sikh Pioneers, and the Madras and Bengal Sappers and Miners were employed in road making at altitudes of 10–15,000 ft (3050–4572 m). 'The results of this exposure to cold and high altitude were chiefly pneumonia, frostbite, and mountain sickness'. Everyone wore green or smoked glass goggles against snow-blindness. 'Mountain sickness was experienced by nearly everyone more or less at high-altitude, in the form of headache and nausea, occasionally with retching and vomiting.' 'There was an undoubted craving for an extra amount of sugar and butter' (Waddell 1905).

Longstaff spent five nights on Mt Gurla Mandhata at altitudes above 19,000 ft (5790 m) in 1905. He says that most of the symptoms he noted seem to have been due to food and fluid lack, poor shelter and 'sun-stroke'. His party spent three days over 23,000 ft (7010 m) and climbed to just over 24,000 ft (7315 m). He noted that the two guides who were with him seemed more or less unaffected by altitude, and considered that the more experienced the mountaineer the less liable he was to mountain sickness. He noted that after a day at high altitude micturition was infrequent and scanty, and considered that the high haemoglobin percentage was due to haemo-concentration. He also observed Cheyne–Stokes respiration to start at about 9700 ft (3000 m); and comments on the value of sugar in the diet. Longstaff recorded, 'that at these altitudes, 15–23,000 ft (4572–7010 m), I have also been conscious of an indefinite deterioration of the physical and mental powers which I can best describe as lassitude and apathy' (Longstaff 1906).

The term 'mountain lassitude' was coined by C. G. Bruce. By this he meant, 'Diminution in the strength of a man due to diminished atmospheric pressure. This weakness is progressive and affects physical, mental and will power'.

Longstaff considered that mountain sickness was due to a

combination of physical exertion, 'want of condition', and poverty of diet. In 1907, he climbed Trisul 23,360 ft (7180 m) ascending from 17,450 ft (5230 m) and climbing 6000 ft (1830 m) in ten hours. He noticed no symptoms of mountain sickness.

A new institute named after Mosso was opened in 1907 at the Col d'Oleu 10,000 ft (2900 m) in the Italian Alps.

In 1909 on the Duke of Abruzzi's expedition to Bride Peak in the Karakoram, twelve Europeans and fifteen coolies lived and worked regularly for about two months at 17,000 ft (5182 m). There was no single case of illness attributable to mountain sickness.

Seven Europeans spent nine days at heights of more than 20,700 ft (6390 m), four of them camping for a night at 21,673 ft (6550 m) and 22,483 ft (6850 m). They made two ascents to 23,458 ft (7160 m) and 24,600 ft (7500 m) 'without exhaustion, without exaggerated breathing, palpitation or irregularity of the pulse; and with no symptoms of headache, nausea or the like'. De Filippi continues

> The atmosphere of these heights did work some evil effect, revealing itself only gradually, after several weeks of life above 17,000 ft (5182 m) in a slow decrease in appetite, and consequent lack of nourishment, without, however any disturbance of the digestive functions. It was possible for the lack of appetite to increase and become almost absolute repugnance to food, if after its appearance one moved and established oneself at a greater height. Perfect adaptation to surroundings is not possible above 17,000 ft (5182 m).

He also comments later that 'the people of Upper Ladakh are averse to descending lower than 10,000 ft (3048 m) and positively refuse to go below 7,000 ft (2134 m) for fear of illness'. He further said 'One would say that mountain sickness, once a necessary evil of mountain climbing, is gradually disappearing, in the same way that scurvy ceased to be an inevitable accompaniment of polar expeditions' (De Filippi 1912).

This height, 24,600 ft (7500 m), remained the highest altitude attained by mountaineers until the first Everest expeditions.

In the meantime controversy had arisen around the physiology of respiratory exchange in the lungs. It began with Muller's declaration in 1870 that the interchange was a secretory process, a position taken up and held consistently by Haldane from 1898 to 1922.

The secretion theory of oxygenation in the lungs gained considerable support from observations made on Pike's Peak (Douglas *et al.* 1913), when the oxygen pressure in arterial blood was 88 mmHg or 35 mmHg higher than the normal resting alveolar Po_2 of 53 mmHg.

The invention by Pfluger in 1869 of the aerotonometer to measure gas tensions enabled the matter to be tested by various investigators and finally in 1915, Krogh with her microtonometer seemed to decide in favour of the physical diffusion. She showed that in an unacclimatised person, diffusion can take care of the oxygen requirement at an altitude of 25,000 ft (7600 m 270 mmHg).

Haldane, however, was still not convinced, and he in competition with Barcroft ascended to higher and higher altitudes, exposing themselves and their companions to progressively lower atmospheric pressures, or to reduced oxygen tension in decompression chambers. Finally Barcroft took an arterial blood sample from an individual who had been kept at an oxygen pressure of 84 mmHg for six days (17,000 ft or 5200 m). Estimation of Po_2 in arterial blood both at work and at rest led to the conclusion that the Po_2 was less in the arterial blood than in the alveolar air.

Further experiments in the Andes in 1921–2 at 14,000 ft (4267 m) and on dogs confirmed this view, whilst other work in 1929 and 1935 failed to confirm the secretion hypothesis.

Finally it became universally agreed that oxygen uptake by the lungs is effected as a result of the difference in partial pressures, and not as an act of secretion of oxygen from air to blood.

In 1910 Barcroft, Douglas and Zuntz went to the Pic of Teneriffe (Alta Vista Hut 11,000 ft (3400 m)). Pike's Peak, in the United States of America, 14,200 ft (4312 m) was used by Schneider and his colleagues in 1907–11 and by Haldane in 1912.

Barcroft was one of the first to see the possibilities of the Andes as a centre for high altitude research, especially as a railway had been built from Lima to altitudes above 13,000 ft (4000 m) at Cerro de Pasco 14,000 ft (4200 m) and Morococha 15,000 ft (4540 m).

A. M. Kellas climbed to 23,600 ft (7210 m) on Mt Kamet in the Garwhal Himal and observed, as have some others, that the altitude at which mountain sickness is met varies with the locality. 'It is met with at 10,000 ft (3000 m) in the Alps and Caucasus, at 13,000 ft (4000 m) in the Andes, and at 16,500 ft (5000 m) in the Himalaya'.

Members of Himalayan and especially Everest expeditions have made a considerable number of observations of the effects of extreme altitude.

In 1921 Mallory (Howard-Bury 1922) commented on how rapidly some mountaineers acclimatised and that they were capable of great exertion between 18,000 and 20,000 ft (5486 and 6100 m). Later he noted that 'the whole machine appeared to be running down'.

In 1922 four men ascended without oxygen to 27,000 ft (8230 m) on Mt Everest. Somervell (Bruce 1923) first used the term high-altitude deterioration. He considered that after a period above 18,000 ft (5486 m) the physical condition of individuals became worse and this process became more rapid with altitude. He commented that appetite was never normal until lower levels were reached and observed gross dehydration above 22,000 ft (6700 m).

Finch in the same year noted the beneficial effect of oxygen, the first time it had been used whilst climbing at high altitude.

In 1924, two men climbed a little higher (to 28,000 ft (8534 m)) without oxygen, whilst Mallory and Irvine were last seen at or above this height. They were both using open circuit oxygen sets. Odell (Norton 1925) in the same year spent eleven consecutive days at or above 23,000 ft (7010 m). He twice climbed to 27,000 ft (8230 m) without exhaustion. He used oxygen once but did not consider that his performance was improved.

Other mountaineers acclimatised to 23,000 ft (7010 m) but deterioration became marked due to cold, lack of sleep and fatigue.

Hingston (Hingston 1925) comments that one mountaineer

did not pass urine for 24 hours after returning from 26,000 ft (7925 m). Two mountaineers who ascended to 28,000 ft (8534 m) were 'parched with thirst'. He also considered that mountaineers lost between 14 and 20 lb in weight whilst above 17,000 ft (5182 m).

Barcroft (1925) commented on his companions' differing ability to adapt to altitude. He recognised that at the end of a period at 14,300 ft (4350 m), they lacked energy and that prolonged concentration was difficult. He also gave a classic description of acute mountain sickness.

In 1928 Carlos Monge described a condition of intolerance to altitude occurring in individuals already well acclimatised and living at considerable altitudes. So far this condition has been described in South America only and it is termed Monge disease (Monge 1928).

Grollman worked in 1930 on Pike's Peak, Hartmann in the Himalaya, and in 1935 a large expedition known as the International High Altitude Expedition went to the Andes. This Expedition spent several months in Peru and concluded that 17,500 ft (5334 m) represented the limit of permanent acclimatisation (Dill 1938).

In 1933, four men climbed to 28,000 ft (8534 m) on Everest without oxygen. One appeared to have suffered from hallucinations. Oxygen was used in 1938 up to 27,000 ft (8230 m) with little obvious increase in climbing rate.

In 1951 a reconnaissance of the Southern or Nepalese side of Everest revealed a possible route. The following spring, two members of the Swiss Everest Expedition reached 28,000 ft (8534 m) using oxygen intermittently. The same year, a British party visited the Everest Region and Pugh worked for three weeks in a tented laboratory at 18,000 ft (5486 m) on the Menlung La. He carried out a number of experiments designed to assess the effects of oxygen on climbing rate. This work together with other investigations into nutrition and clothing formed an essential preliminary to the successful British Everest Expedition in 1953, when the first ascent of this peak was made. In fact without this work it is doubtful if the mountain would have been climbed (Pugh 1952).

On the first ascent in May 1953, Hillary and Tensing used open circuit oxygen. Whilst at rest on the summit 29,002 ft (8839 m) they were able to remove their masks for ten minutes. Since this date Everest has been climbed by a number of routes and on a number of occasions. Oxygen has always been used and the maximum period spent at rest on the summit intermittently without oxygen has been about one hour.

On the American Everest Expedition in 1963 four men bivouacked for between six and seven hours at 28,000 ft (8534 m) on the South Ridge. Because the night was fine and relatively windless, only two were severely frostbitten.

During the winter of 1960–1 a team of medical scientists, physiologists and mountaineers carried out an extensive research programme into the long-term effects of high altitude on man in the Everest Region. Laboratories were placed at Mingbo 13,000 ft (3962 m), the Green Hut 17,500 ft (5334 m), and the Silver Hut 19,000 ft (5791 m) and occupied for four months from December to March.

Following this a party moved twenty miles across the Himalaya to Mt Makalu 27,740 ft (8450 m). Although an attempt on this peak failed due to illness, clinical observation and physiological experiments were carried out at 25,000 ft (7620 m). Two cases of thrombosis—one pulmonary and the other cerebral—occurred at 26,000 ft (7925 m) and 22,000 ft (6706 m) respectively in fit men. In addition it was confirmed that the physical and mental condition of the men deteriorated after long-term residence at 19,000 ft (5791 m) despite comfortable living quarters and adequate food and fluid intake.

Many expeditions to the highest Himalayan peaks have had some research programme, a pattern which has been followed up to the present. This party however was one of the few which had research as its primary aim—although a considerable amount of mountaineering was necessarily carried out at the same time.

Recently Indian observers have made a number of useful contributions as a result of their confrontation with China in certain parts of the Himalaya.

In recent years too, as part of the International Biological

Programme, expeditions have carried out investigations into indigenous high altitude populations in Nepal, Bhutan, Ethiopia, and elsewhere.

Permanent laboratories such as the Jungfraujoch high altitude Research Station have now been built in a number of places. The Institute of Andean Biology has a sea-level station at Lima and a well equipped laboratory at Morococha at 15,000 ft (4540 m). This mining community of 8000 people is only 145 km from Lima by an excellent though tortuous road. The laboratory here owes its conception, design and early management to Alberto Hurtado. The White Mountain Research Station in California consists of three laboratories: Crooked Creek at 10,100 ft (3094 m), the Barcroft Laboratory 12,500 ft (3800 m) and Summit station at 14,200 ft (4343 m). It is operated by the University of California. The Inter-University High Altitude Laboratory on Mt Evans at 14,200 ft (4348 m) is also open during the summer.

Table 2.   The World's highest peaks

Name	Feet	Metres	First ascent
Everest	29,160	8888	1953
K$_2$ (Godwin-Austen)	28,253	8611	1954
Kangchenjunga	25,168	8585	1955
Lhotse	28,028	8525	1956
Makalu	27,790	8470	1955
Cho Oyu	26,904	8200	1954
Dhaulagiri	26,811	8172	1960
Monaslu	26,658	8125	1956
Nanga Parbat	26,658	8125	1953
Annapurna	26,504	8078	1950

References

Barcroft, J. (1925) *The respiratory function of the blood, Part I Lessons from high altitudes.* Cambridge.

Bert, P. (1878) *La pression barométrique.* Masson: Paris.

Bruce, C. G. (1923) *The assault on Mount Everest 1922*. Arnold: London.

Bruhns, C. G. (1872) *Life of Humboldt*. Leipzig.

Calancha, A. (1639) *Cronica moralizada de la orden de San Agustin*. Barcelona.

Conway, W. M. (1894) *Climbing and exploration in the Karakoram Himalaya. Scientific results*. T. Fisher Unwin: London.

De Acosta, J. (1608) *The natural and moral history of the Indies*. Madrid.

De Filippi, F. (1865) *Note di un viaggio in Persia*. Milano.

De Filippi, F. (1912) *Karakoram and Western Himalaya*. Constable: London.

Dill, D. B. (1938) *Life, heat and altitude*. Harvard University: Cambridge, Mass.

Douglas, C. G., Haldane, J. S., Henderson, Y. and Schneider, E. S. (1913) *Proceedings of the Royal Society* Series B **203**, 185.

Egli-Sinclair (1893) *Sur le mal de montaigne. Annales de l'Observatoire Météorologique de Mt Blanc*. Paris.

Freshfield, D. (1869) *Central Caucasus*. Longmans: London.

Gay-Lussac (1816–1846) *Annales de Chimie et de Physique*.

Gerard, A. (1841) *Account of Koonawar*. Ed. Lloyd.

Glaisher, J., Flammarion, C., De Fonvielle, W. and Tissandier, G. (1871) *Travels in the air*. Lippincott: Philadelphia.

Hedin, S. (1913) *Trans-Himalaya*. Macmillan & Co: London.

Hingston, R. W. G. (1925) *Geographical Journal* **65**, 4.

Howard-Bury, C. K. (1922) *Mt Everest. The reconnaissance 1921*. Arnold: London.

Kronecker, C. (1903) *Die Bergkrankheit*. Berlin und Wein.

Longstaff, T. (1906) *Mountain sickness and its probable causes*. Spottiswoode: London.

Mathews, C. E. (1898) *Annals of Mont Blanc*. T. Fisher Unwin: London.

Monge, C. (1928) *La enfermedad de los Andes*. Lima Facultado Medicine.

Mosso, A. (1898) *Life of man on the High Alps*. T. Fisher Unwin: London.

Needham, J. (1954) *Science and civilisation in China.* Vol. 1. Cambridge University Press.

Norton, E. F. (1925) *The fight for Everest.* Arnold: London.

Plutarch (1912) *Alexander and Caesar.* Loeb Classics. Heinemann: London.

Prescott, W. H. (1891) *History of Mexico.* Swan Sonnenschein & Son.

Pugh, L. G. C. E. (1952) *Report on Cho Oyu expedition.* Medical Research Council.

Roborovsky (1896) The Central Asian Expedition of Capt Roborovsky and Lt Kozloff. *Geographical Journal,* **8,** 161.

Von Schlagintweitt, A, H, and R. (1862) *Results of a scientific mission to India and High Asia.* Vol III Trubner & Co.

Tyndall, J. (1906) *The glaciers of the Alps, and mountaineering in 1861.* J. M. Dent: London.

Urteago-Romero (1920) *Hist. Peru.* 2nd series. *Lima Informaciones sobre el Antiguo Peru. Cronicas, 1533–1575.*

Viault, E. (1891) *Compte rendu hebdomadaire des séances de l'Académie des Sciences. Paris.* **112,** 295.

Waddell, L. A. (1905) *Lhasa and its mysteries.* Murray: London.

Whymper, E. (1892) *Travels among the Great Andes of the equator.* Murray: London.

Wise, J. (1873) *Through the air.* To-day Printing and Publishers: Philadelphia.

CHAPTER TWO

The Atmosphere

Barometric Pressure

It has been shown that Man can adapt to oxygen-lack within a range of atmospheric pressure varying from the normal sea-level value to that at 28,000 ft (8534 m), where it is about one third of the sea-level pressure. However he can only live permanently within the range from sea level to 17,500 ft (5308 m) where it is about one half the sea-level figure. At or near sea level, the atmospheric or barometric pressure is about 760 mmHg, the figure depending on meteorological variations.

To be more precise the atmospheric pressure is said to be standard when at a temperature of 0°C, the height of the column in a mercury barometer is 760 mm. This is called 1 atmosphere.

Another unit of measurement used is the number of units of weight per unit of area, e.g. grams per square centimetre or pounds per square inch.

$$
\begin{aligned}
760 \text{ mm mercury (Hg)} &= 29\cdot9 \text{ inch Hg} \\
&= 14\cdot7 \text{ lb/sq inch} \\
&= 1033\cdot3 \text{ g/sq cm} \\
&= 1 \text{ atmosphere} \\
&= 1013\cdot25 \text{ millibars} \\
&= 101\cdot325 \text{ kilopascal}
\end{aligned}
$$

Millimetres of mercury are the accepted standard of pressure measurement in medicine—though it does not relate to the metre–kilogram–second system. The scientific unit of pressure integral with this system is the bar. The bar is equal to 10^5 newtons per square metre. 1 newton is the force required to impart an acceleration of 1 metre per second per second, to a mass of 1 kilogram.

The millibar is 1/1000 of a bar. It is also expressed as a pressure of 1000 dynes per square centimetre, because the dyne is defined as the force required to impart an acceleration of 1 cm per second per second to a mass of 1 gram.

To convert from mmHg to mb, multiply the number of millimetres by 1·333.

To convert from mb to mmHg, multiply the number of millibars by 0·750.

Partial Pressure of Gases

Air is a mixture of gases, mostly nitrogen and oxygen, and their effects depend on their individual—or partial pressures. The composition of air is nitrogen 79 per cent and oxygen 21 per cent. The small quantities of carbon dioxide (0·04 per cent) and other trace elements may be disregarded. This mixture (air) exerts a pressure of 760 mm of mercury and this pressure is shared by nitrogen and oxygen in proportion to the amounts of them present.

Therefore the pressure exerted by nitrogen is 79 per cent of 760 = 600 mmHg, and by oxygen is 21 per cent of 760 = 160 mmHg.

These values are termed the partial pressures of each gas. Therefore the partial pressure of oxygen or PO_2, at sea level is 160 mmHg and the partial pressure of nitrogen, or PN_2, at sea level is 600 mmHg.

The partial pressure represents a measure of the number of molecules of the particular gas striking a unit area in unit time.

Ventilation

Because the volume of a gas changes with temperature, pressure and water vapour saturation, measurement and comparison of gas volumes must be corrected to some standard or uniform state.

The appropriate standard depends on the topic under consideration.

BTPS

To determine lung capacities, gas volumes should be corrected to body temperature, and pressure saturated with water vapour since this is the state of gas in the lungs.

STPD

In metabolic investigations the fundamental interest is in the molecules of a gas rather than its volume as a chemical reaction is a relationship between interacting molecules of various substances and their end products.

Since in the physiological range gases behave approximately ideally, the number of molecules and their volumes are in direct proportion—but this depends on the state of the gas.

By convention the standard state is taken as 0°C (temperature), 760 mmHg (pressure) and dry (no water vapour) in which state one gram-molecule of gas occupies a volume of 22·4 litres.

Properties of Gases and Liquids

Gases and liquids are composed of particles (molecules) in constant motion. They continually collide with each other and with the containing vessel. The pressure exerted by a fluid is simply the consequence of the impacts of the molecules on the confining wall. Local differences in concentration resulting from the mixing of fluids will be more or less rapidly equalised by diffusion (the continued movement of the particles).

In a liquid, molecules have some freedom of movement but they are so close together that they are subject to strong intermolecular forces. The volume of a liquid is independent of its container.

In a gas the individual molecules are so far apart that their attractions for each other are very small. Because of the continuous movement of the molecules a gas will completely fill all the available volume.

Behaviour of Gases

Boyle's Law
The pressure of a gas is inversely proportional to its volume, the temperature being held constant.

The kinetic theory explains this by the fact that decreasing the volume of a gas, increases the number of molecules per unit volume. It therefore increases the rate of molecular bombardment upon the walls of a container.

Charles's Law
The pressure of a gas is directly proportional to its absolute temperature, the volume being held constant.

The kinetic theory explains this by the fact that increasing the temperature of a gas increases the velocity of the molecules and therefore the momentum with which the molecule hits the wall of a container.

Dalton's Law
In a mixture of gases, the pressure exerted by one of these gases is the same as it would exert if it alone occupied the same volume.

Thus if the oxygen was totally removed from a given volume of air at sea level, the remaining nitrogen would exert a pressure of 600 mmHg which is its partial pressure.

Henry's Law
When gases are in contact with a fluid in which they will dissolve, equilibria are set up between the amounts of gases in solution, and the partial pressures of the gases in contact with

the solution. This depends on the temperature of the fluid and the coefficient of solubility of the gas.

Henry's law states that at a constant temperature, the amount of a gas which dissolves in a liquid, with which it is in contact, is proportional to the partial pressure of that gas.

If the partial pressures of gases in contact with body fluids are known, and if the temperature and the coefficients of solubility of the gases in the body fluids are also known, then it will be possible to calculate the amount of each gas that is dissolved, allowing of course for time for equilibrium to be reached.

Barometric Pressure and Altitude

Air has mass and the higher the altitude, the smaller the mass in any given volume—or in other words the atmospheric (barometric) pressure is lower.

If barometric pressure and altitude are plotted against each other it will be seen that the relationship is not a straight line, but exponential. There is in fact progressively less drop in barometric pressure, as the altitude becomes higher. As man ascends to high altitudes not only barometric pressure falls but so also does the partial pressure of oxygen in the atmospheric air. It must be made clear that though the partial pressure, or the number of molecules of oxygen in a given volume of air, falls, the fraction of oxygen in a given volume remains constant at about 21 per cent.

Below 15,000 ft (4572 m) the barometric pressure as calculated (i) from the formula proposed by Zuntz when a mean temperature of $+15°C$ and a sea-level pressure of 760 mmHg were assumed, and (ii) from the internationally adopted altimetric calibration formula, are substantially the same. Above this altitude the barometric pressure obtained from the Zuntz formula exceeds the other by an increasing amount.

Thus on the summit of Everest 29,002 ft (8888 m) the pressure would be 269 mmHg according to the Zuntz formula whilst according to the altimeter scale it would be 236 mmHg.

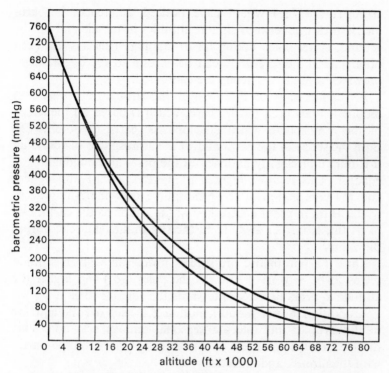

Fig. 1 Curves showing relation of barometric pressure to height. The upper curve is calculated from the formula given by Zuntz, assuming a mean temperature of 15°C. The lower curve is calculated according to the ICAN conventional law, assuming standard conditions (Armstrong 1939).

This difference of 33 mmHg represents a height of between 1000 and 1500 ft.

That a number of observations made on expeditions fall on the Zuntz curve could mean that at an equivalent altitude the mountaineer is at a higher barometric pressure than the airman.

However if differences in barometric pressure at the same altitude in adjacent regions were present, two consequences would result. Air would constantly flow from the region of high to low pressure, and, as the pressure differences may be considerable, there would constantly be winds of great violence. This is not the case. Further, pilots landing at altitudes up to

16,000 ft (4877 m) would have noticed differences in barometric pressure between similar altitudes in the air and on the
ground, either when taking off or landing. This has not been
observed. The discrepancy can be accounted for by the basis
on which aircraft altimeters are calibrated.

An explanation of the changes in barometric pressure in
mountains has been put forward, which is based on the shape
of the atmosphere which envelops the earth (Moore 1972).
Both the shape of the earth and of the atmosphere surrounding
it is oblate or slightly flattened at the poles and bulging at the
equator. This is more marked in the case of the atmosphere
and the contraction of the atmosphere over the Antarctic in
winter is more pronounced than in the Arctic as the earth, due
to its tilt, is farther away from the sun in the Antarctic during
the winter.

Thus the barometric pressure is lower (or a given altitude
seems to be increased) towards the poles (90°) and higher (or
altitude appears decreased) towards the equator (0°).

In addition the north–south motion of the sun over the equator
in the Tropics introduces a seasonal atmospheric tide. This
means that the thickness of the atmospheric envelope varies
with the month, and latitude.

This also means that the 'critical level of altitude'—that level
above which permanent habitation is not possible—will vary
with latitude from about 18,500 to 16,000 ft (5639 to 4877 m).
The altitude (or Po_2) at which acute mountain sickness first
occurs will also vary with latitude and possibly time of year, a
fact already noticed clinically.

That atmospheric pressure at a given altitude does vary considerably has been noted on many occasions (Williams 1958).
During the winter of 1960–1, a range of barometric pressure
from 372 to 384 mmHg, equivalent to an altitude variation of
750 ft (228 m), was observed at the Silver Hut 19,000 ft (5791 m)
in the Everest Region, over a period of three months (Pugh
1962).

Meteorologists are aware that barometric pressure for a given
altitude varies with the season, weather pattern, and latitude
but this variation is often ignored by those living and carrying

out physiological research work at high altitude. It is important to report barometric pressure (Dill 1970).

Cold and Wind

The temperature falls 3°F for every 1000 ft of ascent (1°C for every 150 m). This means that independent of latitude, the higher the altitude the colder it will become. Temperatures of −40°C have been postulated at 27,000 ft (8230 m) in winter.

An additional factor is that of wind—for with increasing wind velocity, the effective temperature at the skin surface falls. This effect—the 'wind-chill factor'—is of great importance on exposed skin-surfaces such as the face, where frostbite may occur due to local skin cooling.

High wind also interferes with movement, may increase oxygen consumption, and may be a contributory factor in fatigue and exhaustion. Winds gusting to about 100 mph are not uncommon in the mountain environment—and certainly a wind of 120 mph has been suggested at the summit of Everest. Few actual measurements have however been taken.

References

Armstrong, H.G. (1939) *Principles and practice of aviation medicine.* Williams and Wilkins: Baltimore.

Dill, D. B. and Evans, D. S. (1970) *Journal of Applied Physiology* **29**, 914.

Moore, T. (1972) *Unexpected effects of the peculiar shape of the envelope of the earth's atmosphere. A physiological study.* Paper presented at the 6th International Biometeorological Congress.

Pugh, L. G. C. E. (1962) *British Medical Journal* **2**, 621.

Williams, E. S. (1958) *Nature* **181**, 1527.

CHAPTER THREE

Man and the Mountain Environment

Mountain Populations

The start of civilisation and the first complex societies was the result of a combination of factors existing simultaneously in ancient river valleys. These were, abundant water supply, easy communication, a good climate and the protection afforded by surrounding lands across which it was difficult to travel.

One such area, the Fertile Crescent, bordered the Mediterranean Sea, stretched between the Tigris and Euphrates rivers, and reached to the Persian Gulf. In this region the Sumerians developed one of the world's first civilisations more than 5000 years ago. They and their successors created rich irrigated farm lands, and later the Babylonian, Assyrian, Phoenician and Hebrew civilisations evolved in this area. Though mountain regions seem to have been occupied long after more favoured areas, the skeleton of a man shown by radioactive carbon studies to be 9000 years old has been found at 14,000 ft (4200 m) at Lauricocha in Peru (Hurtado 1971). Mountain inhabitants may be the remnants of defeated peoples—the Caucasus has been termed the graveyard of nations—and because they are isolated and live in easily defended country their original cultural characteristics will tend to be preserved. The theocracy of Tibet is one such example and the social and economic structure of this civilisation was very akin to that found in the Europe of the Middle Ages (Stein 1972).

Estimates of mountain population are approximate and Weiner (Weiner 1964) gives the total population living in mountainous country as 420 million (12 per cent of the world's population). Individuals living above 10,000 ft (3000 m) have been put at 20–25 million (De Jong 1968).

Tibet, which covers an area of 800,000 square miles with three quarters over 10,000 ft (3000 m) and large areas between 13,000 and 17,500 ft (3960 m and 5334 m) is estimated as having 4–5 million inhabitants. Lhasa 11,600 ft (3500 m) has about 40,000 people and small groups live in scattered villages up to 16,000 ft (4877 m) (Stein 1972, Snellgrove 1961).

In South America large populations have lived at high altitudes since pre-historic times. The Andean (Indian) population at the time of the Spanish conquest (1532–1572) has been calculated as being between 4·5 and 7·5 million. In 1946 the total highland population was about 28 million with Indians making up 4·6 million. Towns such as La Paz 12,000 ft (3658 m) have a population of 350,000 people (Steward 1946).

Effects of the Environment

Low Barometric Pressure

Barometric pressure falls with altitude, the upper limit for permanent habitation being 17,500 ft (5334 m).

The main effect of the adaptive processes is to maintain a high oxygenation of the tissues and use the available oxygen as efficiently as possible. The result is the maintenance of the capacity to survive and reproduce in such a hostile environment.

In a subsistence economy survival means physical fitness and the capacity to perform physical work, and high-altitude natives at high altitude seem as able to perform physical work as lowland natives at low altitudes. The maximum rate of oxygen consumption per unit of body weight in high-altitude natives is equal to that of whites at sea level, and better than that of sea-level residents at altitude (Baker 1968).

Cold

Seasonal and diurnal variations are superimposed on the fall in temperature with increasing height. In tropical latitudes the seasonal change is small, whilst diurnal variation is important: at higher latitudes the seasonal change is larger, whilst the diurnal variation is less important.

As a general rule high-altitude inhabitants seem to withstand cold better than do sea-level residents at altitude. They appear to maintain higher peripheral temperatures with an increased peripheral blood flow, and have an increased metabolism (Baker *et al.* 1966). However protection from cold is achieved more by cultural than physiological means. Clothing is usually made of wool which entraps a layer of air close to the skin as insulation. Boots are stuffed with straw for the same reason, and in Tibet children may be rubbed with fat or butter during cold weather. Individuals keep huddled together, often around a fire, and houses have small windows, often without glass but with wooden shutters. Hay in overhead lofts increases insulation and in many parts of the Himalayas, livestock are wintered on the ground floor, their body heat rising to warm the humans on the floor above.

Terrain

Mountainous country varies widely in form, but there are two main types—the high plateaux (such as occur in Central Asia, and the altiplano of South America) and deep valleys with sides several thousand feet high (Himalaya, Andes).

Plateaux can support large populations and large towns. Valleys, because flat ground is at a premium, tend to have smaller populations. Houses in any one village may be perched on ridges or slopes far removed from one another.

Although large towns can be supported especially in plateau country, they are usually isolated from the major lowland cities with their centres of government, industry and commerce. In mountain valleys, communications are often very difficult and genetic isolation is fairly common. The placing of houses and settlements in sunny positions (adret exposure) will be more difficult than on relatively flat ground and this will add to the isolation.

The energy expenditure for the individual may differ for living on a plateau or in a valley. Any difference in the physiology of exercise between two such individuals may be due to this cause.

Wind

Due to altitude, the lack of windbreaks, the funnelling effect of valleys and other factors, wind velocity may be very great. This may lead to the stunting of vegetation and trees, and in turn population will be restricted to certain areas. Wind also contributes to soil erosion in deforested regions.

Ultraviolet Light

Decreased atmospheric absorption and increased reflection from the snow tends to increase the intensity of ultraviolet light. This will increase the burning effect of sunlight and high-altitude populations have dark skins. However in genetically similar populations in Ethiopia, highlanders did not have darker skins than lowlanders (Harrison *et al.* 1969).

Rain and Snow

Precipitation in mountain regions may be sudden and considerable. This can cause landslides and avalanches, and have catastrophic effects on mountain settlements and communications.

The type of country can greatly influence the amount of precipitation, and thus the form of economy. For instance on the southern slopes of the Himalaya rainfall is considerable, whilst a few miles away on the Tibetan plateau rainfall is low and desert conditions prevail.

In tropical latitudes the snow level is higher than elsewhere though local physical features and other factors produce considerable variations.

Biological factors

Changes in animal and plant life at high altitude will occur as a consequence of the physical environment.

Vegetation changes—the result of cold and lowered oxygen tension—and rainfall will affect the type of agriculture practised and the sort of domestic animal that is herded.

Disease vectors also vary. Mosquitoes are absent above 12,000 ft (3500 m) whilst at this altitude the principal disease vectors are flies and body lice (Buck *et al.* 1968). Bacterial growth may be reduced as a result of solar radiation (Keck and Buchmaiser 1964).

Certain deficiency diseases, such as goitre, the result of the low iodine content of the soil and water following on glacial action, appear to be commoner in mountain areas.

Physical and biological components act on both individuals and on populations—their effects may even be contradictory, cold and wind stunting vegetation, hypoxia stimulating growth.

Population Distribution

Cold seems to be a more important factor in the colonising of high altitude regions than either low barometric pressure or the type of country. However in tropical latitudes, where the summer snow line may be as high as 16,500 to 20,000 ft (5000 to 6000 m) high altitude is more likely to be a factor in population distribution than at higher latitudes.

Within 10° of the equator permanent settlements are usually situated where both timber and pasture can be used, and the upper limit of habitation may be between the two. Further from the equator the upper limit falls below the timber line, as variation in temperature becomes seasonal. Thus the upper pasture lands are available for a semi-nomadic economy, whereas permanent inhabited villages are found at lower levels with isolated groups of houses or shelters on the pastures occupied for the grazing season and evacuated during the winter. Very considerable migration may occur and in some regions part of the population may always be on the move. In regions with permanent snow, habitation consists only of Eskimo settlements, and occasional travellers and explorers.

The distribution of houses within any area will depend largely on the availability of water, so villages tend to follow rivers. Houses will be placed away from areas that can flood and in sunny positions. Protection from avalanches can be afforded by belts of trees, especially those planted in the breakaway zones. Areas swept by landslides will be avoided.

The limiting factors to permanent habitation are frozen soil resulting in insufficient crops or grazing, and altitude, for it appears that above 17,500 ft (5334 m) physical and mental deterioration occurs in man. However dwellings have been placed at higher levels and a house of three rooms has been discovered at 21,650 ft (6600 m) on Cerro Llullaillaco 22,658 ft (6860 m) on the Argentine–Chile border. This is believed to date back to the pre-Columbian period (Guinness 1970).

Those who spend long periods at higher altitudes and above the permanent snowline are essentially mountaineers and skiers. Both involve techniques for movement in mountain country, which have evolved from the necessities of ordinary travel.

Mountaineering originated in the need to cross passes and mountain ridges in order to trade. Aids to movement such as crampons, ice-axes, ropes and the use of guides are centuries old.

Mt Everest has been successfully climbed using supplementary oxygen on a number of occasions. Both high-altitude natives and sea-level visitors have been successful and one man, a Sherpa, has gained the summit on two occasions.

Whether it is possible to climb Everest without supplementary oxygen is a matter for debate, but the high-altitude native would probably be better suited by his generations of adaptation than a sea-level visitor.

In winter, movement across snow is essential for feeding livestock quartered in isolated shelters. Since prehistoric times boards have been placed on the feet to facilitate movement. The earliest references to primitive skis are found in the Nordic Sagas which date back to 3000 BC (Hennings 1966). The earliest mention of skiing on record occurs in Procopius (526–559 AD).

In the United Kingdom skis were used in Cumberland at the start of the nineteenth century. As a modern sport it may be said to date from the first visit of the Telemark peasant to Christiania in 1870 (Lunn 1927).

Economy

Agriculture and Animal Husbandry

Most mountain economies depend on a combination of animal husbandry and agriculture. In some regions one may predominate, for instance Yak herding in Central Asia.

In summer and spring upper pastures are grazed whilst the land round the village is cultivated. In winter the animals are brought to lower levels, and sometimes kept in the houses where they can provide an extra source of heat.

The limiting factor in agriculture is the number of months that the soil remains frozen and a single period of the year lasting only six months may be available for cultivation. The type of crop may influence the size of population. Potatoes introduced into Sola Khumbu in North-east Nepal between 1850 and 1860 resulted in an increase in population from 169 households in 1836 to 596 households in 1957. This increase was due to immigration from Tibet, and individuals freed from 'earning food' took to the religious life and new Bhuddist monasteries were built (Fuhrer-Haimandorf 1964).

A limit to the amount of productive land is the degree of slope, and level land may have to be manufactured in the form of terraces. These are fields built up behind retaining walls of stone, and they range in size from a few square feet to a relatively large area. Usually too small for pasture, manure has to be carried up by the cultivators. Irrigation also may be necessary and the task of building and maintaining terraces is considerable.

The altitude may affect the fertility of animals and the capital of Peru was removed from La Paz 12,000 ft (3600 m) to Lima 500 ft (150 m) because of the relative infertility of animals at the higher level.

Communal pasture land (alps) and terracing involve ownership and maintenance by groups rather than by individuals—the social implications are thus important (Peattie 1936).

The only activity carried on above the highest level of grazing is mining, and this is successfully accomplished at 19,000 ft (5791 m) in South America.

Trade

Highland populations are often strategically placed between areas of prosperous lowland centres. Physiologically too they are more capable of crossing high mountain passes with heavy loads. Thus they play a vital role in trade.

Major mountain passes have been used as arteries for trade, the movement of people and ideas, and have allowed the dissemination of disease. Both the Nangpa La, 19,000 ft (5791 m), between Southern Tibet and North-east Nepal and the Great St Bernard, 8100 ft (2473 m), between Italy and Central Europe have been major trade routes for centuries.

The recent closing of the trade routes between Tibet (China) and Nepal has resulted in many Nepalese highland areas becoming blind ends of communication. The basic pastoral agricultural economy however has been sufficient to prevent any fall in the standards of living or emigration.

Religion

Isolation from modern materialism, together with sudden natural catastrophes, will have contributed to the undoubted leanings that many mountain people have towards the religious life.

Demography

Few comprehensive studies are available.

Comparisons between Amazonian jungle villages and those on the altiplano of Peru have been carried out. The highland villages, at about 11,500 ft (3500 m), had a fairly heavy mortality during the first two decades, but had a higher proportion of both males and females in the 30–50 age range (Buck *et al.* 1968).

In the Himalaya, Gorer (Gorer 1938) gives an age distribution of a Lepcha village in Sikkim at 5300 ft (1600 m), and Kawakita (Kawakita 1953) gives information on a Bhotia village at 11,400 ft (3450 m). The principal difference was that at lower altitudes the proportion of people of both sexes aged over 60 was considerably higher.

In North Bhutan, 340 people out of a total population of over 500 living between 12,000 and 14,000 ft (3658 and 4267 m) were examined (Ward *et al.* 1967). The age and sex distributions were as shown in Table 3.

Table 3. Age and sex distribution of North Bhutanese

Years	Male	Female	Total
0–9	24	39	63
10–19	33	35	68
20–29	20	19	39
30–39	27	25	52
40–49	17	25	42
50–59	13	19	32
60–69	16	9	25
70 and over	4	15	19
Total	154	186	340

The oldest man was 82 and the oldest woman 78.

From questioning it appeared that infection accounted for a high childhood and infant mortality but in the adult population there was a striking absence of infection. In general the health of the population was excellent, possibly for genetic and climatic reasons, and in a community with no medical care only the robust can survive.

Fertility

There seems little doubt that among Andean Indians total fertility (maximum number of children born per woman) is no less than among lowland populations (Cruz-Coke 1968). Census data suggests that in Peru, population growth rate varies little with altitude (Sobrevilla 1968).

The menarche may be delayed in highland populations, but the mean age of the first pregnancy is earlier (Cruz-Coke 1968). In highland women the probability of becoming pregnant remains high throughout the reproductive period.

It appears that in highland villages there is a low rate of loss of foetuses but infant mortality is higher (Cruz-Coke 1968). Abortion rates in the Peruvian highlands do not appear to be greater than in the lowlands (Buck et al. 1968). Data for pregnancy in North Bhutan were compared with Scottish figures. The still-birth rate of 42 per 1000 births compares with 28·4 per 1000 births for Scotland (Thomson 1967). In Ethiopia however the situation appears different. Harrison (Harrison et al. 1969) found that among 53 highland women, for 232 pregnancies there had been 21 abortions. In 49 lowlanders, with 173 pregnancies only one abortion had occurred.

If hypoxia is an important factor in causing abortion, one would expect the rate to be higher in the Andes and Himalaya than in Ethiopia, as the population lives at higher altitude. The time for which populations have lived at their respective altitudes may be important. The Amerindians have lived at an altitude of 13,000 ft (4000 m) for 9000 years and the Central Asians for at least 4000 years, whilst the Amharas have lived in the Ethiopian highlands for a shorter period. As a result of natural selection normal live infants are obviously more likely to be produced in the first two instances than the last.

Neonatal mortality appears to be greater in highland populations, except for Ethiopia (Cruz-Coke 1968). The infant mortality in Bhutan was 189 per 1000 births compared with 50 per 1000 births in recent years in Scotland and 97 per 1000 births fifty years ago (Thomson 1967).

Birth weight is reduced in children born at high altitude (Sobrevilla 1968). The increased number of children of low birth weight—which seems related to slowing of foetal growth in the last three months of pregnancy—may be related to the increased mortality (Grahn and Kratchman 1963).

The effect of altitude on placental weight is as yet not clear. Placentas appear thinner at altitude yet there is no proportionate reduction in size (Sobrevilla 1968).

In high altitude residents there does appear to be a considerable number of deaths before birth, in the neonatal period and in childhood.

Disease Patterns

These have been little studied, but in communities with little idea of preventive hygiene and few medical aids, the incidence of disease may be high and the factors of cold and altitude will be of less importance than those of hygiene.

Most highland regions appear to be freer of infectious disease than lowland areas, and highlanders are often reluctant to descend for long periods especially during the malarial season. Unidentified 'fevers' appear to be less common among highland than lowland populations, though studies of viral serology in North Bhutan revealed antibodies to the following (Gould 1967):

Table 4.   Viral serology of North Bhutanese

Antigen	Percentage positive at serum dilution 1:16
Influenza A	85
Influenza B	50
Influenza C	82
Sendai	80
Adenovirus	80
Lymphogranuloma venereum	82
Q fever	26
Herpes simplex	82
R.S. virus	80
Measles	79
Mumps S	18
Mumps V	82
Lymphocytic chorio-meningitis	0
Mycopneumonia	35

It appeared therefore that exposure of this particular population (34 people) to all these agents except Lymphocytic chorio-meningitis had occurred.

Studies of nasal swabs showed a 4 per cent rate of coagulase positive staphylococci (Selkom 1967) which is considerably lower than the findings of surveys in Western European communities which range from 29 per cent to 46 per cent (Williams *et al.* 1966).

Throat cultures revealed a high frequency of penicillin-sensitive B-haemolytic streptococci (Gould 1967).

Respiratory conditions appear more frequent in some high-altitude communities, though in North Bhutan they seemed rare.

Typhus was found to be more common in one highland village, presumably a correlation with infestation by body lice (Buck *et al.* 1968). A reduction in the incidence of malaria occurs at high altitude, presumably due to lack of resistance of the mosquito to cold. Parasitic infestation of the intestinal tract also seems less common at altitude.

The stress of cold and altitude may result in infection being more severe, and some experimental evidence tends to support this view (Highman and Altland 1950). It has been suggested too that the nature of the immune response may change with altitude, and antibody production appears to be increased in some experimental animals at low barometric pressure (Highman and Altland 1964; Trapani 1964).

On pre-war Everest expeditions the incidence of upper respiratory infections was high, and some individual cases were severe. Somervell at 28,000 ft (8534 m) was nearly suffocated by the sloughing of the mucosa of his nasopharynx (Bruce 1923). On one occasion the party had to descend to lower levels 14,000 ft (4200 m) in order to recuperate (Tilman 1948).

On post-war Everest expeditions this incidence was not so marked. This discrepancy is probably due to the fact that pre-war expeditions travelled across the windy, dry, and dusty plains of the Tibetan plateau to reach the mountain. At Base Camp a new source of infection was introduced by fresh Sherpas from Sola Khumbu in Nepal. These men had crossed the main Himalayan Chain to the northern, Tibetan, side and their arrival seemed to coincide with an exacerbation of intercurrent infection. Post-war parties on the other hand worked with the same

Sherpas from start to finish, and though some infection occurred, its incidence was much less. Other factors were the use of antibiotics, oxygen and the less dusty approach march through the southern, Nepalese valleys.

Long-continued residence at 19,000 ft (5791 m) in high-altitude visitors did not appear to result in a greater tendency to infection. However it was noticeable that in some people respiratory infection appeared to coincide with episodes of high-altitude deterioration, and on descent to 14,000 ft (4267 m) recovery occurred. The introduction of new members from sea level towards the end of this period did not appear to increase the incidence of infection (Ward 1968).

Comparative studies of the incidence of non-infectious disease in highland populations are also rare.

Cancer seemed rare in North Bhutan and no cases of cancer of the breast or thyroid were observed clinically (Ward *et al.* 1967). Obviously cancer must occur in high-altitude populations and some advanced cases have been seen in Sherpa communities.

Chemodectoma appears to be commoner in high-altitude populations in America. This condition has so far not been observed in Asia (Saldana and Salem 1970).

With regard to sickle-cell disease an altitude of about 15,000 ft (4572 m) must be reached before the capillary oxygen tension falls to 10–15 mmHg at rest, which is the level necessary for sickling. It would seem likely that people with this trait are unlikely to reach such an altitude without suffering from symptoms and possible crises.

A slight increase in sickling has been noted and splenic infarction has been reported in people with sickle-cell trait flying in an unpressurised aircraft, and also when crossing passes at 15,000 ft on foot (Sullivan 1950; Rotter *et al.* 1956; Rywlin and Benson 1961; Green *et al.* 1971).

Data from the Andes suggests that blood pressures above 150/90 are rare or unknown (Baker 1968). This was also found in Bhutan.

No evidence of coronary artery disease was found in North Bhutan, and coronary artery occlusion seems rare at altitude (Singh 1968).

In North Bhutan both serum cholesterol and triglyceride levels were low. There was no difference with age group, and no progressive increase with age. This correlates with the absence of clinical and ECG evidence of coronary artery disease. In addition to the relatively low fat diet, the population led an active life.

In both Sherpa and North Bhutanese populations evidence of malnutrition or obesity is rare.

Patent ductus arteriosus appear to be more common, possibly because its patency is maintained by the high pulmonary artery pressure (Almazora *et al.* 1953).

South American studies have shown that people born and living at high altitude have some degree of right ventricular hypertrophy from birth onwards. In North Bhutan however, the Lunana inhabitants showed some degree of right axis deviation, but none of right ventricular hypertrophy (Jackson and Turner 1967).

Monge's disease has not so far been identified in Asian populations.

Goitre

Probably the commonest medical condition found among mountain inhabitants is endemic goitre. In some areas very large percentages of the population are affected, whilst in others with exactly similar living conditions, only a relatively small number have goitre. It is also rare for every member of a particular population to be affected and goitre appears to be commoner in women than men.

Endemic goitre is common in those parts of the world where iodine intake falls below 100 μg per day, and regions where water and soil and consequently foodstuffs are poor in iodine are almost always the site of this condition (WHO 1960).

Sex and heredity

The difference in incidence between men and women has not been adequately explained. It may be due to the increased demands for iodine, and hence stimulation of the gland during pregnancy and with each menstrual period. However, a study made in the northern mountains of Greece where goitre is endemic showed that despite a universally high uptake of radio-active iodine, only certain individuals developed goitre. Since only certain families were affected, and factors other than iodine deficiency were not involved, it was deduced that goitres may have been genetically determined (Malamos *et al.* 1965). Similar evidence has appeared from studies in New Guinea (Choufoer 1963).

Water pollution

The pollution of drinking water with human and animal excreta is known to precipitate goitre in iodine-deficient areas.

In Gilgit, an area in the Karakorum Himalaya, McCarrison (McCarrison 1906, 1908) studied villages situated one below the other on a river from which they drew water and which became more polluted with human and animal excreta as it descended. An increasing goitre incidence occurred with increasing pollution. In the top village it was 11·8 per cent and at the bottom, 45·6 per cent. A nearby village with an independent spring of water was goitre-free. After the polluted water was filtered, twice daily drinks were given to volunteers. In one third, goitre developed after 14 days, reaching maximum size in 30 days. All goitres disappeared after the experiment was finished. No goitres developed in a control group who drank some water with suspended matter after it had been boiled. Seeming confirmation came when McCarrison made a further investigation of a girls' school at Sanawar, also in the Himalaya.

Later work in the same Gilgit valley (Chapman *et al.* 1972) revealed that though the water was grossly contaminated by bacteria, especially faecal coli, there was no correlation between the type of water supply and goitre incidence. Although McCarrison's observations were confirmed, the suggestion that the goitres were due to bacterial pollution was not substantiated.

Calcium

Since earliest times goitre has frequently been noticed to be associated with limestone rocks and drinking water rich in lime (Boussingault 1831). In India drinking hard water and living in areas where the soil is rich in calcium are still regarded as important factors. Experimentally it has been shown in rats on a diet poor in iodine that only if large amounts of calcium are taken does goitre occur (Hellwig 1934). It is possible that in areas where minimal iodine deficiency is present, water hardness may determine the incidence of goitre.

Fluoride

The possible aetiological connection between fluoride and goitre raised by the high incidence of goitre observed in areas of endemic fluorosis has not been substantiated by epidemiological studies carried out in relatively goitre-free regions.

However there may be an association since fluoride fed to animals in large doses produces goitre, and in addition the co-existence of fluorosis and goitre has been noted especially in poor rural populations living on a diet low in protein (Day and Powell-Jackson 1972).

Goitrogens

Certain foods are goitrogenic, and soya bean and vegetables of the genus Brassica, such as cauliflowers, turnips, brussel sprouts and cabbage, have these properties (Chesney et al. 1928).

Variations in the iodine of the diet may account for differences of goitre incidence where these vegetables are eaten.

Certainly many high-altitude populations tend to have a vegetable rather than a meat diet as animals, such as the yak, are more useful alive, even when old. Other animals such as pigs and chickens either do not appear to flourish or may be banned for religious reasons.

No intrathyroidal enzyme defect was found in a Sherpa population living in an endemic goitre area of North-east Nepal (Ibbertson et al. 1971).

It is possible that the additional stress of cold and high altitude affecting thyroid function may contribute to goitre formation in a mountain region with iodine deficiency. Hypothyroidism may be found in endemic goitre patients.

Mild iodine deficiency is usually fully compensated, but more severe deficiency with cretinism may occur. Low normal or low serum PBI occur in supposedly euthyroid individuals. General health and well-being may thus be impaired. A high incidence of dwarfism and mental deficiency has been reported from the highlanders in New Guinea (Gajdusek 1962).

Hyperthyroidism is not common in endemic goitre areas. The relationship between thyroid cancer and endemic goitre has also not been clarified. Pressure symptoms, despite the relatively enormous size of some goitres, seem rare in areas of endemic goitre.

References

Almazora, V., Rotta, A., Battilana, G., Abugattas, R., Rubio, C., Bouroncle, J., Zapata, C., Santa Maria, E., Binder, T., Subira, R., Paredes, D., Pando, B. and Graham, G. (1953) On possible influences of great altitudes on determination of certain cardio-vascular anomalies. Preliminary report. *Pediatrics* **12**, 259.

Baker, P. T. (1968) *Human adaptation to high altitudes. A biological case study of a Quechua population native to the High Andean Region with special reference to hypoxia and cold.* Final progress report. US Army Surgeon General. Contract No. DA-49-193-MD-2260 Department of the Army: Washington, DC.

Baker, P. T., Buskirk, E. R., Picon-Reatequi, E., Kolias, J., Mazes, R. B., Akers, R. F., Little, M. A., Prokop, E. K. and Thomas R. B. (1966) *Altitude and cold. A study of the cold exposure, and thermo-regulatory responses of high altitude Quechua Indians.* Annual progress report. US Army Surgeon General. Contract No. DA-49-193-MD-2260 Department of the Army: Washington, DC.

Boussingault, J. B. (1831) *Annales de chimie et de physique* **48**, 41.

Bruce, C. G. (1923) *The assault on Everest*. Arnold: London.

Buck, A. A., Sasaki, T. T. and Anderson, R. I. (1968) *Health and disease in four Peruvian villages: contrasts in epidemiology*. Johns Hopkins Press: Baltimore.

Chapman, J. A., Grant, I. S., Taylor, G., Mahmud, K., Sardar-ul-Mulk and Shahid, M. A. (1972) *Philosophical Transactions of the Royal Society* Series B **263**, 459.

Chesney, A. M., Clawson, T. A. and Webster, B. (1928) *Bulletin of Johns Hopkins Hospital* **43**, 261.

Choufoer, J. C., Van Rhijn, M., Kassenaar, A. A. H. and Querido, A. (1963) *Journal of Clinical Endocrinology* **23**, 1203.

Cruz-Coke, R. (1968) *Genetic characteristics of high altitude populations in Chile*. WHO/PAHO/IBP. Meeting of investigators on population biology at altitude. Pan-American Health Organisation: Washington, DC.

Day, T. K. and Powell-Jackson, P. R. (1972) *Lancet* **1**, 1135.

De Jong, G. F. (1968) *Demography of high-altitude populations*. WHO/PAHO/IBP Meeting of investigators on population biology of altitude. Pan-American Health Organisation: Washington, DC.

Frisancho, A. R. (1969) *Human growth in a high altitude Peruvian population*. Thesis. The Pennsylvania State University.

Fuhrer-Haimandorf, C. von (1964) *The Sherpas of Nepal. Bhuddhist highlanders*. John Murray: London.

Gajdusek, D. C. (1962) *Pediatrics* **29**, 345.

Gorer, G. (1938) *Himalayan village*. Michael Joseph: London.

Gould, J. C. (1967) In, *Report of IBP expedition to North Bhutan*. *Ed.* Ward, M. P., Jackson, F. S. and Turner, R. W. D.

Grahn, D. and Kratchman, J. (1963) *American Journal of Human Genetics* **15**, 329.

Green, R. L., Huntsman, R. G. and Serjeant, G. R. (1971) *British Medical Journal* **4**, 593.

Guinness book of records (1970) *Ed.* McWhirter, N. and McWhirter, R. Guinness Superlatives Limited.

Harrison, G. A., Kuchemann, C. F., Moore, M. A. S., Boyce, A. J., Baju, T., Mourant, A. E., Godber, M. J., Glasgow,

B. G., Kopec, A. C., Tills, D. and Clegg, E. J. (1969) *Philosophical Transactions of the Royal Society*. Series B **256**, 47.

Hellwig, C. A. (1934) *Endocrinology* **18**, 197.

Hennings, R. (1966) In, *The book of European skiing*. Barker: London.

Highman, B. and Altland, P. D. (1950) *Proceedings of the Society for Experimental Biology and Medicine* **75**, 573.

Highman, B. and Altland, P. D. (1964) In, *The physiological effects of high altitude. Ed.* Weihe, W. H. Pergamon: Oxford.

Hurtado, A. (1971) In, *High altitude physiology. Ed.* Porter, R. and Knight, J. Ciba Foundation symposium. Churchill Livingstone: Edinburgh and London.

Ibbertsen, H. K., Tait, J. and Lim, T. (1971) Abstracts of 4th Asia and Oceanic Congress of Endocrinology, No. 112. University of Auckland: New Zealand.

Jackson, F. S. and Turner, R. W. D. (1967) In, *Report of IBP expedition to North Bhutan. Ed.* Ward, M. P., Jackson, F. S. and Turner, R. W. D.

Kawakita, J. (1953) Ethno-geographical observations in the Nepal Himalaya. In, *Peoples of the Nepal Himalaya. Ed.* Kihara, H. Fauna & Flora Research Society: Kyoto.

Keck, G. and Buchmaiser, R. (1964) In, *The physiological effects of high altitude. Ed.* Weihe, W. H. Pergamon: Oxford.

Lunn, A. (1927) *History of skiing*. Oxford University Press.

McCarrison, R. (1906) *Lancet* **1**, 1110.

McCarrison, R. (1908) *Lancet* **2**, 1275.

Malamos, B., Miras, C., Kostamis, P., Mantzos, J., Kralios, A. C., Rigopoulos, G., Zerefos, N. and Koutras, D. A. (1965) In, *Current topics in thyroid research. Ed.* Cassano, C. and Andreoli, M. Academic Press: New York.

Peattie, R. (1936) *Mountain geography. A critique and field study*. Harvard University Press: Cambridge, Mass.

Rotter, R., Luttgens, W. F., Peterson, W. L., Stock, A. E. and Motulsky, A. G. (1956) *Annals of Internal Medicine* **44**, 257.

Rywlin, A. M. and Benson, J. (1961) *American Journal of Clinical Pathology* **36**, 142.

Saldana, M. and Salem, L. E. (1970) *American Journal of Pathology* **59**, 91a.

Selkom, J. (1967) In, *Report of IBP expedition to North Bhutan*. *Ed.* Ward, M. P., Jackson, F. S. and Turner, R. W. D.

Singh, I. (1968) *Clinical problems at high altitude*. WHO/PAHO/IBP Meeting of investigators on population biology at altitude. Pan-American Health Organisation: Washington, DC.

Snellgrove, D. (1961) *Himalayan pilgrimage*. Cassirer/Faber: Oxford.

Sobrevilla, L. (1968) *Fertility at high altitudes*. WHO/PAHO/IBP Meeting of investigators on population biology at altitude. Pan-American Health Organisation: Washington, DC.

Stein, R. A. (1972) *Tibetan civilization*. Faber: London.

Steward, J. H. (1946) In, *The Andean civilisations handbook of South American Indians*. Vol. 2. Bureau of American Ethnology.

Sullivan, B. H. (1950) *Annals of Internal Medicine* **32**, 338.

Thomson, J. (1967) In, *Reports of IBP expedition to North Bhutan*. *Ed.* Ward, M. P., Jackson, F. S. and Turner, R. W. D.

Tilman, H. W. (1948) *Mount Everest, 1938*. Cambridge University Press.

Trapani, I. L. (1964) In, *The physiological effects of high altitude*. *Ed.* Weihe, W. H. Pergamon Press: Oxford.

Ward, M. P., Jackson, F. S. and Turner R. W. D. (1967) In, *Report of IBP expedition to North Bhutan*.

Ward, M. P. (1968) *Diseases occurring at altitudes exceeding 17,500 ft*. MD thesis. University of Cambridge.

Weiner, J. S. (1964) In, *Human biology*. *Ed.* Harrison, J. A., Weiner, J. S., Barnicot, N. A. and Tanner, J. M. Clarendon Press: Oxford.

WHO monograph series No. 44 (1960) *Endemic goitre*. World Health Organisation: Geneva.

Williams, R. E. O., Blowers, R., Garrod, L. P., Shooter, R. A. (1966) *Hospital infection*. Second edition. Lloyd-Luke: London.

CHAPTER FOUR

Growth

Before birth

The foetus at sea level develops in a hypoxic environment (Barcroft 1933). At high altitude therefore the foetus will be subject to more hypoxic stress than at sea level unless some adaptive response occurs. Peruvian high-altitude populations tend to have low birth weights and relatively greater placental weight than their sea-level counterparts (Frisancho 1970). Reductions in measurements of body size and subcutaneous fat were proportional to the decrease in birth weight.

Studies of the placenta show that at high altitudes the frequency of the 'irregularly shaped' placenta is three times that at sea level. (Rendon 1964). These placentas are thinner and have a much higher cord haemoglobin than at sea level. From experimental work on ewes, pre-natal adjustment to the hypoxia of altitude seems to involve (Barron et al. 1964)

(i) Increased surface area available for diffusion of oxygen between maternal and placental blood.
(ii) Decreased resistance of the placental barrier to the transfer of oxygen.
(iii) A combination of both.

The relative increase in placental weight with a thinner and irregular shaped placenta at high altitude seem to be a compromise increasing the volume and surface area and diminishing the placental barrier, whilst the low birth weight may reduce oxygen requirements.

After birth

Bodily growth

It is generally believed that high-altitude populations are smaller in stature than lowlanders. This however is not invariably the case.

In Ethiopia both male and female adults born at 10,000 ft (3000 m) are heavier than those born at 5000 ft (1500 m). High-altitude females were also taller. Male lowlanders migrating to higher regions were lighter, and highlanders migrating to lowland areas were heavier, than comparable natives (Clegg *et al.* 1970). Studies of growing children and boys particularly show that highlanders were heavier and taller than lowlanders for all ages (Clegg *et al.* 1972). Highlanders tended to grow faster than lowlanders and it would appear that given genetic homogeneity the upland environment was more suitable in terms of physique and growth than the lowland (Harrison *et al.* 1969).

In Asia, certain groups of Tibetans, notably the Khampas, who live on the southern and eastern edge of the Central Asian plateau are tall and well built.

Sherpas, who live up to 14,000 ft (4267 m) appear to be smaller than Europeans, and the typical Sherpa is small and barrel-chested.

In a North Bhutanese population living at similar altitude on the Tibetan border, height, weight, arm and calf circumferences were measured and compared with the British. The Bhutanese appeared to be smaller, their average measurements corresponding to about the 30th percentile of the British. Their proportions however were not dissimilar (Tanner 1967).

In the Andes, the growth of the highlander is retarded by comparison with the lowlander. Differences are most marked at the age of twelve in girls and fourteen years in boys, and persist until age eighteen (Frisancho 1969).

In a high-altitude Peruvian Quechua population at 14,000 ft (4200 m) the pattern of growth showed (Frisancho and Baker, 1969)

(i) A late sexual dimorphism, i.e. after age sixteen.
(ii) Slow and prolonged growth period in body size.
    Termination of growth: male, 22; female, 20.
(iii) Late and poorly defined adolescent spurt in both males and females.
(iv) Accelerated development of chest size and lung volumes when compared to sea-level Peruvian natives.

In addition to retardation of growth, there is also delay in maturation. The adolescent growth spurt was delayed and prolonged until past the age of twenty (Frisancho 1969). Delay in menarche amounting to $1\frac{1}{2}$ years has also been reported (Cruz-Coke 1968).

Data from Bhutan also suggested that menarche was delayed to between eighteen and twenty years as was the adolescent spurt (Tanner 1967).

At altitudes of 13,000 ft (4000 m) and above in Asia and South America, it appears then that there is some retardation of growth and maturation; at 10,000 ft (3000 m) in Ethiopia however the reverse appears to be true.

Heart

At sea level, the right ventricle at birth is slightly larger in size than the left ventricle (Emery and Methal 1961). With adulthood the left ventricle becomes larger than the right. Among high-altitude populations, certainly in South America, the right ventricle in adults is larger than the left (Rotta 1947; Penaloza *et al.* 1961). From anatomical and electrocardiographic studies it has been found that the predominance of the right ventricle begins after the fourth month of post-natal development, and that the enlargement appears to be due to overgrowth of the basal zone (Recavarren and Arias-Stella 1962).

The right ventricular enlargement appears to be related to a high pulmonary blood pressure. In high-altitude natives after the first month of post-natal development there is an increase in muscularity and thickening of the muscular layer of the pulmonary arteries and arterioles (Arias-Stella and Saldana 1962). Together with the high blood viscosity attendant on polycythaemia this results in pulmonary hypertension in children and adults.

In addition there is an increased incidence of patent ductus arteriorus and this may contribute to enlargement of the right ventricle. Of 5000 school-children of both sexes born at high altitudes 0·72 per cent had a patent ductus arteriosus compared to 0·04 per cent at sea level (Penaloza et al. 1964).

After birth, with the interruption of umbilical circulation and expansion of the lungs leading to an increased systemic blood pressure and lowered pulmonary blood pressure, the flow of blood is from the aorta to pulmonary artery (rather than the pre-birth flow from pulmonary artery to aorta) (Assali et al. 1962). Thus if the ductus remains patent it acts as a shunt from aorta to pulmonary artery and the work of the right ventricle is increased. The patent ductus may be a functional response to pulmonary hypertension (Penaloza et al. 1964).

High pulmonary blood pressure may facilitate better perfusion in the lungs and thus greater oxygenation at high altitudes (Grover et al. 1963).

Lung

Lung volume is increased. Despite his smaller stature the high-altitude native has a greater lung volume than his sea-level counterpart.

All compartments of the lung volume are increased in the Peruvian high-altitude natives. The main difference lies in the functional residual capacity (the volume of air remaining in the lung at the end of normal expiration), and that remaining after a forced expiration (residual volume) (Hurtado 1964).

Increased lung volumes in adults are due to accelerated development during childhood and adolescence (Frisancho 1969).

The chest circumference at maximum expiration seems a better predictor than FEV. This suggests that lung size is a function of chest size, rather than stature (Frisancho 1969).

The chest circumference was found to be significantly greater at altitudes above 15,000 ft (4500 m) than at and around 13,000 ft (4000 m) while other measurements of body size remained unchanged. This suggests that accelerated chest development is a specific adaptive mechanism of the chest wall to hypoxia (Frisancho and Baker 1969).

When young (two to sixteen years) sea-level subjects from Peru were acclimatised to 11,500 ft (3400 m) during their period of development, their aerobic capacity and pulmonary ventilation were found to be very similar to those of high-altitude natives—born and bred at that altitude. Sea-level subjects who were acclimatised to similar levels when adult did not attain a ventilation rate and aerobic capacity comparable to high-altitude natives. Essentially the younger the sea-level individual is and the longer he remains at altitude the more likely he is to have ventilation and aerobic capacity similar to that of a high-altitude native (Frisancho *et al.* 1973).

For a Bhutanese population living at 12,000–14,000 ft (3658–4267 m) it was found that the average FVC was significantly greater than for Europeans of the same sex, age and size. The FEVs were somewhat larger but the difference was only significant for women.

If one made allowances however for

   (i) The reduced density and viscosity of respired gas which lowers airway resistance and increases the FEV.
   (ii) The work hypertrophy of the respiratory muscles secondary to hyperventilation which increases the FVC.
   (iii) Minimal atmospheric pollution.

then without these factors the average ventilatory capacity of the Bhutanese would probably be less than for Europeans (Cotes and Ward 1966).

Note: FVC is the Forced Vital Capacity, i.e. the maximum volume of gas that can be expelled from the lung during a forced expiration, starting from total lung capacity (the volume of gas in the lung at the limit of inspiration).

FEV, the Forced Expiratory Volume, is the volume of gas forcibly expired in a given time, usually the first second ($FEV_{1.0}$) following full inspiration.

References

Arias-Stella, J. and Saldana, A. M. (1962) *Medicina Thoracalis* **19**, 484.

Assali, N. S., Seihgal, N. and Marable, S. (1962) *American Journal of Physiology* **202**, 536.

Barcroft, J. (1933) *Lancet* **225**, 1021.

Barron, D. H., Metcalf, J., Meschia, G., Huckabee, W., Hellegers, A. and Prystowsky, H. (1964) In, *Physiological effects of high altitude on man. Ed.* Weihe, W. H. Pergamon Press: Oxford.

Clegg, E. J., Harrison, G. A., Baker, P. T. (1970) *Human Biology* **42**, 486.

Clegg, E. J., Pawson, I. G., Ashton, E. H., Flinn, R. M. (1972) *Philosophical Transactions of the Royal Society* **264B**, 403.

Cotes, J. and Ward, M. P. (1966) *Proceedings of the Physiological Society* **186**, 88pp.

Cotes, J. E. (1968) *Lung function.* 2nd edition. Blackwell Scientific Publications: Oxford.

Cruz-Coke, R. (1968) *Genetic characteristics of high-altitude populations.* WHO/PAHO/IBP Meeting of Investigators on Population Biology at Altitude. Pan-American Health Organisation: Washington, DC.

Emery, J. L. and Mithal, A. (1961) *British Heart Journal* **23**, 313.

Frisancho, A. R. (1969) *Human Biology* **41**, 365.

Frisancho, A. R. (1969) *Human growth in a high-altitude Peruvian population.* Thesis. The Pennsylvania State University.

Frisancho, A. R. (1970) *American Journal of Physical Anthropology* **32**, 401.

Frisancho, A. R. and Baker, P. T. (1970) *American Journal of Physical Anthropology* **32**, 279.

Frisancho, A. R., Martinez, C., Velasquez, T., Sanchez, J. and Montoye, H. (1973) *Journal of Applied Physiology* **34**, 176.

Grover, R. F., Reeves, J. T., Will, D. H. and Blount, S. G. (1963) *Journal of Applied Physiology* **18**, 567.

Harrison, G. A., Kuchemann, C. F., Moore, M. A. S., Boyce, A. J., Baju, T., Mourant, A. E., Godber, M. J., Glasgow, B. G., Kopec, A. C., Tills, D. and Clegg, E. J. (1969) *Philosophical Transactions of the Royal Society* **256B**, 147.

Hurtado, A. (1964) Animals at high altitude–resident man. In, *Handbook of Physiology*. Section 4. *Ed.* Dill, D. B., Adolph, E. F. and Wilber, C. G. American Physiological Society: Washington, DC.

Penaloza, D., Gamboa, R., Dyer, J., Echevarria, M., Gutierrez, E. and Marticorena, E. (1961) *American Heart Journal* **61**, 101.

Penaloza, D., Arias-Stella, J., Sime, F., Recavarren, S. and Marticorena, E. (1964) *Paediatrics* **34**, 586.

Recavarren, S. and Arias-Stella, J. (1962) *American Journal of Pathology* **41**, 467.

Rendon, H. (1964) Thesis. Universidad Nacional de San Agustin Facultad de Medicina: Arequipa, Peru.

Rotta, A. (1947) *American Heart Journal* **33**, 669.

Tanner, J. M. (1967) In, *Report on IBP expedition to North Bhutan. Ed.* Ward, M. P., Jackson, F. S. and Turner, R. W. D.

CHAPTER FIVE

Energy Balance

Introduction

Perhaps the most distinctive feature of a living organism is its utilisation or transformation of energy.

The life of man is made up of a series of events and moments that place him in relationship with his environment. For these events to occur it is necessary to expend energy continually. Bodily movement requires expenditure of energy over and above the basal needs. This must be met by an extra demand for food and oxygen.

In the absence of bodily movement a certain minimum energy is necessary (a basal energy) to support life since man's temperature is normally above that of his environment. This continuous high temperature necessarily means a continuous loss of heat—as heat is a form of energy—and a continuous replacement of heat therefore is essential. This is carried out by assimilation of food and its conversion, usually by oxidation, to substances of lower energy content with a resultant release of energy, which appears ultimately as heat.

The body mechanisms associated with life have a tendency to run down by losing energy. For instance blood loses mechanical energy as it passes through the peripheral circulation and energy is used in the propagation of an action potential down an axon. This energy must be restored to sustain life.

Energy for biological processes could come from many different sources, but conditions in the body are not suitable for the universal conversion of one form of energy to another. A man cannot use electricity, light or heat as sources of bodily energy to keep him alive, but has to rely on food alone.

This food is provided indirectly or directly by plants which use the high energy photons emitted as radiation from the sun.

Man therefore consumes energy as food and emits it mainly in the form of heat for which he has little use if any. As Warburg emphasised, oxygen is not in itself a source of energy, its importance to cell function depends entirely on its ability to liberate energy from foodstuffs.

The energy obtained from food is used in various ways.

About 5 per cent is converted immediately to heat. This leaves 95 per cent available as free energy. The conversion of this free energy in food to high-energy biochemical compounds is not efficient and about 50 per cent is wasted because of biochemical inefficiency.

The remaining 45 per cent is used

   (i) To maintain the structural and biochemical integrity of the body.

 (ii) To maintain internal work. This includes the circulation of the blood, movement of air to lungs, etc. (20–45 per cent).

(iii) To perform external work (0–25 per cent).

That is, the mechanical efficiency of the body is up to 25 per cent.

The end product of the processes concerned with body function is heat unless there is contraction of skeletal muscle when it is heat and external work.

The distribution between heat and work is variable, but at maximal efficiency the distribution is 25 per cent and 75 per cent heat. More usually external work accounts for only a few per cent of the total energy intake, and heat for the rest.

The normal diet consists almost entirely of easily digested foods so that almost all the energy in ingested food is absorbed in a normally functioning gastro-intestinal tract.

The energy content of food, normally measured in kilogram calories, varies. Typical energy contents are, 4 kcal per gram of carbohydrate ingested; 4 kcal per gram of protein ingested; and 9 kcal per gram of fat ingested.

In fact the amount of energy generated does not vary a great deal whatever food is eaten.

A subject at rest, in a steady state, oxidising an average diet generates about 4·83 kcal for every litre of oxygen he consumes. The metabolic rate in kcal is taken to equal the volume of oxygen in litres consumed each minute, multiplied by 4·83.

$$MR = 4·83 \times Vo_2.$$

Assuming a basal oxygen consumption of 250 ml/min, in 24 hours the number of millilitres of oxygen taken in will be $250 \times 60 \times 24 = 360,000$ ml or 360 litre/day. Therefore the metabolic rate in kcal will be $4·83 \times 360 = 1800$ kcal/day.

Or in other words the energy intake each day at rest for a normal person in basal conditions will be 1800 kcal.

As individuals vary in body proportion and weight, and to facilitate comparison, the metabolic rate is usually expressed in terms of energy output per unit area per unit time or kcal/m²/hour.

Various factors influence the metabolic rate.

Factors affecting Metabolic Rate

Physical activity

The level of activity or exercise rate markedly affects the rate of energy output leading to large changes in metabolic rate.

The lowest metabolic rate is whilst asleep, 35 kcal/m²/hour, whilst the maximum steady state energy output is of the order of 350 kcal/m²/hour—or about 10 times the minimum.

Age and Sex

The metabolic rate under resting conditions rises rapidly in the first few weeks after birth. It reaches a peak in early youth; the result of high rates of cell reaction and the rapid synthesis

Table 5.   Energy expenditure for various activities

	kcal/m²/hour
Rest (Sleeping)	35
Light work (Standing)	85
Moderate work	
Housework	140
Walking at 3 mph	140
Heavy work	
Bicycling	250
Skiing	500
Running at 5 mph	570
Walking upstairs	1100
Shivering	250

of cell materials and body growth. The metabolic rate declines with age. Women have a 10 per cent lower rate than men.

Climate

Dwellers in tropical countries have shown a 10–20 per cent lower metabolic rate than inhabitants of Arctic Regions.

The basal metabolic rate (BMR) of Eskimos may be increased by between 23 and 31 per cent in the winter, with a steady decline in the summer months. The current Eskimo generation may have no increase in BMR (Godin and Shephard 1973).

Evidence of effects on visitors to Polar regions is less convincing but rises of up to 5 per cent have been recorded.

Diurnal Variation

The BMR varies diurnally. There is as much as a 10 per cent variation during the day, with peaks at noon and in the evening.

Seasonal Variations

A seasonal variation has been reported from Japanese workers residing in Antarctica. The BMR rose when outside temperature fell and decreased when outside temperature rose (Ohkubo 1973).

Malnutrition

Prolonged malnutrition may decrease BMR by 20–30 per cent. This is a factor to be considered when living for long periods under difficult climatic conditions.

Special Dynamic Action

The taking of food has a stimulating effect on metabolism. This is greatest for proteins and may result in an increase in metabolism of up to 30 per cent. For carbohydrates and fats the increase is less than 5 per cent. On a mixed diet the SDA may be taken to be 10 per cent.

High Altitude

Estimates of basal metabolism at high altitude suggest that it is unchanged (Stickney and Van Liere 1935) or slightly increased (Houston and Riley 1947), or increased transiently in women (Hannon and Sudnam 1973).

A small increase in metabolism at 12,000 ft (3658 m) was attributed to the extra oxygen cost of ventilation (Grover 1963).

Dill (Dill 1966) found no changes in two subjects at 10,500 ft (3100 m) in 1929, yet 34 years later in the same two individuals reported an increase of between 10 and 13 per cent.

Simultaneous exposure to hypoxia (11,000 ft (3353 m)) and cold stress in sea-level visitors for six weeks brought about a rise in basal metabolic rate within a short period. After three weeks, cold stress was withdrawn, and this failed to produce any change.

Acclimatisation to hypoxia alone in this group showed an overall reduction in BMR in the third week, after an initial rise. If cold stress was added during the initial phase, depression of the metabolic rate did not occur. The addition of cold stress in the later stage produced no significant change (Nair *et al.* 1971).

Long-term acclimatisation to great altitude (19,000 ft (5791 m)) may be associated with a raised metabolic rate (Gill and Pugh 1964) and high-altitude natives had a significantly raised basal metabolism in comparison with sea-level visitors (Picon-Reategui 1961, Nair *et al.* 1971).

Discrepancies may be explained by diurnal variation, and only values obtained during the same hour of the day should be used for comparison. The stress of cold is also added to that of high altitude.

Certainly during moderate to severe exercise, a state when more precise regulation occurs than during basal conditions, the oxygen cost for the same work remains identical at different altitudes.

References

Dill, D. B. (1966) US Public Health Service Publication 999–AP 25.

Gill, M. B. and Pugh, L. G. (1964) *Journal of Applied Physiology* **19**, 949.

Godin, G. and Shephard, R. J. (1973) In, *Activity patterns of the Canadian Eskimo. Polar human biology. Ed.* Edholm, O. G. and Gunderson, E. K. E. Heinemann Medical Books: London.

Grover, R. F. (1963) *Journal of Applied Physiology* **18**, 909.

Hannon, J. P. and Sudnam, D. M. (1973) *Journal of Applied Physiology* **34**, 471.

Houston, C. S. and Riley, R. L. (1947) *American Journal of Physiology* **149**, 565.

Nair, C. S., Malhotra, M. S. and Gopinath, P. M. (1971) *Aerospace Medicine* **42**, 1056.

Ohkubo, Y. (1973) In, *Basal metabolism and other physiological changes in the Antarctic. Polar human biology. Ed.* Edholm, O. G. and Gunderson, E. K. E. Heinemann Medical Books: London.

Picon-Reategui, E. (1964) *Journal of Applied Physiology* **16**, 431.

Stickney, J. C. and Van Liere, E. J. (1953) *Physiological Review* **33**, 13.

CHAPTER SIX

Body Composition and Metabolic Aspects

Introduction

Energy output depends on various factors such as physical activity and environmental temperature. Energy intake is determined by the food eaten and absorbed.

Normally the mechanism of hunger maintains the balance between intake and output. When intake is in excess of output the difference is stored as an increase in body fat. When output is excessive there is loss of stored fat which is metabolised to provide the extra energy output. In extreme starvation other constituents of the body and particularly proteins may be metabolised.

The normal daily energy expenditure at sea level is of the order of 2800 kcal for an average person. Studies at sea level suggest that if food intake is restricted to 1500 kcal/day for more than a few days when the energy expenditure is 4000 kcal/day, then morale and performance suffer. Certainly long continued starvation can result in personality change.

Acute Exposure

Acute exposure to altitude results in anorexia, a low calorie intake and loss of weight, a negative nitrogen and water balance

(Consolazio *et al.* 1968; Johnson *et al.* 1969), a decreased resting blood glucose level with lowered glucose disappearance curves (Janoski *et al.* 1969) and changes in electrolyte metabolism have also been observed. These changes are similar to those found in starvation.

More gradual exposure to altitude results in a diminution in the symptoms of mountain sickness, and less nausea and anorexia.

The negative nitrogen balance may be due to decrease in the use of protein, and possibly in its synthesis. A negative water balance has also been observed.

A high carbohydrate diet resulted in a reduction of the severity and duration of symptoms due to acute mountain sickness. Those who are physically fit have fewer symptoms (Consolazio *et al.* 1972). However a sedentary existence associated with a low carbohydrate intake resulted in severe symptoms on acute exposure.

A fall in body weight occurs, though there is less weight loss in those on a high carbohydrate diet, and in those who are able to eat normally. Some loss which is not attributable to body weight also occurs and this is probably due to hypohydration.

During acute exposure, with a daily intake of 50–60 gram of protein, a negative nitrogen balance has been recorded (Surks 1966). However, when adequate calories and protein intake was possible a positive nitrogen balance was obtained (Consolazio *et al.* 1972).

A negative nitrogen balance is therefore probably due to the anorexia which is associated with a reduction in protein intake and deficient calorie consumption, rather than to the effects of hypoxia.

Above 17,500 ft (5334 m)

Continued and prolonged residence at and above this level leads to a blunting of appetite, and resultant decrease in food intake. Weight loss occurs and in severe cases muscle wasting, presumably due to protein breakdown. The emaciated appearance of those members of the successful Everest 1953 Expedition who had been to 26,000 ft (7925 m) and above, even with oxygen, was very marked. One mountaineer in 1933 on Everest commented that after a long period at high altitude, in the course of which he had been to 28,000 ft (8543 m) without oxygen, he could encircle his thigh with the fingers of one hand.

In pre-war Everest expeditions there is evidence that food intake between 17,000 ft (5182 m) and 21,000 ft (6401 m) did not exceed 2000 kcal/day. Above 21,000 ft (6401 m) this fell to 1500 kcal/day.

Table 6.   Energy expenditure on expeditions

Place		Calorie expenditure kcal/24 hours
Approach march	1000–11,500 ft (305–3505 m)	4300
Rest period	15,500–18,000 ft (4725–5486 m)	3200–3700
Climbing	19,000–22,000 ft (5791–6706 m)	3800–4000
	22,000 ft and above (6706 m)	3200
Average climbing day in		
European Alps (i.e. for 10 hours)	10–16,000 ft (3048–4877 m)	6000–7000

The ability to maintain body weight appears to be the best single index of acclimatisation. Poorly acclimatised individuals lose weight due to failure of appetite and an intolerance of fatty foods and possibly intestinal maladsorption.

Good acclimatisation (Ward 1968) is associated with a good appetite and little weight loss, and deterioration with a poor appetite and considerable loss of weight.

At 19,000 ft (5791 m) individuals lost weight over a period of months at an average rate of 1–3 lb/week. Rapid loss during this period was associated with illness, or the sudden deterioration in mental and physical performance that occurred in one or two individuals who did acclimatise well. Descent to 15,000 ft (4572 m) for some days increased weight and appetite.

Long-continued residence at 19,000 ft (5800 m) and above seems unlikely if only for nutritional reasons.

Over four weeks at about 21,000 ft (6401 m) on Everest in 1953, well-acclimatised individuals lost an average of 4 lb, whilst on Cho Oyu in 1952 poorly acclimatised men lost an average of 11 lb at a similar altitude over a similar period (Pugh 1952; Pugh and Ward, 1956).

An initial weight loss may be beneficial by reducing the work of climbing. Recovery from a long period at high altitude however is only complete when the normal body weight is attained.

Dietary Preference

In Polar regions the desire for fat increases. At high altitudes the desire for sugar increases and the desire for fat decreases.

One expedition to Mt McKinley 20,000 ft (6096 m) in Alaska failed because reliance was placed on a diet consisting predominantly of pemmican. This was palatable up to 16,000 ft (4877 m) but not above.

The height at which people avoid fatty foods varies with the individual, the state of acclimatisation and physical fitness. Some are affected as low as 15,000 ft (4572 m) and others not below 21,000 ft (6401 m). Pemmican has been eaten, though not with relish, at 27,000 ft (8230 m).

Table 7.   Fat and carbohydrate intake

Av. fat intake g/24 hours	Av. carbohydrate intake g/24 hours	Altitude
231	453	0–11,000 ft (3353 m)
190	437	18,000 ft (5486 m)
184	478	20,000 ft (6096 m)
54	638	22,000 ft (6706 m)

Sugar tastes less sweet at high altitude and two to three times the normal amount is taken in drinks.

Over a period of three months spent at 19,000 ft (5800 m) a preference for highly spiced meat dishes was noted. This was associated with a craving for fresh rather than tinned or freeze-dried food (Pugh 1965).

Water Metabolism

The changes in water balance at altitude are controversial and as yet unsettled.

A positive water balance of 1·5 litres was reported during the first two days at 11,300 ft (3450 m) (Ullman 1953).

A redistribution of body fluids, with a decrease in plasma volume and an increase in intracellular water, but without dehydration, has been observed (Surks et al. 1966; Hannon et al. 1969).

Other observers have reported absolute dehydration, with large decreases in total body water, plasma, blood volume and a negative water balance (Consolazio et al. 1968; Johnson et al. 1969).

Loss of body weight cannot always be completely accounted for by low calorie intake. Even if calorie intake is adequate, some loss of weight occurs on acute exposure to altitude, and presumably this is due to loss of body water.

Intracellular water falls on acute exposure to altitude, whilst extracellular water remains constant. Total body water therefore fell (Consolazio et al. 1972).

The effect of lower barometric pressure alone however tends to result in a positive fluid balance (Epstein and Saruta 1972).

The maximum period for acute mountain sickness occurred during this period of water shift (Carson 1969).

On initial ascent to high altitude there may be clinical evidence of oedema. A number of cases of gravitational oedema have been recorded—these include orbital and facial oedema noted before rising in the morning. If the individual has been lying on one side unilateral facial oedema with partial closure of the eyelids may occur (Williams 1966; Ward 1968). Clinical oedema is less obvious during a long period at altitude, though it is possible that some water retention occurs even when clinical oedema is absent.

On descent from high altitude, the acclimatised individual after a little delay experiences a diuresis.

Mountaineers have long maintained that the passage of copious urine on arrival at high altitude augured well for the avoidance of acute mountain sickness. A hypoxic diuresis has been noted (Asmussen and Nielsen 1945), and in addition as the temperature falls on ascent cold diuresis may potentiate this effect. Water loss may be an adaptive mechanism to altitude exposure. A fall in total body water may reduce cerebro-spinal fluid pressure and minimise the possibility of cerebral oedema.

Fluid balance over 17,500 ft (5334 m)

Fluid loss at high altitude is higher than at sea level. This is due to a high rate of water loss from the lungs associated with increased respiration, together with heat stress due to a high intensity of direct and reflected solar radiation. Of these two factors the first is probably the more important.

Table 8.   Estimated water loss from respiratory tract at various altitudes (Pugh 1965)

Altitude	Rate of metabolism kcal/24 hours 2000 3000 4000 Water loss, l/24 hours		
Sea level	0·35	0·52	0·69
20,000 ft (6100 m)	0·76	1·15	1·53
24,000 ft (7315 m)	0·94	1·41	1·88
28,000 ft (8530 m)	1·08	1·62	—

An average intake of 3–4 litres per 24 hours has been noted at 17,500 ft (5334 m) and 22,000 ft (6706 m), with a urine output of 1·2–1·5 litres per 24 hours.

On prolonged exposure at an altitude of 19,000 ft (5791 m) in good living conditions, water balance appeared to be normal.

Above 22,000 ft (6706 m) individuals become progressively

dehydrated especially when not using oxygen. The sensation of thirst is blunted, and urine output is diminished. Above 26,000 ft (7925 m) urine output may be of the order of 500 ml daily (Ward 1968).

Kidneys

The kidneys play a part in the haemodynamic changes at altitude. A reduction in plasma flow, a slight reduction in filtration rate and a higher filtration fraction in high-altitude natives have been suggested by studies using insulin and p-aminohippuric acid (Monge *et al.* 1969).

A reduction in creatinine clearance in high-altitude natives (15,500 ft (4710 m)) by comparison with sea-level residents has been attributed to polycythaemia (Rennie *et al.* 1971 (a)). Normal oxygen delivery to and uptake by the kidneys suggested that there was no renal hypoxia in high altitude residents living at 14,000 ft (4300 m) (Rennie *et al.* 1971 (b)).

Exposure to reduced barometric pressure alone without hypoxia results in a progressive decrease in creatinine clearance. After exposure has ceased, recovery occurs (Epstein and Saruta 1972).

Sodium and Potassium Homeostasis

Sodium

Studies on sodium homeostasis have suggested some changes in the handling of sodium ion by the kidneys.

Positive sodium balances were reported during a period in the European Alps in 1911 (Von Wendt 1911). Subsequent studies (Ullman 1953) showed a positive sodium balance during the first two days of exposure to 11,300 ft (3450 m), with a slight negative balance afterwards. Recent work, with control of dietary sodium and potassium intake, has been carried out and during exposure of ten males to 14,100 ft (4300 m) an unaltered sodium balance was reported (Janoski *et al.* 1969). A positive sodium balance occurred during the first two days of exposure at 11,480 ft (3500 m) with a subsequent negative balance, resulting in a mean loss of sodium over a five-day period of 30 meq (Slater *et al.* 1969).

Daily sodium loss in sweat may be fairly high (2·8–6·0 g) in acclimatised subjects (Consolazio *et al.* 1963).

Potassium

The picture for potassium is confused; workers have reported normal (Janoski *et al.* 1969), decreased (Ferguson *et al.* 1957; Gold *et al.* 1961) and increased potassium levels (Jezek *et al.* 1965).

However food intake has been drastically reduced in some studies and this may account for the changes.

A positive balance amounting to 160 meq over a five-day period of exposure at 11,480 ft (3500 m) has been observed (Slater *et al.* 1969). This had previously been demonstrated by estimating the total body content of the naturally-occurring ^{40}K by whole-body counting (Ayres *et al.* 1961).

Both sodium and potassium levels were positive in studies on acute exposure to 14,100 ft (4300 m) (Consolazio 1972).

Reduced barometric pressure by itself may be important as a factor in changes in sodium and potassium homeostasis (Epstein and Saruta 1972).

Inevitably a normal food and fluid intake will maintain a normal electrolyte balance.

Aldosterone

Aldosterone activity has been reported to have decreased at high altitude.

A significant reduction in excretion occurred in individuals during a prolonged stay at 14,300 ft (4360 m) (Ayres *et al.* 1961).

While controlling dietary sodium and potassium intake, a significant decrease in aldosterone secretion occurred following ascent to 11,500 ft (3500 m). On return to sea level, aldosterone returned to normal levels. The decrease was real, and due neither to an alteration in renal excretion of acid labile aldosterone metabolite nor to a change in metabolism (Slater *et al.* 1969).

A small increase in aldosterone secretion was observed following 7–9 days exposure to reduced barometric pressure alone which suggests that decreased excretion may be due to hypoxia, hypocapnia, or some other mechanism rather than reduced barometric pressure (Epstein and Saruta 1972).

There is some evidence that a mechanism for suppressing aldosterone secretion may be present in the right atrium, for when the atrium was stretched secretion diminished. At high altitudes it is likely that stretching of the right atrium occurs in association with right ventricular hypertrophy (Anderson *et al.* 1959).

Changes in intravascular volume may also play a part in control.

As hypersecretion of aldosterone causes hypertension, a decrease at high altitude may provide protection and could be implicated in the low incidence of hypertension in high-altitude natives (Williams 1966).

Renin

Studies of the renin–angiotensin mechanism have been carried out mainly in animals. These suggest some increase in plasma renin during the initial period at high altitude (Gould and Goodman 1970).

In a man decompressed to the equivalent of 14,000 ft (4279 m) an increase in serum renin activity was reported (Tuffley *et al.* 1970). Unfortunately the subjects were not in a steady state of sodium balance at the time of the 'ascent'. On the first 'ascent' the heart rate was increased considerably whereas on the second, three hours later, there was a lesser increase in plasma renin and only a slight change in heart rate.

Adrenal Cortex and Medulla

Stress causes the median eminence of the hypothalamus to release a hormonal factor, the corticotrophin-releasing factor.

This is thought to be transported by way of the pituitary portal venous system to the anterior lobe of the pituitary which acts to accelerate the release of adrenocorticotrophic hormone (ACTH).

Under hypoxic stress a marked increase in electrical activity limited to the posterior hypothalamus has been observed.

In the absence of the hypothalamus, i.e. after hypophysectomy no lymphopenia occurred in rats decompressed to the equivalent of 28,000 ft (8534 m). This suggests that no ACTH activation occurred.

On acute exposure to high altitude plasma cortisol was found to be increased.

At altitudes of about 17,500 ft (5334 m) stimulation of the adrenal cortex occurs. The initial activity is apparent from the increased urinary excretion of 17-hydroxycorticosteroids, 17-ketosteroids and eosinopenia (Timiras *et al.* 1957).

Medullary activity is also stimulated during the early stages of acclimatisation to altitude. An increase in urinary excretion of noradrenaline was observed in men taken from sea level to 12,460 ft (3800 m). During fourteen days' stay at this altitude noradrenaline excretion doubled. No change in adrenaline excretion was recorded (Pace *et al.* 1964).

After about two or three weeks at altitudes probably not exceeding 14,000 ft (4300 m) the adrenal gland in sea-level visitors appears to return to normal activity. (Moncloa *et al.* 1965 (a)).

The response of the adrenal cortex to ACTH was much the same in the high-altitude natives and sea-level residents. A higher titre of ACTH may have been necessary to maintain normal cortical activity at high altitude (Siri *et al.* 1966; MacKinnon *et al.* 1963; Hornbein 1962).

Normal medullary activity seems to occur in high-altitude natives. No significant difference occurred between plasma catecholamines of high-altitude natives at 14,900 ft (4500 m) and at sea level (Moncloa *et al.* 1965 (b)).

During 30–40 days spent at and above 21,000 ft (6400 m)

the excretion rate of 17-hydroxycorticosteroids, 17-ketosteroids and catecholamines was not significantly different from sea-level values.

Abnormally high 17-hydroxycorticosteroid urine levels were found with exposure to extreme altitude—one from a climber who bivouacked at 28,000 ft (8534 m) and who was severely frostbitten, the other from a member who spent a night at 27,000 ft (8230 m) (Siri *et al.* 1969).

After long periods at altitudes above 17,500 ft (5334 m) some clinical deterioration does occur. Adequate studies of adrenal gland activity have not been made. However a reduction in total neutral 17-ketosteroids and 17-ketogenic steroids was noted after a 60-day period at 19,000 ft (5791 m) (Pugh 1962).

Disappearance of circulatory eosinophils after a long and arduous mountain ascent at Alpine pace was noted in two men after about three months at 19,000 ft (5791 m), suggesting that the adrenal gland was capable of responding to stress (Ward 1968).

Although little evidence of adrenal exhaustion has been found biochemically all mountaineers who spend prolonged periods at high altitudes would agree that stress is considerable especially above 23,000 ft (7010 m) and when maximum physical work is carried out for long periods.

Two cases of exhaustion at 20,000 ft (6096 m) were examined in 1953 on Everest and low blood pressures were recorded in both (Pugh and Ward 1956).

In a case of Addison's disease of about nine months duration in a high-altitude native resident at 12,000 ft (3658 m) it was noted that the heart shadow was smaller, the haematocrit was lower (46·5 per cent) and the total red cell volume lower than the normal findings at that altitude. The electrolytes were within normal limits (Moncloa *et al.* 1964).

This suggests that tolerance to hypoxia may exist with no significant blood change and hypofunction of the adrenal cortex. As the electrolytes were normal it appears that there was a minimal deficiency in mineralocorticoids.

Thyroid

The results of thyroid function studies in experimental animals exposed to the stress of hypoxia and high altitude are contradictory.

In men exposed to high altitude, elevated free and total thyroxine concentrations have been reported within three days (Surks *et al.* 1967; Kotchen *et al.* 1973).

An elevated PBI was reported in one individual during exposure for four days to 16,400 ft (5000 m) (Siri *et al.* 1966).

An increased rate of thyroxine degradation within the first three days was reported by Surks (Surks *et al.* 1967).

Lack of raised TSH suggests that thyroxine secretion is not raised at a simulated altitude of 12,000 ft (3658 m). The percentage of T_3 uptake, which is an indirect measure of the effect of modification in plasma proteins upon certain indices of thyroid function, remained unaltered at simulated altitude but this may be affected by many factors. On return to 'sea level' all thyroid function changes returned to normal on the second day (Kotchen *et al.* 1973).

A lower prevalence of goitre has been noted among populations living at higher altitudes (over 3000 m) (Fierro-Benitez *et al.* 1969). It has been suggested that a lower peripheral utilisation of iodine may result in a decreased thyroid activity and hence a lower prevalance of goitres.

Many mountain areas are relatively iodine deficient and this fact must be taken into account when assessing thyroid function tests.

Fertility

Although lowered fertility was reported by the Spanish Conquistadores at high altitudes in South America, no alteration in the urinary excretion of gonadotropin was observed in sea-level natives acutely exposed to altitudes of 14,000 ft (4267 m).

High-altitude natives excreted the same amount of gonadotropin and the fertility of the high-altitude natives seemed unimpaired (Sobrevilla *et al.* 1967).

Blood Sugar

Inconstant changes in fasting blood sugar and glucose tolerance curves have been reported in high altitude visitors.

Increased glucose tolerance curves (Forbes 1936) and a faster rate of glucose utilisation in high-altitude residents have been observed (Picon-Reategui 1962).

More recent work at 14,100 ft (4300 m) has shown normal fasting blood sugar levels and glucose tolerance curves at altitude, when food intake and glucose utilisation were normal (Consolazio *et al.* 1972).

References

Anderson, G. H., McCally, M. and Farrell, G. L. (1949) *Endocrinology* **64**, 202.

Asmussen, E. and Nielsen, M. (1945) *Acta physiologica scandinavica*, **9**, 75.

Ayres, P. J., Hurter, R. C., Williams, E. S. and Rundo, J. (1961) *Nature* **191**, 78.

Carson, R. P., Evans, W. O., Shields, J. L. and Hannon, J. P. (1969) *Federation Proceedings. Federation of American Societies for Experimental Biology* **28**, 1085.

Consolazio, C. F., Johnson, H. L. and Krzywicki, H. J. (1972) Body fluids, body composition and metabolic aspects of high altitude adaptation. Desert and mountain. In, *Physiological adaptation. Ed.* Yousef, M. K., Horvath, S. M. and Bullard, R. W. Academic Press: New York and London.

Consolazio, C. F., Matoush, L. O., Nelson, R. A., Harding, R. S. and Canham, J. E. (1963) *Journal of Nutrition* **79**, 407.

Consolazio, C. F., Matoush, L. O., Johnson, H. L. and Daws, T. A. (1968) *American Journal of Clinical Nutrition* **21**, 154.

Epstein, M. and Saruta, T. (1972) *Journal of Applied Physiology* **33**, 204.

Ferguson, F. P., Smith, D. C. and Barry, J. Q. (1957) *Endocrinology* **60**, 761.

Fierro-Benitez, R., Wilson, P., De Groot, L. J. and Ramirez, I. (1969) *New England Journal of Medicine* **280**, 296.

Forbes, W. H. (1936) *American Journal of Physiology* **116**, 309.

Gold, A. J., Barry, J. Q. and Ferguson, F. P. (1961) *Journal of Applied Physiology* **16**, 837.

Gould, A. B. and Goodman, S. A. (1970) *Laboratory Investigation* **22**, 443.

Hannon, J. P., Chinn, K. S. K. and Shields, J. L. (1969) *Federation Proceedings. Federation of American Societies for Experimental Biology* **28**, 1178.

Hornbein, T. F. (1962) *Journal of Applied Physiology* **17**, 246.

Janoski, A. H., Whitten, B. K., Shields, J. L. and Hannon, J. P. (1969) *Federation Proceedings. Federation of American Societies for Experimental Biology* **28**, 1185.

Jezek, V., Ourednik, A., Daum, S. and Krouzkoa, L. (1965) *Acta medica scandinavica* **177**, 175.

Johnson, H. L., Consolazio, C. F., Matoush, L. O. and Krzywicki, D. H. J. (1969) *Federation Proceedings. Federation of American Societies for Experimental Biology* **28**, 1195.

Kotchen, T. A., Mougey, E. H., Hogan, R. P., Boyd, A. E., Pennington, L. L. and Mason, J. W. (1973) *Journal of Applied Physiology* **34**, 165.

Krzywicki, H. J., Consolazio, C. F., Matoush, L. O., Johnson, H. L. and Barnhart, R. A. (1969) *Federation Proceedings. Federation of American Societies for Experimental Biology* **28**, 1190.

MacKinnon, P. C. B., Monk-Jones, M. E. and Fotherby, K. (1963) *Journal of Endocrinology* **26**, 555.

Moncloa, F. J., Donayre, L. A., Sobrevilla, L. A. and Guerra-Garcia, R. (1965) *Journal of Clinical Endocrinology and Metabolism* **25**, 1640.

Moncloa, F., Gomez, M. and Hurtado, A. (1965) *Journal of Applied Physiology* **20**, 1329.

Moncloa, F., Guerra-Garcia, R., Lara, A., Mayor, M. and Paitan, J. (1964) *Journal of Clinical Endocrinology* **24**, 1328.

Monge, C., Lozano, R., Marchena, C., Whittembury, J. and Torres, C. (1969) *Federation Proceedings. Federation of American Societies for Experimental Biology* **28**, 1199.

Pace, N., Griswold, R. L. and Grunbaum, B. W. (1964) *Federation Proceedings. Federation of American Societies for Experimental Biology* **23**, 521.

Picon-Reategui, E. (1962) *Metabolism: Clinical and Experimental* **11**, 1148.

Pugh, L. G. C. E. (1952) *Report on Cho Oyu expedition.* Medical Research Council.

Pugh, L. G. C. E. and Ward M. P. (1956) *Lancet* **271**, 1115.

Pugh, L. G. C. E. (1965) *High altitude* in *Exploration medicine. Ed.* Edholm, O. G., Bacharach, A. L. and Wright, J. Bristol.

Pugh, L. G. C. E. (1962) *British Medical Journal* **2**, 621.

Rennie, D., Marticorena, E., Monge, C. and Sirotsky, L. (1971(a)) *Journal of Applied Physiology* **31**, 257.

Rennie, D., Lozano, R., Monge, C., Sime, F. and Whittembury, J. (1971(b)) *Journal of Applied Physiology* **30**, 450.

Siri, W. E., Cleveland, A. S. and Blanche, P. (1969) *Federation Proceedings. Federation of American Societies for Experimental Biology* **28**, 1251.

Slater, J. D. H., Tuffley, R. E., Williams, E. S., Beresford, C. H., Sonksen, P. H., Edwards, R. H. T., Ekins, R. P. and McLaughlin, M. (1969) *Clinical Science* **37**, 311.

Sobrevilla, L. A., Romero, I., Moncloa, F., Donayre, J. and Guerra-Garcia, R. (1967) *Acta endocrinologica (Copenhagen)* **56**, 369.

Surks, M. I., Chinn, K. S. K. and Matoush, L. O. (1966) *Journal of Applied Physiology* **21**, 1741.

Surks, M. I. (1966) *Journal of Clinical Investigation* **45**, 1442.

Surks, M. I., Beckwitt, H. J. and Chidsey, C. A. (1967) *Journal of Clinical Endocrinology* **27**, 789.

Timiras, P. S., Pace, N. and Hwang, C. A. (1957) *Federation Proceedings. Federation of American Societies for Experimental Biology* **16**, 340.

Tuffley, R. E., Rubenstein, D., Slater, J. D. H. and Williams, E. S. (1970) *Journal of Endocrinology* **48**, 497.

Ullman, E. A. (1953) *Journal of Physiology* **120**, 58.

Von Wendt (1911) *Skandinavisches Archiv für Physiologie* **24**, 247.

Ward, M. P. (1965) *Diseases occurring at altitudes exceeding 17,500 ft.* M.D. Thesis. University of Cambridge.

Williams, E. S. (1966) *Proceedings of the Royal Society. Series B* **165**, 266.

CHAPTER SEVEN

Respiration: the Gas Phase

At high altitude the main responses to changes in barometric pressure are those concerned with the effects of hypoxia, though low barometric pressure itself, apart from hypoxia, may contribute to these adjustments.

Changes occur at each stage in the transport of oxygen from the ambient air to the tissues.

In its widest sense, respiration may be divided for the sake of simplicity into three phases in each of which the effects of altitude appear.

Gas phase. This comprises two components:

The flow of air in and out of the lungs through the airway.

The gas exchange mechanism—or arterialisation within the lungs.

Here facilities for free diffusion of gases in either direction are provided.

Fluid phase. This is formed by blood and interstitial fluid. The main function of this phase is the rapid transfer of gas from the lungs to the tissues.

Tissue phase. This controls the migration of oxygen molecules from the interstitial fluid to the respiratory cytochromes, flavoproteins, and pyrimidine molecules, which are the main components of the mitochondria of the cell.

This chapter deals with the first of these three phases.

Oxygen Transport

The composition of atmospheric air and alveolar air differs for a number of reasons:

(i) Dry atmospheric air that enters the lung is humidified before it reaches the gas exchange area.

(ii) Alveolar air is only partially replaced by atmospheric air with each breath.

(iii) Oxygen is constantly being absorbed from the alveolar air.

(iv) Carbon dioxide is constantly diffusing from the pulmonary capillaries to the alveoli.

At each breath the amount of alveolar air replaced by fresh atmospheric air is only about 15 per cent of the total. Even when the alveolar ventilation is twice normal, only half the total volume is removed in eight seconds.

This slow replacement of alveolar air is important in preventing sudden changes in gas concentration in the blood. This stabilises the control of respiration and helps to prevent sudden and excessive changes in tissue oxygenation.

Water Vapour

At body temperature, the partial pressure of water vapour in fully saturated air is 47 mmHg. This is independent of the barometric pressure and there is thus no change with altitude. The lower the barometric pressure (or the higher the altitude) the larger is the relative percentage of alveolar air that water vapour forms.

Because the total pressure of alveolar air cannot rise above 760 mmHg, the addition of 47 mmHg of water vapour to the atmospheric air at sea level as it enters the lung and is humidified, results in the partial pressure of oxygen being reduced from about 160 to 150 mmHg and of nitrogen from about 600 to 560 mmHg.

The oxygen concentration in the alveoli is controlled by the rate of absorption of oxygen in the blood and the rate of entry of oxygen into the lungs.

Similarly, the carbon dioxide concentration in the alveoli is controlled by the rate of excretion of carbon dioxide from blood to the alveoli and the rate of removal of carbon dioxide from the lungs by ventilation.

Thus the concentration of oxygen and carbon dioxide depends on the rate of absorption and excretion of each gas and the degree of alveolar ventilation.

Ambient air. The total atmospheric pressure is 760 mmHg. Of this, 20·9 per cent is oxygen, so Po_2 in ambient air is 20·9 per cent of 760 mmHg = 159 mmHg.

Inspired air. As air is inhaled it becomes saturated with water vapour at body temperature. The partial pressure of water vapour is 47 mmHg. Therefore the Po_2 of inspired air is 20·9 per cent of $760 - 47$ mmHg = 149 mmHg.

Alveolar air. Because oxygen is being continuously removed from inspired air and carbon dioxide added, the Po_2 of alveolar air is less than that of inspired air. A balance is struck between the rate at which oxygen is removed and the rate at which it is replenished. The Po_2 is about 100 mmHg. If alveolar ventilation falls the alveolar Po_2 falls, and if it is increased the alveolar Po_2 rises.

Thus even in a perfect oxygen transport system one third (150 mmHg reduced to 100 mmHg) of the Po_2 is lost before the oxygen reaches the arterial blood (see Table 9).

Table 10 shows the partial pressure and composition of inspired and alveolar air at varying altitudes up to 25,700 ft (7830 m).

Table 9.   Changes in the composition of air during respiration at sea level

Gas*	Atmospheric air	Humidified air (inspired)	Alveolar air	Expired air	Arterial blood	Venous blood
Nitrogen	597·0	563·4	569·0	566·0	547·0	570
Oxygen	159·0	149·3	104·0	120·0	96·0	40·0
Carbon dioxide	0·3	0·3	40·0	27·0	40·0	46·0
Water	3·7	47·0	47·0	47·0	47·0	47·0
Total	760·0	760·0	760·0	760.0	760·0	760·0

* Gas tensions in mmHg.

Table 10.   Composition of inspired and alveolar gas at various
altitudes from sea level to 25,700 ft (7830 m)

Altitude	Barometric pressure mmHg	$P_{I}\,O_2$ mmHg	$P_{Alv}\,O_2$ mmHg	$P_{Alv}\,CO_2$ mmHg
Sea level	750	150	110	38
19,000 ft (5800 m)	380	69	45	22
21,000 ft (6400 m)	344	62	38	21
24,400 ft (7440 m)	300	53	34	16
25,700 ft (7830 m)	288	50	33	14

Oxygen Gradient at Altitude

Plotting the oxygen pressure at various stages in its transport
from ambient air to mixed venous blood, and then comparing
the gradient between sea level and 19,000 ft (5791 m) brings out
two points. The gradient is steeper at sea level, and there is only a
10 mmHg difference between the P_{O_2} of mixed venous blood
both at rest and during exercise, suggesting that the mechanisms
of adaptation are remarkably efficient.

The curve in Fig. 2 may be analysed in three sections.

(i) Inspired to alveolar air. At high altitude the main part of
the curve where the slope is less steep is that between inspired
and alveolar air. This is due to the increased ventilation that
occurs within a few hours of arrival and increases rapidly during
the first week. It is, initially, the main clinical feature.

The effect of the increased ventilation at high altitude is to
reduce the gradient of oxygen pressure between the ambient air
and alveoli. There is a difference between acclimatised and unacclimatised individuals.

The alveolar P_{O_2} will fall with altitude in individuals at rest
and acutely exposed to high altitude but there is no measurable
increase in ventilation with resultant fall of P_{CO_2} until a level
of about 15–18,000 ft (4572–5486 m).

In acclimatised visitors however the ventilation is increased
at a much lower altitude or higher P_{O_2}. The Rahn–Otis diagram

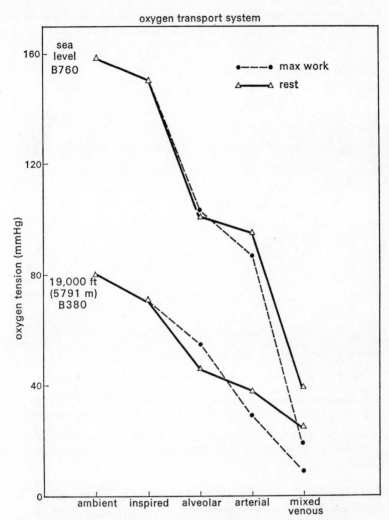

Fig. 2   Oxygen tension at various stages in the oxygen transport system at rest and for maximum exercise for subjects at sea level and at 19,000 ft (5800 m) in the acclimatised state (Pugh 1965).

which plots $PAlv.O_2$ against $PAlv.CO_2$ illustrates this point (Rahn and Otis 1949) (Fig. 3).

If one further adds lines along which the alveolar value at any given altitude must lie at a given alveolar exchange rate of

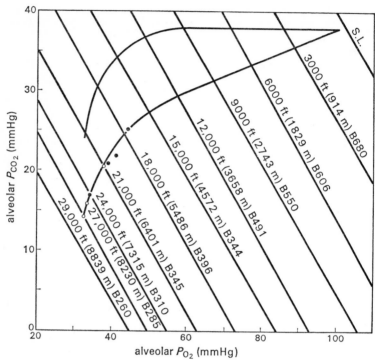

Fig. 3 The CO_2–O_2 diagram showing alveolar P_{CO_2} and P_{O_2} in un-acclimatised persons acutely exposed to altitude (upper curve) and in acclimatised persons chronically exposed to altitude (lower curve). The plotted points represent mean values of Haldane end expiratory samples taken on Himalayan expeditions. The oblique lines are lines along which the alveolar values at any given altitude must lie at a given alveolar exchange ratio of 0·85. (Pugh 1965.)

0·85, it can be seen that at a given altitude of say 12,000 ft (3658 m) the $P_{Alv}.O_2$ in unacclimatised man is about 50 mmHg, whereas in acclimatised visitor it is about 60 mmHg.

In other words the $P_{Alv}.O_2$ of the acclimatised visitor is higher—and his haemoglobin is better saturated.

Further points are that

(a) between the altitudes of 9000 and 15,000 ft (2700 and 4600 m) the gain in $P_{Alv}.O_2$ in acclimatised individuals is up to about 10 mmHg. This corresponds to an altitude of 3–4000 ft

(900–1200 m) or the acclimatised man is at a 'lower altitude' than the unacclimatised with regard to his PAlv.O_2.

(b) Above 15,000 ft (4600 m) the gain in PAlv.O_2 with acclimatisation becomes less until above 27,000 ft (8230 m) the acclimatised and unacclimatised mountaineer are in the same situation with regard to their PAlv.O_2.

(ii) Alveolar to arterial. Increased ventilation reduces the P_{O_2} gradient between the alveoli and the arterial blood. The normal difference is about 10 mmHg, at sea level, whereas at rest at 14,000 ft (4267 m) it is about 2 mmHg (Dill 1938; Houston and Riley 1947).

This is due to an improved distribution of ventilation in underventilated parts of the lung; improved distribution of perfusion due to an increased artery pressure; a raised ventilation perfusion ratio, secondary to increased ventilation (Hurtado 1964); and the reduction at low P_{O_2} of the O_2 gradient associated with the venous admixture effect.

During exercise diffusion may become a limiting factor and increase the alveolar–arterial gradient.

Diffusing capacity does not change at altitude in visitors, but is higher in high-altitude natives.

(iii) Arterial to venous blood. The remaining part of the oxygen transport system, where the gradient is less steep at high altitude, is between the arterial and venous points. This is due (a) to displacement of the oxygen uptake to the steep part of the oxygen dissociation curve. In this part of the curve (P_{O_2} 80–40 mmHg) the relatively small change in pressure results in a large change in oxygen content of the blood. This is an inherent property of haemoglobin and not an adaptive response to altitude, nevertheless it is important in man's ability to live and exercise at altitude; (b) to an increased oxygen capacity of blood; (c) the gradient also depends on the cardiac output.

Mechanics of Respiration

Three structures are involved: the chest wall, the lungs and the respiratory muscles.

The chest wall has an elasticity (chest elasticity) for which there is a 'position of rest'—that is, if the chest wall is compressed or expanded it returns to this position of rest. The position of rest for the empty chest cage is such that if it occupied this position in the living body the lungs would contain about 60 per cent of a maximal inspiration (or 60 per cent of the vital capacity).

The lungs have elasticity or a tendency to collapse (lung elasticity). When the lungs are in the chest cage and the respiratory muscles are collapsed or paralysed, the lungs contain about 40 per cent of the vital capacity.

It is from this base-line, which is the balance between chest elasticity and lung elasticity, that normal respiration occurs.

In normal inspiration the diaphragm and intercostal muscles are primarily involved. The diaphragm increases lung volume downwards, and the intercostal muscles expand the chest cage upwards and outwards. When these muscles relax, the lung and chest elasticities both tend to 'collapse' until the normal balance in the position of rest is reestablished. Inspiration is a muscular effort, expiration is the elastic recoil of lung and chest wall. Normally it is passive. For respiration up to 50 litres per minute (minute volume), only the diaphragm and intercostals are active.

Accessory Muscles of Respiration

Over 50 litres per minute the accessory muscles of respiration, the sterno-mastoids and extensors of the spine, may come into action, as also will the pectoral muscles. In expiration there is no evidence that the intercostals are active—except possibly during the early part, when they act as a braking effect on the elastic recoil. In forcible expiration the muscles of the abdominal wall may also be actively employed.

The use of the accessory muscles of respiration can be seen clearly when climbing at altitude.

Initially it is only necessary to stop and pant whilst standing—sometimes with the hands fixed. In fact many people walk uphill at moderate altitudes with their hands on their hips. Probably in this instance the pectoral muscles are acting as accessory muscles of respiration. After greater exertion, an ice-axe is often placed in the slope above the climber who places his hands on it and leans forwards, thereby fixing the arms and scapulae more firmly.

After extreme exertion, in addition to the hands or arms being placed on a support, the head may be rested on it as well. This fixes the skull, cervical spine, both scapulae and humeri, so that the muscles which have their origins on these bones and the thoracic cage may be used in respiration. They include the scaleni, sterno-mastoids, rhomboids, trapezii, pectorals and serratus anterior. After periods of great effort, the muscles of respiration have been observed to ache in much the same way as the arm or leg muscles after taking severe exercise.

Table 11.   Respiratory muscles active during inspiration and expiration at various minute volumes

Mild activity Min. vol. less than 50 l/min	Moderate to severe activity Min. vol. more than 50 l/min

Inspiration
  Diaphragm
  Internal intercostals
  Scalene muscles occasionally
	Diaphragm, scalene muscles,
	Sterno-mastoid, extensors of neck.

Expiration
  Passive
	Internal intercostals,
	  transverse and oblique
	  abdominal muscles.

The Work of Breathing

In respiration work is done to overcome the elastic resistance of the lungs and the thoracic cage (the compliance), the airway resistance and the viscosity of pulmonary tissues.

Elastic Resistance

The elastic properties of the lungs are caused by the surface tension of the fluids lining the alveoli and the elastic fibres in the lung itself. The elastic properties of the thoracic wall are due to the natural elasticity of the muscles, tendons and connective tissue.

The expansibility of the lungs and thorax is called the compliance.

To overcome this resistance in the lung and chest wall, work has to be carried out.

Airway Resistance

A certain amount of energy is needed to move air along the airways.

In quiet respiration the amount required is slight but if there is any resistance, as in asthma or emphysema, a large amount of extra energy may be needed by the respiratory muscles.

Air flow in the respiratory tract is partly streamlined and partly turbulent. Turbulence increases as the rate of flow increases. The resistance offered to a turbulent flow is much greater than to a streamlined flow—therefore as respiration increases so does turbulence and the work required to maintain the flow rate. At high altitude lowered viscosity and air density will offset this to a certain extent.

Expiration is believed to be passive in normal breathing but it may be active in voluntary hyperpnoea and increased respiratory exertion during exercise.

At extreme altitude clinical observation suggests that expiration is often active, especially on severe exertion.

Viscosity of Pulmonary Tissues (or Non-elastic Tissue Resistance)

A certain amount of work is required to rearrange the molecules in the tissues of the lungs and thoracic cage in order to change them to new dimensions. This means slipping molecules over each other and this constitutes a type of resistance.

When the lungs are oedematous or have lost most of their elastic properties because of fibrotic changes, this resistance is greatly increased and the work output is greater. The oxygen cost of breathing is increased and under the extreme conditions of hypoxia this may be serious.

Oxygen Cost of Ventilation at Altitude

The work cost of breathing is the amount of oxygen used by the respiratory muscles, which have a rather low efficiency.

Inspiration is an active process and the work mainly results from inhaling the tidal volume of air against resistance and expanding the lungs against the elasticity of the lungs and chest walls.

At rest the average consumption of oxygen by the respiratory muscles is from 1–3 per cent of the total oxygen used by the body, that is, 1–3 per cent of 250 ml = 2·5–7·5 ml/min. The percentage rises at high ventilation rates and the oxygen cost of ventilation increases considerably.

Since the oxygen available for work other than breathing is the difference between the total oxygen uptake and the oxygen cost for breathing, the oxygen used for breathing results in a reduction in that available for other work. Studies at the extreme limits of exercise in athletes suggests that a point may be reached where any increase in ventilation may so increase the oxygen cost of breathing that most of the increased oxygen uptake would be used by muscles involved in respiration. However such a situation is probably encountered only in those who have been trained to exercise to the absolute limit of their maximal oxygen uptake.

A similar situation may well occur at extreme altitudes without supplementary oxygen; however, because of the reduced viscosity and density and therefore lower airway resistance the oxygen cost of breathing may not be as high as expected.

At 12,000 ft (3800 m) work requiring an oxygen uptake of 2·2 litres/min can be sustained for about the same oxygen cost as at sea level. At a higher altitude and a higher level of work a higher oxygen uptake was found, and this suggests that the oxygen cost of ventilation was higher.

In high-altitude visitors at 19,000 ft (5791 m) the oxygen cost of ventilation when working at 300 kg m/min would be of the order of 25 ml/min.

At ventilation volumes of over 150 litres/min, which at 19,000 ft (5791 m) is equivalent to a work rate of 900 kg m/min, and at 21,000 ft (6401 m) equivalent to 6–700 kg m/min, the oxygen cost rises steeply.

During exercise a critical level of about 140 litres/min ventilation seems to occur. Above this level a further increase in ventilation makes no more oxygen available to the muscles, without a lowering of Po_2.

At 24,500 ft (7450 m) this level of ventilation is reached when working at 600 kg m/min which is maximal for sea-level visitors at this altitude. This critical level—140 litres/min—will vary with the individual.

High-altitude natives enjoy a considerable advantage by being able to supply oxygen to the muscles at a lower oxygen cost because of lower ventilation rates (Pugh *et al.* 1964).

Alveolar Pco_2 is therefore higher, and the pH of arterial blood decreased, in comparison with high-altitude visitors. Their diffusing capacity is higher and the same amount of oxygen is extracted from the air with less work by the muscles of respiration. As the maximum heart rate is higher than in high-altitude visitors, the cardiac output may also be higher.

At very high ventilation rates, the respiratory work is such that the oxygen gained is all used by the respiratory muscles; at very high altitude therefore the Sherpa (high-altitude native) is at a distinct advantage (Lahiri and Milledge 1966).

Upper Respiratory Tract and Lungs

In the upper respiratory tract under normal circumstances expired air is fully saturated with water vapour. The volume of water lost in this manner is extremely variable. Any figure quoted (5 ml/hr/sq. metre is very approximate) will be affected by the ambient temperature and humidity. At high altitude when ventilation is greatly increased, loss of water from the upper respiratory tract is an important factor in dehydration (see Chapter 6). The drying of the mucosa which is associated may predispose to severe upper respiratory tract infection and sloughing of the mucosa of the nasopharynx with partial suffocation has been recorded at 28,000 ft (8534 m).

The protection of the respiratory tract by the ciliary system of the cells lining the bronchi seems very efficient, removing dirt by carrying it on a moving blanket of mucus.

The bronchial tree exists to conduct air to the alveolar surface. The bronchi and bronchioles are concerned with air conduction alone. The remaining part is concerned with air conduction and gas exchange, the latter becoming more important as the system is followed distally. The last purely conducting structure is the terminal bronchiole. That portion of the lung distal to this is the gas exchanging area and is termed an acinus. It is made up of respiratory bronchioles, alveolar ducts, atria, alveolar sacs and the alveoli themselves. The alveolar sac is the terminal blind end of the respiratory passage.

The total cross-sectional area gradually increases after an initial narrowing in the main, lobar and segmental bronchi. It is this increase in area which is responsible for the low resistance to air flow in the small airways.

There are about 300 million alveoli in each average sized adult lung, or 600 million in the normal adult. The total alveolar surface area is related to body length and varies between 40–100 sq. metres or about 50 times the skin surface of the body. Some loss occurs with increasing age.

The overall thickness of the respiratory membrane through which gas exchange occurs varies from 1·0 microns to less than 0·1 microns. This separates a total volume of blood in the lung capillaries of between 60 and 100 ml, from a total volume of air in the gas exchange area of about 3 litres. Thus gas exchange is rapid and easy, despite the blood being exposed for only 0·8 seconds and being replaced up to about 100 times per minute.

The average diameter of a pulmonary capillary is about 7 microns. As the average diameter of a red blood cell is 8 microns it must be squeezed and the wall of the red blood cell and the wall of the capillary must be in contact. The red blood cell is basically a bag whose peripheral diameter is 2·0 micron, and with a central diameter of 1·0 micron. It can be deformed, and this deformation and its contact with the capillary wall aids the rapidity of oxygen and carbon dioxide diffusion.

Below are given some useful magnitudes.

The total lung gas volume at the end of normal expiration (functional residual volume) is between 2500 and 3000 ml.

The total volume of air in the conducting airways is about 150 ml (anatomical dead space).

The total volume of blood undergoing gas exchange in the pulmonary capillaries is about 70 ml.

Assuming the tidal volume (or air breathed in and out in a single respiration) is 500 ml, and the number of breaths each minute is 15, the total volume of inspired air each minute is $15 \times 500 = 7500$ ml/minute (the minute volume).

Of each 500 ml of tidal volume, 150 ml remains in the conducting airways and takes no part in gas exchange. The remainder, 350 ml, is concerned with gas-exchange as alveolar air.

Thus the alveolar ventilation is $350 \times 15 = 5250$ ml/min.

The cardiac output at rest is about 5 litre/minute and the total amount of blood brought to the alveolar membrane is approximately the same.

Adaptations in the Lung

In high-altitude natives the following are increased

(i) Total lung capacity (or total lung volume), which is the amount of gas contained in the lung at the end of a maximal inspiration.

(ii) Functional residual capacity (the volume of gas remaining in the lungs at the resting expiratory level).

(iii) The residual volume (or volume of gas remaining in the lungs at the end of maximal expiration) (Hurtado 1964).

The direction of the ribs in the high-altitude native is more horizontal than in visitors. The average slope as measured by Barcroft was 13°, as against 21° in visitors. This suggests a relatively larger A–P diameter of the chest (Barcroft 1925).

Table 12.   Adaptations in the lung

	SL resident at sea level	HA native resident at 15,000 ft (4540 m)
Total lung capacity	6·5	6·96
Vital capacity	5·0	4·88
Inspiratory capacity	3·23	3·16
Functional residual capacity (Expiratory capacity + residual volume)	3·26	3·80
Expiratory capacity	1·76	1·73
Residual volume	1·50	2·07

The chest circumference has been found to be significantly greater at altitudes exceeding 15,000 ft (4500 m) than at and around 13,000 ft (4000 m) whilst other measurements of body size remained unchanged. This suggests that accelerated chest development is a specific adaptive mechanism of the chest wall to hypoxia (Frisancho and Baker 1969). The change means that a greater volume of air, in dilated alveoli, is in contact with the pulmonary capillaries. This, with the associated dilatation of the pulmonary capillary bed, produces conditions which favour gas exchange between alveoli and circulating blood.

Respiratory Membrane

The respiratory membrane is composed of (a) a monomolecular layer of surfactant which covers the surface of (b) a thin layer of fluid lining the lung alveolus; (c) the epithelium of the alveolus; (d) the interstitial space between the alveolar epithelium and (e) the basement membrane of a lung capillary; and (f) the capillary endothelium (Fig. 4).

The rate at which a gas will pass through the respiratory membrane will depend on a combination of the thickness of the whole membrane, the surface area of the membrane, the diffusion coefficient of the gas in water and the difference in partial pressure of the gas between the two sides of the membrane.

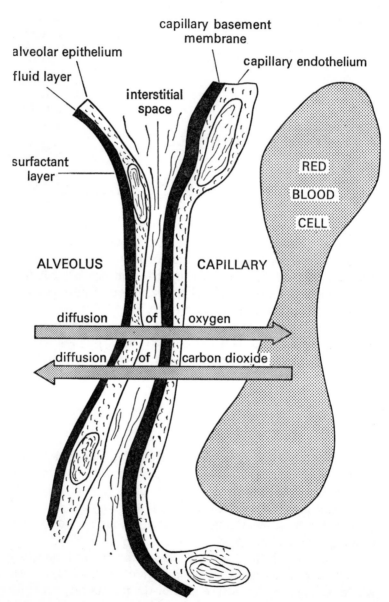

Fig. 4 Ultrastructure of the respiratory membrane.

Thickness of membrane. This will increase with (a) oedema fluid in the interstitial space, (b) fluid in alveoli (i.e. infection, or pulmonary oedema from other causes) and (c) increased thickness of alveolar walls due to fibrosis of the lung following disease. As the rate of diffusion is inversely proportional to thickness, any factor which increases thickness by more than 2 or 3 times can markedly interfere with gas exchange. This occurs in high-altitude pulmonary oedema, or any lung disease at altitude.

Decreasing surface area. Surface area may be decreased by removal of part or all of a lung, or by disease putting certain parts out of action, either temporarily or permanently. On extreme exercise even the smallest decrease in surface area may be detrimental to exchange. This will be more marked at altitude.

Diffusion coefficient. This depends on the solubility of the gas and its molecular weight. Thus carbon dioxide diffuses twenty times as rapidly as oxygen, and oxygen diffuses twice as rapidly as nitrogen and at the same rate as helium.

Pressure difference. The partial pressure of a gas in the respiratory membrane represents a measure of the number of molecules of that gas striking a unit area of the alveolar surface of the membrane and a similar measure applies to the partial pressure of the gas in blood.

Diffusing Capacity of the Respiratory Membrane

The diffusing capacity represents the ability of the respiratory membrane to allow a gas to pass between the alveolus and the lung capillaries. It is measured by the volume of gas that diffuses through the membrane each minute for a pressure difference of 1 mmHg. (It is usual to use carbon monoxide to measure the diffusing capacity.)

In the adult at rest the total oxygen diffusing through the respiratory membrane is about 250 ml (resting oxygen consumption). As about 21 ml per mmHg of oxygen diffuses through each minute, then the pressure difference during quiet breathing is about 11 mmHg.

For perfect gas exchange the ratio of air and blood should be even in all lung units, as clearly if all the blood went to one part of the lungs and all the air to another there would be no gas exchange at all. This is termed the $\dot{V}/\dot{Q}$ ratio, where $\dot{V}$ equals volume of air shifted per minute in and out of the lung, and $\dot{Q}$ equals blood flow (litres/min) in and out of the lung. Even in the normal upright lung there is a degree of unevenness of air and blood flow, and due to gravity blood flow is higher in the lower part of the lung. Ventilation is also slightly higher in the lower zones but the differences are less marked than in the case of the blood flow.

During exercise the diffusing capacity for oxygen increases in young adults up to 65 ml/min or three times the resting value. This increase is the result of (a) opening up of previously closed pulmonary capillaries, thereby increasing the surface area of blood with which the oxygen can diffuse; (b) dilatation of all those pulmonary capillaries which are already open; (c) stretching the respiratory membrane: this increases the surface area and decreases the thickness of the membrane; (d) improvement in the even distribution of $\dot{V}/\dot{Q}$ ratio. Cardiac output is increased, as is pulmonary blood flow. As a result lung perfusion is evened out in the upper and lower part of the lung, hence the $\dot{V}/\dot{Q}$ ratio becomes less uneven, with a consequent increase in diffusing capacity. High altitude has a similar effect due to pulmonary hypertension.

Carbon dioxide diffuses so rapidly through the respiratory membrane that the difference in P_{CO_2} between the pulmonary capillaries and the alveoli is about 1 mmHg.

Diffusion Capacity at High Altitudes

High-Altitude Natives
An increased diffusing capacity has been found in Andean highlanders at 12,000 ft (3700 m) and at 15,000 ft (4500 m) (Remmers and Mithoefer 1969) and in Caucasians at 10,000 ft (3100 m) (De Graff et al. 1970).

An increase in membrane component and an increase in

pulmonary capillary blood volume was also recorded (De Graff *et al.* 1970).

High-Altitude Visitors

Work by West at 19,000 ft (5800 m) and at 24,400 ft (7400 m) showed no significant difference in the diffusing capacity between measurements made at sea level and at 15,300 ft (4672 m). A small but significant rise in diffusing capacity was noted after seven to ten weeks' residence at 19,000 ft (5800 m). This increase however could be explained by the increased rate of reaction of carbon monoxide with haemoglobin due to hypoxia, and by the increased blood haemoglobin concentration.

Thus there was no evidence of any acclimatisation change in the lung itself (West 1962).

Uptake of Oxygen by Pulmonary Capillaries

In the alveolar space the Po_2 is about 104 mmHg and at the arterial end of the pulmonary capillary 40 mmHg (Fig. 5).

Thus the difference in pressure between the alveolar space and pulmonary capillary at the arterial end is 64 mmHg (104–40). Therefore oxygen diffuses from the alveoli to the capillary.

Before reaching the mid-point of the pulmonary capillary the Po_2 in the capillary is approaching 104 mmHg, which is equal to the alveolar Po_2 or the Po_2 at the venous end.

Up to twenty times the normal oxygen requirement may be needed during exercise but the increase in cardiac output means that the time spent by the blood in the pulmonary capillary is decreased. Oxygen uptake might suffer because of the short time that blood is in contact with the alveolar space and the larger quantities of oxygen that are needed.

However despite these factors blood is saturated with oxygen because the diffusing capacity of the capillaries is increased by three times, which comes about by opening up new capillaries and the dilatation of existing capillaries, and also under normal conditions blood is completely saturated with oxygen by the time

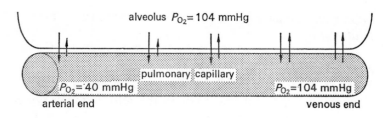

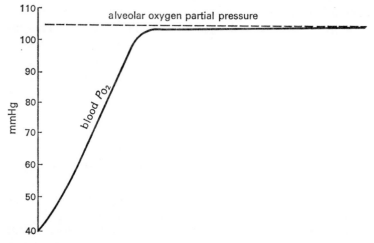

Fig. 5   Uptake of oxygen by the pulmonary capillary blood (Guyton 1971).

it is one third of the way along the capillary, or in other words it stays in the capillary three times longer than is necessary. Thus even if the diffusing capacity is not increased, there is a factor of three in reserve for full oxygenation alone.

Effects of High Altitude

In conditions of alveolar hypoxia, such as occur at high altitude, the alveolar Po_2 may be only 50 mmHg, and Po_2 of mixed venous blood 20 mmHg.

There is thus a pressure difference of only 30 mmHg and the rate of oxygen movement across the respiratory membrane is slower. By the time the pulmonary blood has reached the end of the pulmonary capillary its Po_2 may be well short of 50 mmHg.

If, in addition, the subject is exercising the time available for diffusion will be less and this exaggerates the diffusion defect. The Po_2 in the arterial blood may then be around 40 mmHg or less.

This mechanism is responsible for some of the severe hypoxaemia found in normal acclimatised subjects at high altitude when exercising.

Another factor is the shape of the oxygen dissociation curve.

At sea level, when the Po_2 is high, the curve is flat. This means that a large driving gradient is maintained between the arterial and venous points.

At altitude (19,000 ft (5791 m)) the curve is steeper and consequently the driving gradient is smaller between the arterial and venous points (see Fig. 6).

Pulmonary Circulation

The pulmonary circulation acts as a reservoir. The normal total blood volume is 5–6 litres, and a mean value of 10–12 per cent of this—about 500 ml—are in the pulmonary circulation but this can vary from 250 to 1000 ml. About 70 ml of this is in the capillaries and the remainder is divided between the arteries and veins.

The mean pulmonary artery pressure is 13 mmHg, and the mean left atrial pressure is 4 mmHg. Unfortunately no direct measurements of the pulmonary capillary pressure have been made but it will lie between these two and closer to the venous value. It is probably about 7 mmHg.

When the cardiac output is normal the blood passes through the pulmonary capillaries in about one second. Increasing the cardiac output may decrease this time to 0·4 seconds. The opening of normally collapsed pulmonary capillaries plays a part in accommodating this increase in blood flow.

The rate of pulmonary blood flow is equal to the cardiac output except for the 1–2 per cent that goes through the bronchial circulation.

Hydrostatic factors affect the pressures in the lungs. When the person is standing, the pulmonary vascular pressure at the

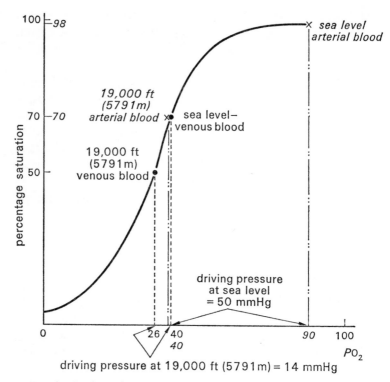

Fig. 6   Gradient for oxygen pressure between venous and arterial blood at sea level and 19,000 ft (5791 m).

apex of the lungs (3 mmHg), is 10 mmHg lower than it is in the middle of the lungs (13 mmHg) at cardiac level. At the bottom of the lung the pressure is 10 mmHg higher (23 mmHg).

There is thus a difference in blood flow between the upper and lower lung. Blood flow and blood volume at the lung bases are much greater than in the middle of the lung. At the apices blood flows only during systole. However, greater lung ventilation occurs at the bases. The effect of this together with regional differences of ventilation and gas exchange has been discussed previously.

When lying down a different pattern of blood distribution occurs with extra blood volume and flow in the more dependent parts.

Exercise partially overcomes the maldistribution because the pressure in the pulmonary artery rises high enough to give a reasonably good flow even at the apices.

When PAlv.O_2 becomes very low the adjacent pulmonary vessels constrict and the vascular resistance may double. The effect of this is to distribute blood to where it is most effective. When alveoli are poorly ventilated and their Po_2 is low the local vessels constrict. This causes blood to flow through other better aerated portions of the lung, and provides an automatic system for distributing blood flow. In lung disease such as pneumonia, where areas of the lung are either not ventilated or under-ventilated, this mechanism is helpful in matching blood flow to the ventilated areas.

At high altitude this mechanism causes a rise in pulmonary artery pressure which may be marginally beneficial in reducing the uneven perfusion of the lung due to gravity. In certain individuals however it may be detrimental by causing a great increase in pulmonary artery pressure and may be a factor in the production of high altitude pulmonary oedema (Chapter 21).

Normal Fluid Exchange at Pulmonary Capillaries

The forces tending to move fluid out of the capillary are

   (i) Pulmonary capillary pressure   7·0 mmHg
  (ii) Interstitial colloid osmotic pressure   4·5 mmHg
 (iii) Negative interstitial fluid pressure in
        the lungs   17·0 mmHg
                  Total   28·5 mmHg

The force tending to move fluid into the capillary is the plasma colloid osmotic pressure of 28 mmHg.

There is thus a slight net outward force with a tendency to drive fluid from the capillaries into the lung alveoli.

This excess returns to the circulation by means of the lymphatic channels of the lungs.

Another mechanism by which the alveoli are kept 'dry' is the negative pressure of the interstitial fluid, which 'pulls' fluid from the alveoli through the respiratory membrane into the interstitial space. The pulmonary interstitial space is extremely narrow as it is 'squeezed' by the 17 mmHg force exerted by the normal interstitial fluid which tends to 'pull' the alveolar epithelial membrane and the capillary membrane together. This results in the distance between the air in the alveoli and the blood in the capillaries being minimal. It averages less than 0·4 micron which aids diffusion of gases.

Pulmonary Oedema

Pulmonary oedema means excessive quantities of fluid in the alveoli or interstitial spaces.

The commonest cause is a greatly raised pulmonary capillary pressure, the result of left ventricular failure and back pressure in the lungs. However the pulmonary capillary pressure has to rise to about 30 mmHg (the colloid osmotic pressure is 28 mmHg) before oedema occurs. Another safety factor is the extremely rapid run-off provided by the pulmonary lymphatics.

A mild degree of pulmonary oedema is limited to an increase in interstitial fluid whilst more severe oedema results in intra-alveolar fluid.

References

Barcroft, J. (1925) *The respiratory function of the blood. Lessons from high altitude.* Cambridge.

De Graff, D. C., Grover, R. F., Johnson, R. L., Hammond, J. W. and Miller, J. M. (1970) *Journal of Applied Physiology* **29**, 71.

Dill, D. B. (1938) In, *Heat, life, altitude.* Harvard University Press: Cambridge, Mass.

Frisancho, A. R. and Baker, P. T. (1969) *American Journal of Physical Anthropology* **32**, 279.

Guyton, A.C. (1971) *Textbook of medical physiology.* W.B. Saunders: Philadelphia.

Houston, C. S. and Riley, R. L. (1947) *American Journal of Physiology* **149**, 565.

Hurtado, A. (1964) *Animals at high altitude—resident Man*. In, *Handbook of Physiology*. Section 4. Adaptation to environment. *Ed*. Dill, D. B., Adolph, E. F. and Wilber, C. G. American Physiological Society: Washington, DC.

Lahiri, S. and Milledge, J. S. (1966) *Federation Proceedings*. *Federation of American Societies for Experimental Biology* **25**, 1392.

Pugh, L.G.C.E. (1965) High altitude. In, *Physiology of human survival*. *Ed*. Edholm, O. and Bacharach, A.L. Academic Press: New York and London.

Pugh, L. G. C. E., Gill, M. B., Lahiri, S., Milledge, J. S., Ward, M. P. and West, J. B. (1964) *Journal of Applied Physiology* **19**, 431.

Rahn, H. and Otis, A. B. (1949) *American Journal of Physiology* **157**, 445.

Remmers, J. E. and Mithoefer, J. C. (1969) *Respiratory Physiology* **6**, 233.

West, J. B. (1962) *Journal of Applied Physiology* **17**, 421.

CHAPTER EIGHT

Respiration: The Fluid Phase

Oxygen Transport from Lungs to Tissues

At sea level, at rest, 5 ml of oxygen are transported from the lungs to the tissues for every 100 ml of blood. If the normal cardiac output is 5000 ml/min the total quantity of oxygen transported to the tissue each minute is 250 ml.

This corresponds to an oxygen intake of 250 ml/min.

During exercise this rate can be increased fifteen-fold. This is because of the ability of haemoglobin to give up three times the normal amount of oxygen (or more) that is, a three-fold increase in the coefficient of utilisation, together with an increase in cardiac output to 25,000 ml/min or five times normal.

The rate of oxygen transport and possible usage is therefore raised to 15 × 250 or 3750 ml/min. Special adaptation and training may increase this even further by (a) increasing the haemoglobin, which at high altitude can reach 20 grams per cent, and (b) increasing the maximum cardiac output. Levels of 4·5–5·0 litres/minute can be obtained by trained athletics. This is twenty times the normal resting level.

Effect of Haematocrit on Oxygen Transport

An increase in haematocrit will increase blood viscosity and therefore diminish cardiac output. The increase in the oxygen-carrying capacity of the blood will not compensate for this so the amount of oxygen carried to the tissues will decrease.

At high altitude with some desaturation the amount of oxygen carried can be maintained up to about 15,000 ft (4572 m) by increasing the oxygen-carrying capacity through a raised haematocrit. The price paid is increased viscosity and therefore increased load on the heart. Above about 20 grams per cent the viscosity increases very considerably and haemoglobin values much above this level are seldom found.

Diffusion of Oxygen from Capillaries to Interstitial Fluid

The Po_2 is 95 mmHg in arterial blood and 40 mmHg in interstitial fluid. Therefore the pressure difference at the arterial end of the capillary is 55 mmHg.

Most of the diffusion occurs before blood has passed very far along the capillary. The Po_2 in the capillary drops until it reaches 40 mmHg at the venous end.

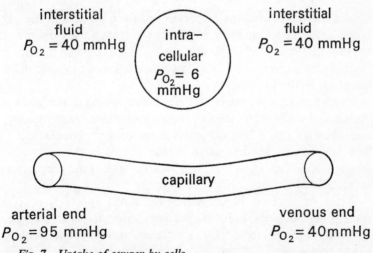

interstitial fluid
$P_{O_2} = 40$ mmHg

intra–cellular
$P_{O_2} = 6$ mmHg

interstitial fluid
$P_{O_2} = 40$ mmHg

capillary

arterial end
$P_{O_2} = 95$ mmHg

venous end
$P_{O_2} = 40$ mmHg

Fig. 7   Uptake of oxygen by cells.

Tissue Po_2 is determined by a balance between the rate of oxygen transport by the blood and the rate of oxygen utilisation by the tissues.

Diffusion of Oxygen from Interstitial Fluid to the Cells

Intracellular Po_2 is always lower than interstitial Po_2 because oxygen is always being used by the cells.

Intracellular Po_2 often approaches interstitial Po_2 as oxygen diffuses rapidly through the cell membrane. However a considerable distance may separate the capillaries and the cells, permitting intracellular Po_2 to range from 40 mmHg to 6 mmHg. Only a 1–5 mmHg pressure is necessary for metabolism. Mitochondrial Po_2 may be as low as 0·1 mmHg.

Under basal conditions, 5 ml of oxygen are extracted for every 100 ml of blood passing through the tissue capillaries.

For 5 ml of oxygen to be released from 100 ml of blood the Po_2 must be about 40 mmHg, so the tissue capillary Po_2 does not normally rise above this value.

On exercise, the Po_2 in the tissue capillaries falls and larger quantities of oxygen are released.

Oxygen Transport in the Blood

Under normal conditions 97 per cent of the oxygen is in the red blood cells. The remaining 3 per cent is transported dissolved in the plasma. Under conditions of high oxygen pressure (hyperbaric oxygen), relatively large quantities of oxygen can be dissolved in the plasma.

Oxygen combines loosely with the haem portion of the haemoglobin molecule. When the Po_2 is high it combines more readily, and when the Po_2 is low, oxygen is released by the haemoglobin. The oxygen dissociation curve illustrates this in the form of a graph, where the Po_2 in mmHg is plotted against the percentage saturation of haemoglobin with oxygen.

When oxygenated blood leaves the lungs at a Po_2 of 100 mmHg the haemoglobin is 97 per cent saturated with oxygen. When the venous blood leaves the tissues at a Po_2 of 40 mmHg, the haemoglobin is 70 per cent saturated or less.

The blood of a normal person contains approximately 15 gram of haemoglobin in each 100 ml. As each gram of haemoglobin can bind with 1·34 ml of oxygen, then in 100 ml of blood there are about 20 ml of oxygen. This can be expressed as 20 volumes per cent, and the oxygen dissociation curve redrawn with volumes per cent rather than oxygen saturation.

The total oxygen in 100 ml of arterial blood leaving the lungs ($Po_2 = 95$ mmHg and 97 per cent saturated) will be 19·4 ml or 19·4 vol per cent.

The total oxygen in 100 ml of venous blood leaving the tissue capillaries ($Po_2 = 40$ mmHg and 75 per cent saturated) will be 14·4 ml or 14·4 vol per cent.

Therefore 5 ml of oxygen will have been given off to the tissues for every 100 ml of blood.

Oxygen Dissociation Curve

The shape of the oxygen dissociation curve is remarkably constant in any one person, but may differ from that found in another; also, it is a little more sigmoid in the female. The differences may be due to individual variations in carbon dioxide tensions, pH values and body temperature.

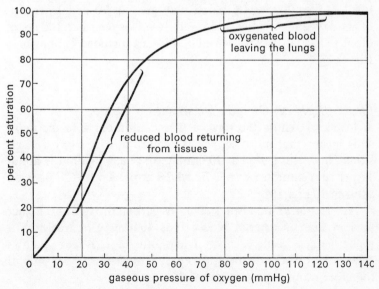

Fig. 8   The oxygen–haemoglobin dissociation curve (Guyton 1971).

Because the oxygen dissociation curve flattens at the top there may be a considerable fall in oxygen tension with a relatively small change in oxygen content at that level.

This is of major importance in maintaining the oxygen content of arterial blood, for when the P_{O_2} is 60 mmHg, equivalent to an ascent to a medium altitude, the haemoglobin is still about 90 per cent saturated and each 100 ml of blood contains about 18 ml of oxygen.

In other words the tissue P_{O_2} hardly changes over a $P_{Alv.O_2}$ range from 100–70 mmHg. Thus the atmospheric P_{O_2} may vary considerably without the tissue P_{O_2} changing more than a few mmHg.

As the P_{O_2} falls from 70 to 40 mmHg, which is the steeper part of the curve, a rapid fall in oxygen saturation of haemoglobin occurs.

A large amount of the oxygen carried by the haemoglobin is lost to the tissues for a relatively small change in oxygen tension, which is an advantage for normally active tissues.

Below 40 mmHg, the normal venous P_{O_2}, the curve still descends steeply. Thus during severe exercise when the P_{O_2} may fall to 15 or 20 mmHg, blood may give up 70 or 80 per cent of its oxygen (or between 14 and 16 ml oxygen per 100 ml of blood). The curve with various altitudes included is shown in Fig. 9.

Effect of pH on Oxygen Dissociation Curve

A lower pH shifts the oxygen dissociation curve to the right. This means that more oxygen is evolved at lower oxygen tension. Thus with a P_{O_2} of 20 mmHg, the haemoglobin is about 17 per cent saturated at pH 7·2 whilst at pH 7·4 it is 20 per cent saturated (Fig. 10).

The venous blood always contains carbon dioxide at a higher tension than in arterial blood. It is 46 mmHg at rest and at higher values during exercise. The pH therefore is *lower* than in arterial blood—the dissociation curve is shifted to the right and therefore more oxygen is given off.

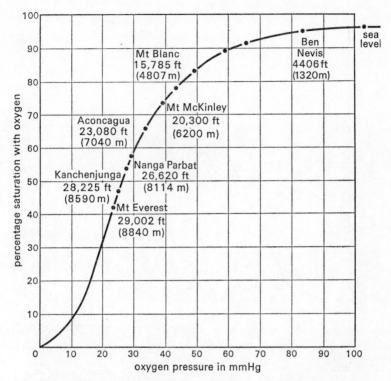

Fig. 9 Oxygen dissociation curve. The curve of alveolar oxygen tensions for altitudes corresponding to a number of well-known mountains shows that up to 10,000 ft (3000 m) the blood is almost fully saturated with oxygen. At 15,000 ft (4500 m) the percentage saturation is starting to fall; whilst at 20,000 ft (6000 m) the curve is steepening rapidly. At 29,000 ft (8800 m) the blood is 40 per cent saturated—or below the venous point for rest at sea level (Ruttledge 1937).

Effect of Temperature on the Oxygen Dissociation Curve

A rise in temperature shifts the curve to the right, and more oxygen is given off for a similar oxygen tension.

At a Po_2 of 40 mmHg, the haemoglobin is 50 per cent saturated at 42°C and 70 per cent saturated at 38°C (Fig. 11).

This is an advantage during muscular work when an increase in local heat will mean that more oxygen is evolved at a low Po_2.

Presumably it will be a disadvantage in hypothermia when less oxygen will be given off.

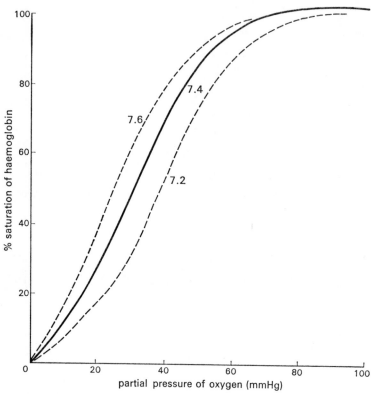

Fig. 10   Effects of variations in pH on the oxyhaemoglobin dissociation curves.

Effect of High Altitude on the Oxygen Dissociation Curve

Barcroft (Barcroft 1925) showed that there was a tendency for the oxygen dissociation curve to shift to the left, which could be explained by a decrease in acidity during acclimatisation. Later studies (Dill *et al.* 1931) did not confirm this.

It has recently been established that the concentration of an organic phosphate, 2,3-diphosphoglycerate (DPG), in the red blood cells can reduce the affinity that haemoglobin has for oxygen. This will facilitate the unloading of oxygen to the tissues. The formation of DPG is stimulated when the amount of reduced haemoglobin in the blood is increased.

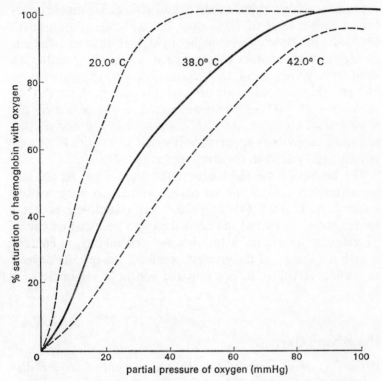

Fig. 11 Effect of temperature variation on the oxyhaemoglobin dissociation curve.

A rapid rise of DPG occurs within 24 hours of ascent to 15,000 ft (4572 m) (Lenfant *et al.* 1968), and it is associated with a rightwards shift of the oxygen dissociation curve. This effect is brought about either by direct action or by lowering intracellular pH (Bohr effect). Although this is one mechanism for regulating the oxygen affinity of the red blood cell, other factors, such as mean corpuscular haemoglobin and dissolved carbon dioxide, play a significant role. The rightward shift is not nearly so important an adaptation as the increase in ventilation. It disappears rapidly in both high-altitude visitors and high-altitude natives on return to sea level, and is proportional to altitude (Lenfant *et al.* 1971).

Studies on high-altitude natives and visitors in America confirm a higher level of DPG than in plainsmen (Eaton *et al.* 1969) and the Bohr effect is higher in high-altitude natives than in high-altitude visitors (Morpurgo *et al.* 1970), possibly an evolutionary adaptation. In Asia, the 2-3,DPG content of both Sherpas (high-altitude natives) and Europeans (high-altitude visitors) at 14,760 ft (4500 m) was raised to approximately the same extent. However, the right-ward shift of the oxygen dissociation centre was apparent neither in high-altitude natives nor high-altitude visitors (Morpurgo *et al.* 1972).

The benefit of the rightward shift becomes less as altitude increases because the arterial oxygen content is progressively reduced. At 15,000 ft (4572 m) the Po_2 of mixed venous blood approximates to that of the normal oxygen dissociation curve. Therefore when arterial saturation and arterial oxygen content is high the shift is of the greatest benefit. If the arterial oxygen saturation is below 70 per cent the benefit is minimal (Luft 1972).

Hyperbaric Oxygen

If the Po_2 rises above 100 mmHg, the amount of oxygen dissolved in the plasma will increase.

The effect on the tissues is as follows. At twice the atmospheric pressure the amount of oxygen dissolved in plasma is 4·2 ml. The total oxygen in 100 ml of blood is therefore 19·5 + 4·2 = 23·7 ml compared with 19·5 + 0·3 = 19·8 when breathing air at ordinary pressure. At four times the atmospheric pressure the total oxygen content of 100 ml blood is 29 ml (vol per cent). Only 4 ml is given off in the tissues, leaving 24 ml. The tissue Po_2 is about 1200 mmHg.

Cyanosis

Cyanosis is caused by excessive amounts of reduced haemoglobin in the blood vessels of the skin. The intense blue of the reduced haemoglobin is seen through the skin.

Because the red colour of oxyhaemoglobin is weak by comparison with the blue of reduced haemoglobin, the oxyhaemoglobin has relatively little colouring effect when the two are mixed.

Definite cyanosis appears whenever arterial blood contains more than 5 gram of reduced haemoglobin per 100 ml (about 30 per cent by weight) and it cannot occur in severe anaemia, whilst cyanosis is very common in polycythaemia because of the large amount of haemoglobin in the blood.

When mountaineering at high altitudes a practical point enters into the detection of cyanosis. Since most tents are coloured and inside a tent a person's skin will always have a tinge of the tent colour, whilst outside, dark glasses are worn above the snow line, which also 'tints' the skin, people are seldom seen in a normal light and cyanosis may not be noted until it is severe.

The capillary blood determines the skin colour. The blueness of the blood is determined by the concentration of reduced haemoglobin in arterial blood entering the capillaries and the amount of reduction that occurs during the passage of blood through the capillaries.

If the blood flow is slow, as in cold conditions, marked desaturation occurs and causes cyanosis. This is a form of stagnant hypoxia. Thus marked cyanosis can occur at high altitude, in cold conditions, or in combination.

In those with very thin skin, and in particularly vascular parts of the body such as the lips and fingernails, cyanosis is more obvious.

Carbon Dioxide Transport

Cells to Tissue Capillaries

Cell metabolism results in the continuous formation of carbon dioxide. The intracellular carbon dioxide tension rises. As carbon dioxide diffuses twenty times more easily than oxygen, it reaches the interstitial fluid and the capillary blood without difficulty.

The intracellular P_{CO_2} is 46 mmHg, whilst the interstitial and venous capillary P_{CO_2} is 45 mmHg—a pressure gradient of 1 mmHg. Arterial blood has a P_{CO_2} of 40 mmHg, and as it passes through the capillaries it rises to 45 mmHg at the venous end, where it reaches equilibrium with the interstitial fluid.

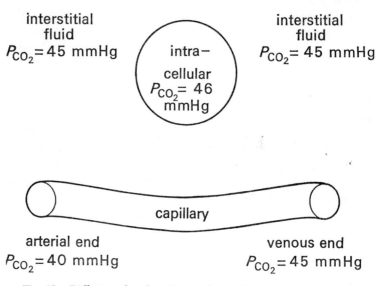

Fig. 12   Diffusion of carbon dioxide from cells.

Effect of Tissue Metabolism and Blood Flow on Interstitial P_{CO_2}

Blood-flow and tissue metabolism affect tissue P_{CO_2} in exactly the same way as they effect P_{O_2}. A decrease in blood flow increases tissue P_{CO_2} and vice versa.

An increase in metabolic rate, especially if the blood flow is reduced, increases the tissue P_{CO_2} to very high levels. Reducing the rate of metabolism reduces the tissue P_{CO_2}.

Transport of Carbon Dioxide in Body Fluids and Blood

Carbon dioxide diffuses out of the cell in simple solution, and not as bicarbonate. This is because the cell membrane is less permeable to bicarbonate ion than to the dissolved carbon dioxide.

It enters the tissue capillary and is transported in the blood partly in the plasma and partly in red blood cells (RBCs) in three main forms: (a) as dissolved carbon dioxide (7 per cent); (b) as bicarbonate ion (60–90 per cent); and (c) in combination with haemoglobin and plasma protein (5–10 per cent).

The total carbon dioxide content of the plasma is about three times that of the red blood cells.

Carbon Dioxide Dissociation Curves

The behaviour of carbon dioxide in the blood can be followed by determining its content in the blood at different carbon dioxide pressures.

By plotting the volume of carbon dioxide in ml per 100 ml of blood against the tension in mmHg, a dissociation curve may be obtained.

Curves may be obtained for oxygenated blood (i.e. in lungs, $Po_2 = 100$ mmHg) and reduced blood (i.e. in tissues, $Po_2 = 40$ mmHg).

In Fig. 13, point A shows that at a normal Pco_2 in tissues of 45 mmHg, about 52 vol per cent of carbon dioxide is combined in the blood.

On entering the lungs the Pco_2 falls to 40 mmHg while the Po_2 rises to 100 mmHg.

If the carbon dioxide dissociation curve remained the same (i.e. dotted line), the CO_2 content of the blood would fall to 50 vol per cent so only 2 vol per cent would be given off.

However the increase in Po_2 in the lung shifts the carbon dioxide dissociation curve downwards (i.e. from the dotted to solid line). The carbon dioxide content of the blood falls to about 48 vol per cent (point B), that is, an extra 2 vol per cent of carbon dioxide are given off making 4 vol per cent in all.

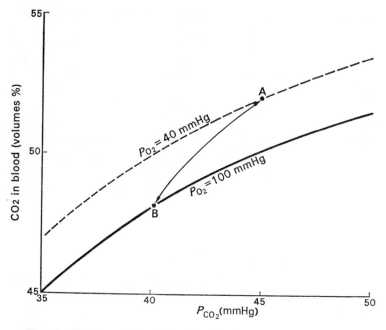

Fig. 13 Portions of the carbon dioxide dissociation curve when the Po_2 is 100 mmHg and 40 mmHg, respectively. The arrow represents the Haldane effect on the transport of carbon dioxide (Guyton 1971).

So, at any given pressure of carbon dioxide, reduced blood takes up a larger volume of the gas than oxygenated blood and, conversely, oxygenation of the blood leads to evolution of carbon dioxide.

Haldane Effect

There is some degree of interaction between the uptakes of oxygen and carbon dioxide.

An increase in Po_2 tends to displace carbon dioxide from the blood due to the combination of oxygen with haemoglobin, which makes the haemoglobin more acid, decreasing the affinity of carbon dioxide for haemoglobin. The increased acidity of haemoglobin means an increase in acidity of both the water in the red blood cells and of the plasma. Consequently, bicarbonate ions are converted to carbonic acid, which dissociates and leaves carbon dioxide in the blood. This is known as the Haldane effect.

Bohr Effect

Essentially, the Bohr effect is complementary to the Haldane effect: when P_{CO_2} rises, the pH of the blood falls and there is an increased combination of carbon dioxide with haemoglobin.

This reduces the affinity of haemoglobin for oxygen so that oxygen dissociates from the haemoglobin. Quantitatively speaking, this is much less important than the Haldane effect.

Blood pH

Normal arterial blood has a pH of about 7·40. As blood acquires carbon dioxide in the tissues, the pH falls to about 7·36 (venous blood has a pH of 7·36). The reverse occurs in the lungs.

The decrease in pH in the peripheral blood may be by as much as 0·4, that is, to pH 7·0. This occurs during exercise, when metabolic activity is high, or when blood flow is decreased. The limits of pH compatible with survival are approximately pH 7·0 and 7·8.

Removal of Carbon Dioxide from the Lungs

On arrival at the lungs the P_{CO_2} of venous blood is 45 mmHg whilst in the alveolus it is 40 mmHg.

Because the coefficient of diffusion of carbon dioxide is twenty times that of oxygen, the pressure gradient is towards the alveolus, and carbon dioxide is transferred to the alveoli.

Almost all the carbon dioxide has been removed within one quarter of the distance along the pulmonary capillary.

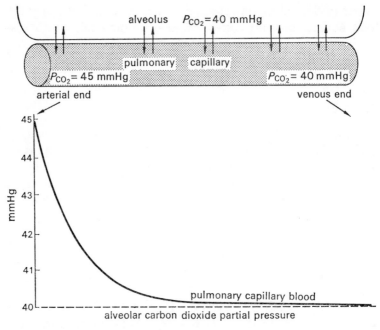

Fig. 14   Diffusion of carbon dioxide from pulmonary blood into the alveolus (Guyton 1971).

The decrease in P_{CO_2} in the red blood cells reverses all reactions that occur on tissue uptake of carbon dioxide.

Carbonic acid dissociates to water and carbon dioxide, carbaminohaemoglobin releases carbon dioxide and chlorides return to the plasma from the red cells.

Effects of High Altitude

The blood of partially acclimatised high-altitude visitors contains less carbon dioxide at a given P_{CO_2} than the blood of sea-level residents. This is due to the excretion of bicarbonate by the kidneys.

High-altitude natives have even less carbon dioxide and the bicarbonate values are less than for high-altitude visitors. This suggests that renal compensation is even greater which is confirmed by the fact that the pH of arterial blood is 7·37 for high-altitude natives and 7·45 for visitors.

A given rise of P_{CO_2} causes a slightly smaller fall of pH in the blood of high-altitude natives than in the blood of sea-level dwellers. Therefore despite a relatively low plasma bicarbonate, the buffering power for carbon dioxide is greater at altitude than at sea level. This is the result of the increase in haemoglobin concentration.

In the carbon dioxide dissociation curve for fully oxygenated blood plotted on log–log scale, the upper line represents the blood of normal adults living at sea level, the lower line represents high-altitude natives (South American miners) living at 17,500 ft (5300 m) and working each day at 19,000 ft (5800 m) and the middle line represents the blood of high-altitude visitors who lived and worked at 19,000 ft (5800 m) for a period of three months in 1960–1. (See Fig. 15.)

Acid–base Balance at High Altitude

At 16,000 ft (4880 m), the CSF pH of a high-altitude visitor was higher, pH 7·374, than that of a high-altitude native (Sherpa), pH 7·328 (Lahiri and Milledge 1967).

It is now recognised that changes in CSF pH are small over a wide range of change in blood pH. Around the middle range of blood pH (7·3–7·5) some maintain that the CSF pH remains at about 7·32 (Severinghaus *et al.* 1963), whilst others believe that CSF pH changes continuously (Fencl *et al.* 1966).

At altitude, hypoxia itself may influence the acid–base regulation particularly in high-altitude visitors. Hypoxic drive at altitude increases ventilation but alkalosis resulting from hyperventilation, and the associated arterial desaturation, lessens the full effect.

According to earlier views, with acclimatisation and compensation of respiratory alkalosis by the excretion of bicarbonate, the hypoxic drive decreased and the increased ventilation was maintained by increased sensitivity of the respiratory centre to carbon dioxide. Recent investigations however show

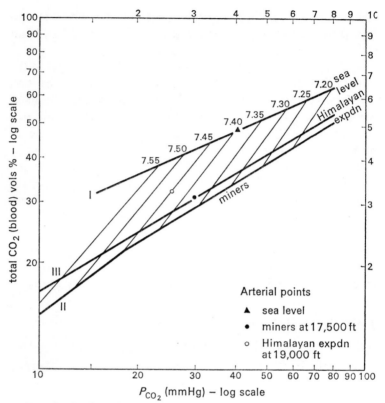

Fig. 15 (*Dill et al. 1937a, 1937b; Pugh 1965*).

that hypoxic drive does not decrease in recently acclimatised man (Astrand 1954; Michel and Milledge 1963). The current view is that the respiratory drive due to P_{CO_2} and H^+, particularly in the CSF and blood, is maintained at a normal level, and that increased ventilation is due to hypoxia (Mitchell and Severinghaus 1965).

Results on high-altitude natives—both Sherpas and Andean—showed that they had normal sea-level values for CSF and blood pH, therefore the respiratory drive from CO_2 and H^+ acting on the medullary and peripheral chemoreceptors could be considered normal.

The lower ventilation in high-altitude natives must be due to a lowered hypoxic drive via the peripheral chemoreceptor.

CSF and blood pH in high-altitude natives were lower than in high-altitude visitors acclimatised to the same altitude. In both high-altitude visitors and natives at altitude the response to carbon dioxide was similar and higher than their response at sea level (Lahiri and Milledge 1965; Milledge and Lahiri 1967).

At altitude the CSF HCO_3^- is less than normal; therefore, a given increase in PCO_2 will increase H^+ more and result in a stronger medullary drive to respiration (Michel and Milledge 1963; Mitchell and Severinghaus 1965). The carbon dioxide response of high-altitude natives should be larger because the CSF HCO_3^- and pH is lower than in high-altitude visitors. However, the carbon dioxide response seems a variable factor and it may be assumed that the medullary drive was similar in both high-altitude natives and visitors.

Alveolar PCO_2 is less at altitude than at sea level, and in Sherpa subjects at 4880 m $PAlvCO_2$ was about 26 mmHg by comparison with 28 mmHg for high-altitude visitors (Lahiri and Milledge 1967; Chiodi 1957).

Although high-altitude natives (Sherpas) have a lower sensitivity to hypoxia, their blood and CSF H^+ were similar to those found at sea level. The recently acclimatised high-altitude visitor with a normal sensitivity to hypoxia was found to have a higher blood and CSF pH. The time taken for recent arrivals to acquire the characteristics of high-altitude natives is not known—and possibly 'complete' acclimatisation to altitude never occurs in sea-level man.

Blood Morphology

Changes on Ascent and Descent

The first adjustment to high altitude to be clearly recognised was an elevation of the red cell and haemoglobin content of the blood (Viault 1891). This finding has been demonstrated repeatedly amongst both high-altitude natives and high-altitude visitors.

The polycythaemia of high altitude is the consequence of hyperactivity in the formation of red blood cells. In high-altitude visitors and natives, the mean corpuscular volume of $97\mu^3$ is a little higher than at sea level. The cells are normally filled with haemoglobin (M.C.H.C. 32–34 per cent). The number of reticulocytes in the peripheral blood is increased, but the number of platelets and leucocytes in both high-altitude visitors and natives remains at the normal sea-level value (Hurtado 1964; Pugh 1964). In the bone marrow there is hyperplasia of the erythroid elements. The myeloid cells and megakaryocytes are normal both in number and maturation (Merino and Reynafarje 1949).

In the new-born at high altitude bone-marrow hyperplasia is no greater than in the new-born at sea level. Erythropoietic activity starts a few days after birth, showing that the hypoxic stimulus is absent or ineffective during intrauterine life (Reynafarje 1959).

From the early hours of exposure to high altitude of a sea-level resident, red blood cell production exceeds destruction. As the mechanism which controls erythropoiesis is very sensitive to hypoxia red cell iron turnover rate is increased after only two hours. The highest increase takes place seven to fourteen days after exposure, and at this time erythropoietic activity is about three times normal. After six months there is still an elevated red cell iron turnover and equilibrium between red cell destruction and formation is not reached even at eight months.

A gradual increase in red cell mass continues until about eight months after exposure. After a year, the red cell mass is similar in size to that found after eight months; however neither the total blood volume nor any of its components reach the level found in high-altitude natives.

The life span of red cells in newcomers exposed to high altitude is normal (Reynafarje 1962).

A rise in haemoglobin concentration of between 10 and 15 per cent occurred on rapid ascent to an altitude of 14,000 ft (4267 m) (Barcroft 1925). This was attributed to a reduction in plasma volume and fluid shifts (Asmussen and Consolazio 1941). A slow rise for the next two months followed this rapid increase until the level finally levelled off.

Blood volume and plasma volume fall during the first two to four months at high altitude but subsequently rise. The blood volume reaches a level 10 to 20 per cent above the normal sea-level value. Plasma volume remains a little below the sea-level value.

The haemoglobin concentration is constant after about two months though the red cell mass rises. Thus haemoglobin concentration depends to some extent on plasma volume (Pugh 1965).

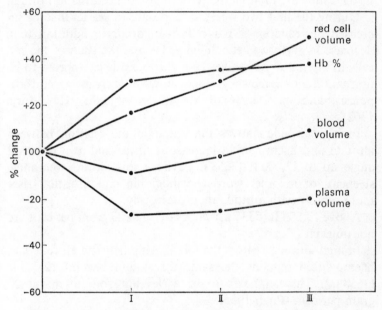

Fig. 16   Average changes in haemoglobin concentration, red cell volume, plasma volume and blood volume in four subjects during eight months on a Himalayan expedition: (I) after eighteen weeks at altitudes between 13,000 ft (4000 m) and 19,000 ft (5791 m); (II) after three to six weeks at 19,000 ft; and III after nine to fourteen weeks at or above 19,000 ft. (Pugh 1965.)

High-altitude natives living at high altitude have a daily red cell production about 30 per cent higher than that of sea-level subjects at sea-level. As blood destruction is proportionately higher, an equilibrium between destruction and formation must exist.

When high-altitude natives are exposed to sea level a progressive decrease in red cell iron turnover rate is found. This reaches its lowest level from the third to the fifth week, and during this period it is only one third of its initial value. A diminution in red cell production and red cell mass therefore occurs. This is followed by a gradual return to normal (Reynafarje *et al.* 1959).

The red cell volume reaches a level which is lower than normal after three months at sea level—thus a true anaemia occurs—but in the following months the red cell volume returns to normal.

During the first two weeks of exposure to sea level some increased destruction of red cells may occur in addition to a decrease in erythropoietic activity, but the life span of the red cells in high-altitude natives brought to sea level appears to be normal. Bone-marrow cytology shows a decrease in erythropoiesis, and the degree of reticulocytosis falls (Reynafarje 1962).

In high-altitude natives the graph of the relation between altitude and haemoglobin increase is linear and at a constant angle up to 12,000 ft (3658 m). Above this altitude the angle steepens, or in other words haemoglobin concentration rises more rapidly with altitude than previously.

Above 17,500 ft (5334 m) values of up to 23 gram per cent are not unusual (Fig. 17).

In high-altitude visitors the relationship between altitude and haemoglobin remains the same up to and beyond 12,000 ft (3658 m). There appears to be a 'levelling off' at about 20 gram per cent (Pugh 1965).

Oxygenation of Arterial Blood

In both high-altitude natives and high-altitude visitors, the oxygen saturation at rest falls to about 76 per cent at 17,500 ft (5334 m). Above this altitude it continues to fall until at 20,500 ft (6300 m) it is down to 65 per cent in high-altitude visitors at rest.

In high-altitude natives the oxygen capacity remains higher than in high-altitude visitors up to 17,500 ft (5300 m). At this altitude, the high-altitude native has an oxygen capacity of 30·5 ml/100 ml, whereas the acclimatised high-altitude visitor has only 25 ml/100 ml—a difference of 10 per cent, and also has an oxygen capacity which is greater than at sea level.

At between 17,500 and 21,500 ft (5300 and 6500 m) the high-altitude visitor has an average oxygen capacity of 27·4 ml/100 ml.

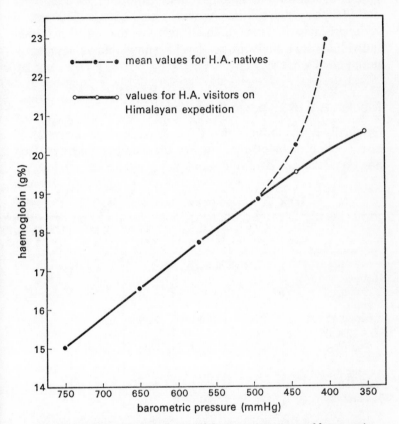

Fig. 17   Relation between haemoglobin concentration and barometric pressure in native residents and acclimatised visitors at various altitudes (Pugh 1965).

The oxygen content of arterial blood at 17,500 ft (5300 m) is higher in high-altitude natives than in high-altitude visitors. In high-altitude natives the oxygen content is higher at high altitude than at sea level. In high-altitude visitors the oxygen content at 17,500 ft (5300 m) is either equal to or a little lower than at sea level.

It is interesting that there has never been any correlation between physical working capacity and oxygen content of arterial blood (as shown by oxygen saturation and haemoglobin concentration) amongst both European mountaineers and Sherpas—high-altitude natives—over 17,500 ft (5300 m).

Surprisingly in some high-altitude populations occasional individuals are found with sea-level haemoglobin values and an unimpaired work capacity.

Mechanism of Hypoxic Stimulus

Originally it was thought that this mechanism was the result of direct action of blood P_{CO_2} or P_{O_2} on the bone marrow. This however was not confirmed and the presence of a humoral,

Table 13. Blood oxygenation (Pugh 1965)

	Sea level	7500 ft (2300 m)	15,000 ft (4500 m)	17,500 ft (5300 m)	16,000 ft (5800 m)	17,500–21,500 (5300–6500 m)
High-altitude native						
Haemoglobin, gram per cent		17·7	20·1	22·9		
O₂ Capacity, ml/100		23·8	26·9	30·5		
Arterial O₂ content, ml/100		21·3	22·6	23·2		
% Saturation		91	80	76		
High-altitude visitor (acclimatised)						
Haemoglobin, gram per cent	14·5		19·5	18·9	19·6	20·5
O₂ Capacity, ml/100	19·5		24·8	25·1	26·2	27·4
Arterial O₂ content, ml/100	18·9		19·7	18·9	17·5	17·8–19·2
% Saturation	97		80	75	67	65–70

erythropoietic, factor was sought, especially as such a factor had been suggested earlier in the century (Carnot and Deflandre 1906).

Plasma from high-altitude natives produced a moderate increase in reticulocytes when injected into normal subjects at sea level. By contrast plasma from sea-level subjects produced no such effect (Merino 1956). The degree of stimulus is important in determining the degree of polycythaemia, and the degree of polycythaemia, at least in high-altitude natives, is dependent on the altitude at which they live (Hurtado 1960).

There is evidence from animal experiments that erythropoiesis is regulated by renal excretion of erythropoietin, which is a hormone taken up by the erythropoietic tissue, and that the kidney is the site of production. Erythropoietin acts on the marrow cell that precedes the recognisable erythroblast (Krantz and Jacobson 1970). When there is a sudden demand for red cell formation, the circulating erythropoietin increases for a few hours. Once the erythropoietic tissue has increased its activity the hormone almost disappears from the blood. Plasma erythropoietin concentration reached a maximum after 19–39 hours hypoxia at 14,300 ft (4300 m) and then decreased rapidly. By the tenth day at this altitude erythropoietic levels had decreased to pre-hypoxia values (Abbrecht and Littell 1972).

In high-altitude natives brought down to sea level there is a decrease in red cell mass and depression of erythropoiesis. This could be brought about by an inhibitory hormonal factor. It is

Table 14.   Blood composition of native residents (Hurtado 1964)

	Sea level	15,000 ft (4540 m)
Total blood volume, litres	4·77	5·70
Total plasma volume, litres	2·52	2·23
Total red cell volume, litres	2·25	3·41
Red blood cells million/cub mm	5·11	6·44
Haematocrit %	46·6	59·5
Haemoglobin g/100 cc	15·6	20·13
Reticulocyte thousands/cub mm	17·9	45·5
Platelets, thousands/cub mm	406	419
Leucocytes, thousands/cub mm	6·68	7·04

possible that it does not act directly on erythropoiesis but blocks the action of erythropoietin. Inhibitors of erythropoietin have been found in the urine in these subjects (Lindemann 1971).

Iron Adsorption

Hypoxia acts through the erythropoietic factor and stimulates erythropoiesis. In consequence, the iron turnover rate and intestinal iron absorption rate increase. Whether this is due to the direct effect of erythropoietic factor or whether it works through a mechanism depending on erythrocyte activity is not known.

In sea-level subjects taken to high altitude (15,000 ft (4540 m)) iron adsorption was increased three to four times during early exposure, the maximum rate being reached after one week. On return to sea level, iron adsorption decreased, reaching one fifth of its normal value in three weeks (Reynafarje and Ramos 1961).

In high-altitude natives, permanently resident at altitude, there was no significant difference in iron adsorption in comparison with people born and living at sea level. It appears then that it is not the direct action of Po_2 at intestinal level which is the stimulus to iron adsorption but the demand of the bone marrow.

Blood Changes during Exercise

From the haematological point of view there was no difference between work performed at sea level and at high altitude. Although there were slight increases in haematocrit and haemoglobin, this is probably explained by a redistribution of red cells and there was no obvious increase in erythropoietic activity due to exercise as a quick return to normal values occurred. An increase in leucocytes was noted and this is probably also explained by a redistribution of cells, normally out of the active circulation (Reynafarje 1962).

References

Abbrecht, P. H. and Littell, J. K. (1972) *Journal of Applied Physiology* **32**, 54.

Asmussen, E. and Consolazio, C. F. (1941) *American Journal of Physiology* **132**, 555.

Astrand, P. O. (1954) *Acta Physiologica Scandinavica* **30**, 343.

Barcroft, J. (1925) *Respiratory function of the blood*. In, *Lessons from high altitude*. Cambridge University Press.

Carnot, P. and Deflandre, C. (1906) *Comptes rendu hebdomadaire des séances de l'Académie des Sciences* **143**, 432.

Chiodi, H. (1957) *Journal of Applied Physiology* **10**, 81.

Dill, D. B., Edwards, H. T. and Consolazio, W. V. (1937(a)) *Journal of Biological Chemistry* **118**, 635.

Dill, D. B., Edwards, H. T., Folling, A., Oberg, S. A., Pappenheimer, A. M. and Talbott, J. H. (1931) *Journal of Physiology* **71**, 47.

Dill, D. B., Talbot, J. H. and Consolazio, W. V. (1937(b)) *Journal of Biological Chemistry* **118**, 649.

Eaton, J. W., Brewer, G. J. and Grover, R. F. (1969) *Journal of Laboratory and Clinical Medicine* **73**, 603.

Fencl, V., Miller, T. B. and Pappenheimer, J. R. (1966) *American Journal of Physiology* **210**, 459.

Guyton, A.C. (1971) *Textbook of medical physiology*. W.B. Saunders: Philadelphia.

Hurtado, A. (1964) Animals at high altitude–resident man. In, *Handbook of Physiology*. Section 4. Adaptation to environment. *Ed*. Dill, D. B., Adolph, E. F. and Wilber, C. G. American Physiological Society: Washington D.C.

Hurtado, A. (1960) *Annals of Internal Medicine* **53**, 247.

Krantz, S. B. and Jacobson, L. O. (1970) *Erythropoietin and the regulation of erythropoiesis*. University of Chicago Press.

Lahiri, S. and Milledge, J. S. (1965) *Proceedings of the 23rd International Congress of Physiological Science, Tokyo*, p. 319.

Lahiri, S. and Milledge, J. S. (1967) *Respiratory Physiology* **2**, 323.

Lenfant, C., Torrance, J. D., English, E., Finch, C. A., Reynafarje, C., Ramos, J. and Faura, J. (1968) *Journal of Clinical Investigation* **47**, 2652.

Lenfant, C., Torrance, J. D. and Reynafarje, C. (1971) *Journal of Applied Physiology* **30**, 625.

Lindemann, R. (1971) *Israel Journal of Medical Science*, **7**, 1007.

Luft, U. C. (1972) In, *Physiological adaptations. Desert and Mountain. Ed.* Yousef, M. K., Horvath, S. M. and Bullaro, R. W. Academic Press: New York and London.

Merino, C. F. and Reynafarje, C. (1949) *Journal of Laboratory and Clinical Medicine* **34**, 637.

Merino, C. F. (1956) *The plasma erythropoietic factor in the polycythaemia of high altitudes.* Report 56–103 School of Aviation Medicine ASAF.

Michel, C. C. and Milledge, J. S. (1963) *Journal of Physiology* **168**, 631.

Milledge, J. S. and Lahiri, S. (1967) *Respiratory Physiology* **2**, 310.

Mitchell, R. A. and Severinghaus, J. W. (1965) *Physiology for Physicians* **3**, 1.

Morpurgo, G., Berinini, L., Battaglia, P., Paolucci, A. M. and Modiano, G. (1970) *Nature* **227**, 387.

Morpurgo, G., Battaglia, P., Carter, N. D., Modiano, G. and Passi, S. (1972) *Experientia* **28**, 1280.

Pugh, L. G. C. E. (1965) High altitude. In, *The physiology of human survival. Ed.* Edholm, O. and Bacharach, A. L. Academic Press: New York and London.

Pugh, L. G. C. E. (1964) *Journal of Physiology* **170**, 344.

Reynafarje, C. (1959) *Journal of Pediatrics* **54**, 152.

Reynafarje, C. (1962) Haemotologic changes during rest and physical activity in man at high altitude. In, *The physiological effects of man at high altitude. Ed.* Weihe, W. H. Pergamon Press: London.

Reynafarje, C., Lozano, R. and Valdivieso, J. (1959) *Blood* **14**, 433.

Reynafarje, C. and Ramos, J. (1961) *Journal of Laboratory and Clinical Medicine* **57**, 848.

Ruttledge, H. (1937) *Everest. The unfinished adventure.* Hodder and Stoughton: London.

Severinghaus, J. W., Mitchell, R. A., Richardson, B. W. and Singer, M. M. (1963) *Journal of Applied Physiology* **18**, 1155.

Viault, E. (1891) *Comptes rendu hebdomadaire des séances de l'Académie des Sciences* **112**, 295.

CHAPTER NINE

Respiration: The Tissue Phase

A number of discrepancies between the adjustments to oxygen uptake and transport at altitude have suggested that other adjustments at tissue level may be of equal or more importance. For instance there appears to be no definite correlation between haemoglobin concentration and therefore oxygen content of the blood and physical performance. In addition the physical performance of high-altitude natives always appears to be better than that of high-altitude visitors. Also newcomers to altitude always acclimatise more slowly than those who have previously been to altitude, despite many other comparable features of adaptation.

Changes at tissue level therefore which involve an increase in tissue capillaries, together with other processes, may be of importance equal to or greater than changes in the oxygen transport mechanism.

There is no clear understanding as to whether the energy requirements of the organism are reduced—or whether the tissues acquire an ability to utilise oxygen more efficiently. For instance, aerobic metabolic activity seems to be increased. However reduced lactic acid production has been reported at high altitude during exercise (Edwards 1936). Presumably too high a production of acid would interfere with acid–base balance (Cerretelli 1967).

At tissue level four mechanisms for adaptation to hypoxia appear to be present: increase in capillary density, an increase in myoglobin, an increase in the number of mitochondria, and changes in enzyme levels and the biochemical aspects of cell metabolism.

Tissue Capillaries

Despite various adaptive mechanisms, it appears that the tissues at altitude would still be functioning at a Po_2 lower than the sea-level value, especially during exercise. The level of Po_2 in the tissues below which the mitochondria cannot operate may therefore have been reduced.

The critical Po_2 of mitochondria is of the order of 1–3 mmHg (Chance *et al.* 1964). As pressure at the venous end of the capillary is around 30 mmHg the diffusion pressure is about 30 mmHg between the venous end of the capillary and the mitochondria.

Normally a cylinder of tissue surrounds a capillary. As the Po_2 drops from the arterial towards the venous end, so the diffusion pressure gradient will be lower at the venous end. Thus a drop of 15 mmHg in the Po_2 in the venous end of the capillary would jeopardise the cells in the periphery of the cylinder of tissue surrounding the capillary, unless diffusion was made easier.

Reduction in the distance for diffusion between capillary and tissue could be effected by increasing the number of capillaries. In acclimatised animals this appears to be the case, and increased capillary counts have been recorded (Valdivia 1958).

Changes at tissue level therefore include an increased density of capillaries in muscles and also permanent dilation of the capillary bed in the lungs.

A greater calibre of the blood vessels of the retina has been observed in high-altitude subjects, and post-mortem reports at high altitude often comment on the degree of capillary congestion found in all viscera (Valdevelland 1951).

There is indirect evidence that blood flow through active

muscles is greater in high-altitude natives than in acclimatised visitors. This is inferred from the observation that the cardiac output is higher in high-altitude natives at the same work rate.

As high-altitude natives have lower blood lactic acid values than acclimatised visitors after submaximal exercise, it could be considered that their muscles have a greater diffusing capacity for oxygen. This would be associated with a greater number of open capillaries and a higher blood flow.

Myoglobin

Myoglobin, which takes up oxygen at low tissue tensions for storage, and also enhances oxygen diffusion, has been found to be increased in the heart and skeletal muscles of high-altitude animals (Hurtado *et al.* 1937).

Myoglobin is a protein containing haem which is found in muscles, especially those that show repeated contraction such as the heart and leg muscles. Oxygen combines with it loosely and reversibly and it holds oxygen in combination in muscle as a reserve store which is available during activity.

The affinity of oxygen for myoglobin is greater than for haemoglobin, especially at low pressures of oxygen. Myoglobin therefore remains well saturated with oxygen even when the Po_2 is very low and it is as a result well adapted to taking up oxygen at low interstitial fluid Po_2 and making it available to the cells: e.g. at a Po_2 of 40 mmHg, myoglobin is 95 per cent and haemoglobin is 75 per cent saturated with oxygen; at a Po_2 of 10 mmHg myoglobin is 70 per cent and haemoglobin is 10 per cent saturated with oxygen.

The speed of combination of oxygen with myoglobin is very rapid and it will therefore be able to deliver oxygen when the blood flow to a muscle decreases during contraction.

Both myoglobin and haemoglobin are able to increase the diffusion rate of oxygen. Therefore an increase in quantity and activity of myoglobin may be an important factor in adaptation to high altitude.

Probably the most essential factor in producing changes in

myoglobin content is hypoxia of sufficient intensity and duration.

In general there is an increase in the concentration of myoglobin in experimental animals adapted to hypoxia over a period of months. Increases occurred in myoglobin content of the heart, diaphragm and some skeletal muscles. On return to sea level the myoglobin content fell to normal. (Tappin and Reynafarje 1957; Vaughan and Page 1956).

Mitochondria

An increase in the number of mitochondria in the heart of high-altitude cattle has been reported (Ou and Tenney 1970).

Changes in Enzyme Levels and Biochemical Aspects of Cell Metabolism

Reference should be made to chapters by Barbashova (1964) and Harris (1971).

References

Barbashova, Z. I. (1964) Cellular level of adaptation. In, *Handbook of Physiology. Adaptation to environment.* American Physiological Society: Washington D.C.

Cerretelli, P. (1967) In, *Exercise at altitude. Ed.* Margaria, R. Excerpta Medica Foundation: Amsterdam.

Chance, B., Schoener, B. and Schindler, F. (1964) In, *Oxygen in the animal organism. Ed.* Dickens, F. and Neil, E. Macmillan: New York.

Edwards, M. T. (1936) *American Journal of Physiology* **116**, 367.

Harris, P. (1971) Some observations on the biochemistry of the myocardium at high altitude. In, *High altitude physiology.* Ciba Foundation Symposium. *Ed.* Porter, R. and Knight, J. Churchill-Livingstone: Edinburgh and London.

Hurtado, A., Rotta, A., Merino, C. and Pons, J. (1937) *American Journal of Medical Science* **194**, 708.

Ou, L. C. and Tenney, S. N. (1970) *Respiratory Physiology* **8**, 151.

Tappin, D. V. and Reynafarje, B. D. (1957) *American Journal of Physiology* **190**, 99.

Valdivia, E. (1958) *American Journal of Physiology* **194**, 585.

Vaughan, B. E. and Pace, N. (1956) *American Journal of Physiology* **185**, 549.

CHAPTER TEN

Respiratory Control

Respiratory Centre

The medullary centre is a widely dispersed group of neurones situated bilaterally in the reticular substance of the medulla oblongata and pons.

It is normally divided into the medullary centre and the apneustic and pneumotaxic areas.

Medullary Centre

This is found beneath the lower part of the floor of the 4th ventricle in the medial half of the medulla. Inspiratory and expiratory neurones intermingle in this centre.

When respiration increases both inspiratory and expiratory neurones are excited above the normal, transmitting an increased number of impulses to the inspiratory muscles during inspiration and an increased number of expiratory impulses during expiration.

A basic rhythm is established in the medullary centre and normally inspiration lasts for about two seconds, expiration for about three.

The medullary centre is not by itself capable of producing a smooth pattern of respiration. If it functions alone the pattern of respiration is short inspiration and prolonged expiration occurring in gasps.

Signals entering from the spinal cord, cerebral cortex, mid-brain and pneumotaxic centre all modify the respiratory rhythm and contribute to the normal pattern of respiration.

A mechanism explaining the rhythmicity of the medullary centre has been postulated. This is based on two oscillating circuits, one for inspiration and the other for expiration. These cannot oscillate simultaneously because they inhibit one another. When the inspiratory neurones are active the expiratory ones are inactive and vice versa. A rhythmic alternation between inspiratory and expiratory signals is thus set up, causing the act of respiration.

Apneustic Area and Pneumotaxic Areas

These areas are found in the reticular substance of the pons.

When the apneustic area is connected to the medullary centres but not the pneumotaxic area, stimulation produces a prolonged inspiration and short expiration.

If the pneumotaxic area is left connected to the medullary centre, the pattern of respiration becomes essentially normal with a reasonable balance between inspiration and expiration.

Stimulation of this area produces a change in rate, hence its name.

Chemosensitive Area of the Brain Stem

A small chemosensitive respiratory area has been identified on each side of the medulla at approximately the entry of the 8th, 9th and 10th cranial nerves.

This area seems to be very sensitive to changes in H^+ ion concentration in the cerebrospinal fluid. An increase in H^+ ion (decrease in pH) increases activity and vice versa.

Carbon dioxide diffuses easily and rapidly from the blood to the cerebrospinal fluid but H^+ ions do not. The carbon dioxide combines with the water of the cerebrospinal fluid to form carbonic acid and this dissociates to increase the concentration of hydrogen ions in the fluid. These ions stimulate the respiratory centre.

Therefore, in fact, it is the carbon dioxide concentration in the blood which in this indirect fashion stimulates the chemosensitive area of the medulla.

The 'respiratory centre' is affected by impulses from other parts of the nervous system.

Spinal Cord

Facilitatory impulses from the spinal cord play an important part in keeping the respiratory centre active. Even when the respiratory centre is so depressed that respiration has almost ceased it is possible to stimulate it by a peripheral impulse, e.g. applying cold water to the skin or slapping the skin may often revive respiration.

Herring–Breuer Reflex

Stretch receptors are present in the visceral pleura, bronchi, bronchioles and alveoli.

On inspiration, the lungs expand and these receptors transmit impulses via the vagus nerves to the tractus solitarius of the spinal cord and then to the respiratory centre. Respiration is inhibited and over-distension of the lungs is prevented.

A similar deflation reflex occurs via compression receptors during expiration. This reflex is however much less active.

The Herring–Breuer reflex is important in maintaining a rhythmic respiration.

Emotional States

Fear characteristically stimulates respiration and heart rate.

Chemical or Humoral Control

As the main purpose of respiration is to regulate the concentration of oxygen, carbon dioxide and hydrogen ions in the body fluids it responds to small changes in concentration of any of these substances.

Carbon dioxide and hydrogen ions act primarily on the respiratory centre in the brain, while lack of oxygen acts on the peripheral chemoreceptors.

Carbon Dioxide and Hydrogen Ions

Providing all other factors are constant

  (i) an increase in carbon dioxide concentration can increase the rate of alveolar ventilation by as much as seven times.
  (ii) an increase in H^+ ion (decrease in pH) also increases the alveolar ventilation by the same amount.

However under normal conditions in the body, carbon dioxide affects respiration more than the H^+ ion concentration.

Oxygen

Various peripheral chemoreceptors are sensitive to changes in oxygen, carbon dioxide and H^+ ion concentration.

From the carotid bodies impulses pass via the glossopharyngeal nerve, and from the aortic bodies via the vagus nerve, to the medulla oblongata.

A low oxygen tension (Po_2) may depress the respiratory centre directly.

A lowered Po_2 in arterial blood stimulates the respiratory centre—indirectly—through the chemoreceptors. The number of nerve impulses is greatly increased in the Po_2 range 30–60 mmHg. This is the range in which the oxygen saturation of haemoglobin decreases rapidly.

An increase in carbon dioxide and H^+ concentration also stimulates the chemoreceptors and thus indirectly increases respiration, but the direct effect of both is so much more powerful that this indirect effect may be disregarded.

Effect of Arterial Po_2

So long as the arterial Po_2 is above 100 mmHg there is very

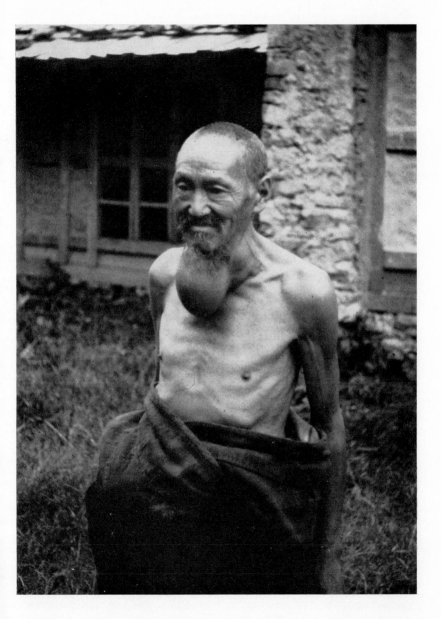

Plate 1.   Large pendulous goitre.

Plate 2. Frostbite of feet showing patchy gangrenous areas and blisters.

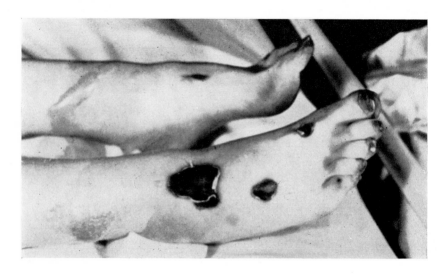

Plate 3. The feet of a pilgrim who was able to walk barefoot in the snow without local cold injury.

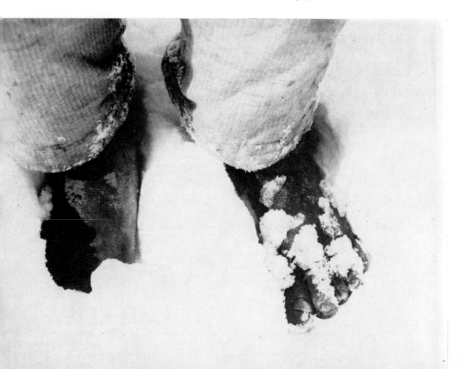

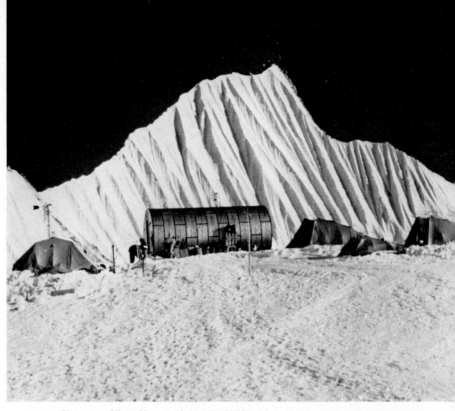

Plate 4. Silver Hut at 19,000 ft. (5791 m) in the Everest region. This was occupied throughout the winter of 1960–1.

Plate 5. Bicycle ergometer, used for studying maximal work rates and oxygen uptake.

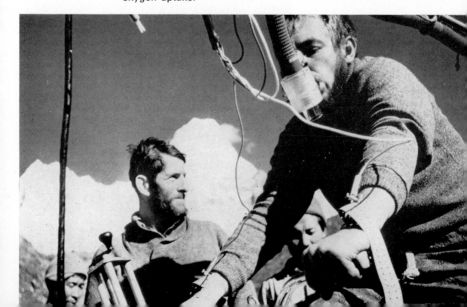

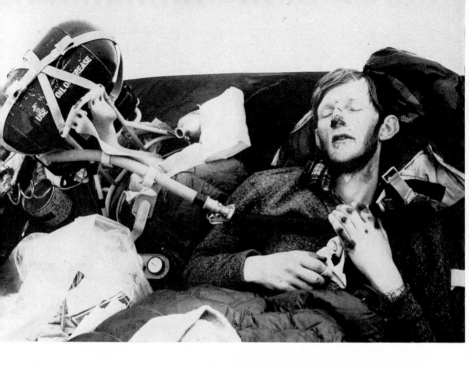

Plate 6. Exhaustion, and frostbite of nose and fingers. This patient also had a pulmonary thrombosis at 26,000 ft (7925 m).

Plate 7. Climbing in the winter 1960–1 at 21,000 ft (6400 m). Showing protective clothing.

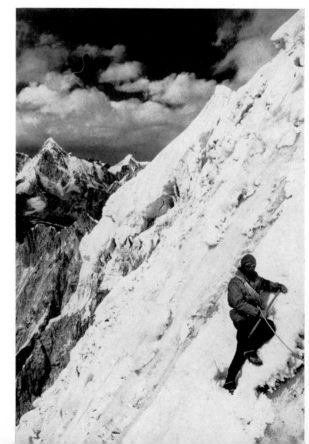

little effect on alveolar ventilation. As it falls, alveolar ventilation increases.

Each of the individual factors, carbon dioxide, H^+ ion and oxygen, can produce very powerful effects on alveolar ventilation, provided the other two are kept at normal levels.

In fact this does not occur and carbon dioxide is the main regulating factor in alveolar ventilation.

Carbon Dioxide

As carbon dioxide is one of the end products of tissue metabolism its concentration affects the chemical reactions of the cells. The tissue fluid P_{CO_2} therefore must be accurately regulated. This regulation is carried out by the alveolar ventilation so the feedback via the respiratory centre is important in maintaining the tissue concentration.

An increase in P_{CO_2} stimulates the respiratory centre: this in turn increases alveolar ventilation and reduces the alveolar P_{CO_2} and the tissue P_{CO_2} returns to normal.

The Carotid Bodies

These are two reddish-brown ellipsoidal structures situated one on each side of the neck in close relation to the carotid sinus.

Each is about 5 mm in height and 2·5 mm in width. They vary in position and may (a) lie deep to the bifurcation of the common carotid artery; (b) be completely or partially wedged between the origins of the internal and external carotid artery; or (c) be attached to or partially embedded in the fibrous coat of the arteries.

Each is surrounded by a fibrous capsule and divided by fibrous septa into lobules. Each lobule contains a mass of large polyhedral epithelioid (glomus cells) and supporting cells with a network of sinusoidal blood vessels.

The cells are closely applied to the endothelium lining the sinuses and contain granules which give a positive reaction to catecholamines.

Abundant nerve fibres permeate the epithelioid cells, and

numerous sensory endings are present in relation to them and the sinusoids.

One group of nerve fibres end in terminal bulbs invaginated into the surface of the glomus cells. These endings are packed with mitochondria and they may be oxygen tension receptors, the mitochondrial oxygen consumption maintaining a constant level against which environmental changes are measured.

The nerves are derived mainly (a) from the carotid branch of the glossopharyngeal nerve but also from (b) the superior cervical ganglion of the sympathetic; and (c) the inferior cervical ganglion of the vagus.

The carotid body is developed from the mesenchyme of the 3rd pharyngeal arch, appearing as a condensation of the mesenchyme around the 3rd pharyngeal pouch artery, and its nerve supply is mainly from the nerve of that arch—the glossopharyngeal.

The blood supply to the carotid body is rich—the flow is 2000 ml/100 gram per minute—which is 30 times larger than to the brain or heart.

The oxygen consumption is 9 ml/100 gram per minute, which is three times that of the brain.

Other small bodies, aortic bodies, with a similar structure, are found in relation to the arteries of the 4th and 6th pharyngeal arches.

They lie close to the arch of the aorta, the ductus arteriosus and the right subclavian artery.

Their histological structure is identical with the carotid body. Innervation is by branches of the vagus nerve. Their functions are identical with those of the carotid body and the two sets of chemoreceptors behave as a unit.

Increase in carbon dioxide causes hyperpnoea, whether or not the carotid and aortic bodies are denervated. This is because of the effect of a raised P_{CO_2} acting directly on the central respiratory mechanism.

Systemic hypoxia causes hyperpnoea in the intact animal, but if both the carotid and aortic bodies are denervated, hypoxia depresses the respiration directly.

Thus hypoxia directly depresses the central respiratory mechanism but indirectly—acting via the chemoreceptors—causes stimulation.

Carotid Bodies at High Altitude

It appears that the carotid bodies of subjects exposed to high altitude in the Andes are larger than those of people living on the Peruvian coast (Arias-Stella 1969). A similar finding is reported in animals born and living at high altitude (Edwards 1971).

A generalised hyperplasia has been reported in man.

It is considered that there are three kinds of light cell (type I) and one of these secretes erythropoietic substance.

The chief cells probably have a chemoreceptor function. They contain catecholamines.

The type II cells have a 'supporting' function.

The relative hyperplasia of light type I cells (with decrease in number of dark cells) in high-altitude guinea pigs and rats suggest that this is the cell that responds specifically to hypoxia.

A pronounced vacuolation of these cells was also noted in high-altitude animals. The degree of vacuolation may indicate increased activity associated with hypoxia (Edwards 1971).

A correlation between the weight of the carotid body and the degree of right ventricular hypertrophy has been observed in patients dying with cardiopulmonary disease associated with chronic hypoxia (Heath *et al.* 1970).

No definite conclusion on the relationships between structure and function of the carotid bodies at high altitude can yet be drawn.

Chemodectoma

Chemodectoma are tumours of the carotid bodies and similar chemoreceptors.

Incidence

Seventy-five per cent of tumours have been in patients of between 30 and 60 years—the mean age is about 42 years old. Many are known to be of long duration, up to 35 years or longer—so that the actual age at onset is usually early adult life in most cases. Males and females are equally affected.

With rare exceptions the growth is unilateral, though bilateral tumours have been recorded.

Carotid body tumours have been reported wherever chemoreceptor tissue is found, i.e. the aortic bodies, glomus jugulare, ganglion nodosum, and in the pineal gland, urinary bladder and nasal cavities. The most frequent site is the glomus jugulare which is associated with invasion of the middle ear.

Simultaneous tumours of the carotid body and one or more of the other chemoreceptors have been reported.

A high frequency of chemodectoma especially of the head and neck has been reported in individuals born and living at altitudes from 6500–14,500 ft (2000–4350 m) in Peru, Colorado and Mexico. In general they were benign, but one tumour of the glomus jugulare was malignant. There was also a preponderance of females (Saldana *et al.* 1970, 1973).

Cases from Ethiopia and Asia have not so far been reported.

Chronic hypoxia is a stimulus for carotid body hyperplasia, an effect found in animals (Edwards *et al.* 1971), and in man at sea level in conditions of chronic hypoxia (Heath *et al.* 1971).

Chemodectoma occur at sea level as a familiar disease and these are unlikely to have been caused by hypoxia. Therefore the predominance of the disease at high altitude may merely indicate a population trait, possibly a response to chronic hypoxia.

Structure

The chemodectoma is known as the 'potato tumour'.

It is smooth, lobulated, firm, homogeneous, and greyish-white in colour. It usually envelops the artery at the bifurcation of the common carotid—or the vessels lie in a groove in the tumour.

It varies from 2–6 cm in diameter.

Under the microscope it is seen to consist of masses of epithelioid cells resembling those of the carotid body, separated by strands of connective tissue or blood vessels. Plentiful nerve fibres may be present.

The cells are large, polyhedral and irregular with an indefinite outline—often with vacuolated cytoplasm.

Adrenaline is usually not found in the tumour although noradrenaline-secreting tumours have been reported. Physiological effects have not been reported.

In general these tumours are benign, growing slowly, remaining circumscribed, and producing no metastases. Tumours of the glomus jugulare, though growing slowly, invade the surrounding bone; metastases in lymph nodes and liver have been reported (Willis 1967).

References

Arias-Stella, J. (1969) Abstract 150. Program and Abstracts of the 66th Annual Meeting of the American Association of Pathologists and Bacteriologists.

Edwards, C. W. (1971) In, *High altitude physiology*. *Ed.* Porter, R. and Knight, J. Ciba Foundation Symposium. Churchill Livingstone: Edinburgh and London.

Edwards, C., Heath, D., Harris, P., Castillo, Y., Kruger, H. and Arias-Stella, J. (1971) *Journal of Pathology* **104**, 231.

Heath, D., Edwards, C. W. and Harris, P. (1970) *Thorax* **25**, 129.

Saldana, M. and Salem, L. E. (1970) *American Journal of Pathology* **59**, 91a.

Saldana, M., Salem, L. E. and Travezan, R. (1973) *Human Pathology* **4**, 251.

Willis, R. A. (1967) *Pathology of tumours*. Butterworths: London.

CHAPTER ELEVEN

Ventilatory Response to Hypoxia

Clinically the most obvious change on ascending to high altitude is an increase in the rate and depth of respiration.

The initial change appears to be in the depth (tidal volume) rather than the rate of respiration.

There is a difference of opinion as to the level of inspired oxygen tension, or altitude, at which an increase in rate first occurs.

On acute exposure in unacclimatised man an increased rate of ventilation does not occur until the alveolar Po_2 is about 50–60 mmHg, or at 12,000–13,000 ft (3658–3962 m). However, individual variation is very great and in some people an increase in respiration occurs as low as 3000–4000 ft (900–1200 m) or at a Po_2 of 70 mmHg.

In experimental subjects at rest the minute volume increases with altitude above about 12,000 ft (3658 m), whereas the rate of respiration does not seem to increase significantly until 20,000–22,000 ft (6096–6706 m).

During exercise all complained of increased respiration (both in rate and depth) above the normal level.

Even mild exercise produced a marked change in the rate of respiration in comparison with that at sea level.

It may take some weeks before a normal pattern of respiration occurs.

Table 15. Respiration and altitude at rest (Rahn and Otis 1947)

Altitude ft	m	Minute volume l/min	Rate per min
sea level		8·85	12
12,000	3658	9·71	14
18,000	5486	11·06	12
22,000	6706	15·31	15

In acclimatised visitors to high altitude the minute volume (STPD) at rest tends to be constant and independent of altitude, so that the reduced density of the air is compensated. However individual variation is considerable (Pugh 1957; Gill and Pugh 1964).

High-altitude natives, however, at 13,000–15,000 ft (3962–4572 m) ventilated less than acclimatised or partially acclimatised visitors (Chiodi 1957).

Table 16. Effect of exercise on respiratory rate (Schneider 1932)

Place	Sea level	14,000 ft (4267 m)
Bed	17	17
Standing	17	20
Walking (5 mph)	20	36

High-Altitude Visitors

In sea-level residents ascending to altitude the change in Po_2 acts via the chemoreceptors (carotid and aortic bodies) on the respiratory centre. This effect becomes more marked when the Po_2 falls to about 60 mmHg with a resulting increase in the number of impulses in the glossopharyngeal and vagus nerves.

This hypoxic stimulus to breathing leads to an increase in alveolar ventilation, and carbon dioxide is washed out of the lungs. The Pco_2 falls and to restore the normal H^+ concentration, HCO_3^- has to be reduced since H^+ concentration is proportional to Pco_2/HCO_3^-.

When the P_{CO_2} is low the provision of H^+ ions for the renal tubular cells is inadequate, bicarbonate is not well absorbed and some HCO_3^- ions are excreted to give an alkaline urine. Thus by removal of HCO_3^-, the H^+ concentration is readjusted.

Although this response does occur, it is sluggish and takes weeks or months to make itself manifest.

It has been noted too that in a number of individuals on first ascending to 18,000 ft (5486 m) the urine is more acid than alkaline. This seeming paradox may be explained by the fact that many suffer from acute mountain sickness, anorexia, and loss of weight. Therefore excretion of acetone bodies may occur, the result of low food intake making the urine acid and masking the sluggish renal compensation (Warren 1936; Ward 1953).

A more plausible hypothesis has been put forward by Severinghaus and others who studied a number of subjects acutely exposed to 12,470 ft (3800 m).

After 24 hours hyperpnoea developed. Arterial P_{CO_2} fell from 40 to 30 mmHg while arterial pH rose from 7·43 to 7·48. In addition, P_{CO_2} in the cerebrospinal fluid (CSF) fell from 49 to 39 mmHg, but its pH remained steady at its sea-level value of 7·32, whereas it would have been expected to rise to 7·43.

Thus the bicarbonate content of the CSF must have been reduced by some means. Measurements showed that it had in fact fallen by 5 mequiv per litre. This was not due to renal excretion of bicarbonate because the plasma bicarbonate fell by only 1–2 mequiv per litre.

The conclusion drawn was that active transport of HCO_3^- out of the CSF had occurred (Severinghaus et al. 1963).

The mechanism of respiratory regulation can be envisaged as follows.

On initial exposure to altitude, the peripheral chemoreceptors, which are sensitive to low P_{O_2}, cause increased ventilation. This results in lowered alveolar, arterial, interstitial fluid and CSF P_{CO_2}. The decreased P_{CO_2} of the CSF (decreased H^+ concentration) tends to inhibit the peripherally induced hyperventilation— that is, it reduces the hypoxic drive by direct action on the medullary centres. The decreased H^+ concentration of the CSF results in increased transport of bicarbonate out of the CSF and interstitial fluid, so that the H^+ concentration is brought back to normal balance.

This adjustment takes time and therefore respiratory adjustment takes a few days.

Once the CSF has returned to its normal pH, the inhibition of the peripheral chemoreceptors is removed and ventilation increases.

As the CSF bicarbonate is low, any change in P_{CO_2} will be mirrored by a change in the pH of the CSF and result in a change in ventilation.

From work carried out at 19,000 ft (5791 m) it appears that after acclimatisation in a sea-level visitor there was an increased sensitivity to carbon dioxide. This was a gradual change taking place within one month at 19,000 ft. The response threshold to carbon dioxide at varying oxygen pressures was decreased from 38 mmHg at sea level to 24 mmHg after a week at 19,000 ft (5791 m). Even after many weeks at altitude subjects were still responding primarily to the hypoxic drive via the carotid bodies. Sensitivity to hypoxia did not appear to be changed after twelve weeks at 19,000 ft (Milledge 1963).

Lowlanders who live for years at high altitude do not in general seem to lose their sensitivity to low P_{O_2}. However in one study of sea-level natives who had moved to 15,000 ft (4540 m) 75 per cent developed a low sensitivity to hypoxia after nine months (Severinghaus 1971).

High-Altitude Natives

High-altitude natives appear to be relatively insensitive to hypoxia, and therefore show a relatively small increase in ventilation with low P_{O_2}, by comparison with sea-level visitors at altitude (Milledge and Lahiri 1967). This applies at rest, during work, and in response to hypoxic stimuli.

The high-altitude native does hyperventilate at high altitude, possibly because of the low pH of the cerebrospinal fluid. This may result from increased anaerobic glycolysis in the brain (Sorensen and Milledge 1971).

The respiratory sensitivity to carbon dioxide at high altitude was no different from lowlanders. On returning to sea level, the blunted hypoxic response persisted for six weeks at least. The carbon dioxide sensitivity also seemed to decrease at sea level, possibly the result of decreased ventilation (Lahiri *et al.* 1969).

It is now generally accepted that this relative insensitivity persists even after the high-altitude native has lived at sea level for long periods. This suggests that there is some irreversible factor present.

This blunted response to hypoxia could be the result of de-sensitisation of the peripheral chemoreceptors, the result of chronic exposure to hypoxia. Alternatively it could be a process of natural selection which results in a decreased sensitivity being a genetic characteristic of high-altitude natives.

Genetic factors appear to be unlikely. Caucasians living permanently in Kashmir at 11,500 ft (3500 m) and in Colorado at 10,000 ft (3000 m), and natives of Asia and South America, of Mongoloid origin, all show a blunted response.

Long-continued hypoxia from the pre-natal to post-natal period may be a possible cause.

Studies on sea-level individuals with long-standing hypoxia associated with congenital cyanotic heart disease showed some blunting of the response to hypoxia. Although the mechanism need not necessarily be the same as in high-altitude natives, this does indicate that hypoxia from early life exerts an important effect on ventilatory control (Edelman 1970).

Studies on animals born and rasied at high altitudes however showed no blunting of the hypoxic response. Similar results were obtained in sea-level animals (goats) born and raised in an altitude chamber at an altitude equivalent of 16,500 ft (5000 m) (410 mmHg) (Lahiri 1971).

These findings suggest that in animals some peculiarity other than lifelong hypoxia is necessary for blunting to develop.

Observation on man suggests that hypoxia during neonatal life may contribute to this blunted response.

Before birth the human foetus at sea level has an arterial Po_2 between 32 and 36 mmHg (Bartels 1968). At high altitude this is presumably a little lower (Dawes 1968). In the newly born child at sea level this hypoxia disappears, whereas at high altitude it persists.

The effect of transient hypoxia on neonates is to depress the respiration after a period of 2–3 minutes. The blunted hypoxia response of the high altitude natives could well be a combination of this response (Lahiri 1971).

However, loss of hypoxic ventilatory drive did not occur in the neonatal period in a group of children born and bred at 10,100 ft (3100 m) by comparison with those born and bred at 5000 ft (1600 m). This indicates that the change is acquired over many years (Byrne-Quinn *et al.* 1972).

These results do not suggest that more severe hypoxia (say at 13,000 ft (4000 m) could not cause a blunted response at an earlier age.

Suprapontine Influence

Respiratory centres are found in the pons and medulla. How-ever it is common knowledge that respiratory movements can be controlled for a limited period, and that stimulation of certain parts of the cerebral cortex affects breathing.

Acute hypoxia in the intact animal produced a high degree of cortical arousal but if the peripheral chemoreceptors are dener-vated this does not occur.

Hypoxia excites the medullary centres, (a) by the direct action of the peripheral chemoreceptors on the medulla, and (b) by the action of the peripheral chemorecopters on the cortex via the reticular activating mechanism.

The descending cortical influences exerted directly on the medullary centres are essentially inhibitory but when mediated by the diencephalon, are facilitatory.

Thus the final effect of the suprapontine influences would be a balance between the two, and the degree of influence would depend on severity and time of exposure to hypoxia.

It is suggested from work on cats that acute hypoxia is attended by sympathetic discharge and adrenal response, which is not sustained in the acclimatised state.

Therefore, early in acclimatisation cortical arousal working via the reticular activating mechanism could account for the origin of symptoms, i.e. irritability and insomnia.

Later the inhibitory influence of the cortex develops slowly, but eventually in high-altitude natives it overrides the diencephalic facilitatory influence and blunting to hypoxia occurs.

It has also been suggested that if in acute hypoxia there is sympathetic vasoconstriction of the vessels of the carotid body, then in chronic anoxia this response (even to acute hypoxia) might be lost. Then the output of impulses from the carotid body to the medullary centres would be less than expected and blunting would occur (Tenney *et al.* 1971).

Periodic Breathing

During the initial phase of ascent to high altitude the breathing may become disordered. This is commonly called Cheyne–Stokes respiration. Possibly the first description was given by Hippocrates (Major 1932) and certainly John Hunter recorded a lucid account in his case-books in 1781 (Ward 1973), over thirty years before Cheyne's paper (Cheyne 1818).

Hunter's description of Mr Boyde is as follows

> …but his breathing was very particular: he would cease breathing for twenty or thirty seconds and then begin to breathe softly, which increased until he breathed extremely strong, or rather with violent strength, which gradually died away until we could not observe that he breathed at all (Hunter 1781).

Mosso (1894) was the first person to investigate disordered breathing at altitude, and this was carried out at the Cabana Regina Margarita 15,000 ft (4560 m) on the Punta Gniffeti, one of the summits of the Monte Rosa, the highest mountain in Switzerland.

He however quotes a French physician, Dr Egli-Sinclair, who

had described an irregularity of respiration 'of the Stokes type' at altitude some years previously (Egli-Sinclair 1893).

However a Mr Hirst commented of his friend Professor J. Tyndall who was sleeping exhausted near the summit of Mt Blanc 15,800 ft (4807 m) in 1857, that he did not appear to breathe at all for periods. (Tyndall 1906).

Presumably this was the 'apnoeic phase' of Cheyne–Stokes respiration.

Another type of disordered respiration, Biot's respiration, has been recorded in cases of meningitis. Biot's account has been translated

> This irregularity of the respiratory movements is not periodic, sometimes slow, sometimes rapid, sometimes superficial, sometimes deep, but without any constant relation of succession between the two types, with pauses following irregular intervals, preceded and often followed by a sigh more or less prolonged (Biot 1876; Editorial *J.A.M.A.* 1957).

Essentially this type of breathing is jerky and irregular.

A personal impression is that both types of irregular respiration are present at altitude but the Cheyne–Stokes variety is very much commoner and therefore more readily recognised.

Cheyne–Stokes breathing may occur at rest or whilst asleep and has been recorded as low as 8,000 ft (2438 m). It tends to pass off as the subject becomes better acclimatised but even so it may persist for a long period whilst at high altitude.

Considerable discomfort may occur at night as the periods of dyspnoea are associated with feelings of suffocation and claustrophobia which cause the subject to partially wake and then return to sleep.

Clinically, Cheyne–Stokes breathing consists of three phases:

Hyperventilation. Usually 3–5 respirations with a progressive increase in tidal volume. This is followed by

Diminution. A decreasing depth of respiration.

Apnoea. This is either absolute or partial and lasts for about 10 seconds. Each cycle of periodic breathing lasts about 15–20 seconds.

Changes occurring during the different phases are as follow.

During hyperpnoea, heart rate slows, cardiac output increases, cerebral perfusion is high, P_{ArtO_2} is lower, P_{ArtCO_2} is higher and arterial pH is lower.

During apnoea, heart rate increases, cardiac output decreases, cerebral perfusion is low, P_{ArtO_2} is high, P_{ArtCO_2} is low and arterial pH is higher.

At the end of apnoea, cyanosis may occur (Dowell et al. 1971).

In high-altitude visitors, Cheyne–Stokes respiration may persist for several months at high altitude, but it does not seem so marked in high-altitude natives. This may be due to the decreased sensitivity of their respiratory centre to hypoxia in these individuals.

Possible Mechanism

Theoretically, in a normal person if the respiration becomes more rapid and deeper than usual, this causes the P_{CO_2} in the pulmonary blood to decrease, and the decreased P_{CO_2} inhibits respiration. The P_{CO_2} in the pulmonary blood then gradually increases, and in another few seconds this blood, with its increased P_{CO_2} arrives at the respiratory centre and respiration is stimulated. The individual then starts over-breathing again.

An increase or decrease in blood P_{O_2} could also account for the feedback necessary to produce periodic respiration. However even after denervation of the chemoreceptors periodic respiration occurs illustrating that oxygen lack is not a necessary feature.

Therefore as the basic mechanism for Cheyne–Stokes respiration is present in every individual, this type of breathing should be present continuously in normal life.

The fact that it is not the normal pattern of respiration may be due to the damping of the feedback mechanism. The total body fluid contains very large quantities of stored gases, and it takes a long period of hyper- or hypo-ventilation to change the concentration of these gases to any significant extent. In normal respiration before significant changes in the P_{CO_2} or P_{O_2} can occur, the respiratory centre readjusts the breathing towards normal. The extreme changes in P_{CO_2} and P_{O_2} necessary to cause Cheyne–Stokes breathing are thus prevented. The stabilising capacity of the tissues for P_{O_2} and P_{CO_2} have therefore an important damping effect in preventing Cheyne-Stokes breathing in normal people.

However even in normal people a certain degree of this normal non-damped feedback mechanism is present.

For instance when an individual voluntarily over breathes for a minute or two, a period of apnoea will follow, and then one or two cycles of Cheyne–Stokes respiration, before normal involuntary breathing is regained. The forced breathing washes out carbon dioxide from the alveoli and when the alveolar P_{CO_2} falls to about 17 mmHg, the subject stops ventilating. During the period of apnoea P_{CO_2} rises until at about a P_{CO_2} of 38 mmHg breathing restarts. A few breaths are taken and then a second apnoeic period occurs—in other words the breathing becomes periodic with shorter periods of apnoea until normal breathing occurs. The period of apnoea is due to the inhibitory effect of the low alveolar P_{CO_2} on the medullary chemoreceptors.

During apnoea the alveolar P_{O_2} falls to a level where it acts as a respiratory stimulant—and the subject may in the meantime become cyanosed. A few breaths then occur, the alveolar P_{O_2} rises, and the hypoxic stimulus is reduced, and apnoea occurs again because the respiratory centres are still inhibited by lowered alveolar P_{CO_2}.

At high altitude hypoxia causes over-breathing, and in addition a general instability in the feedback mechanism for respiration (i.e. changes in P_{O_2}, P_{CO_2}, and pH, and in the CSF, arterial and venous systems. In addition, redistribution of blood from the peripheral to central circulation occurs). Thus the whole system of respiratory control becomes unstable and oscillation in a rhythmical, self-sustaining manner, i.e. Cheyne–Stokes respiration, occurs (Dowell *et al.* 1971).

References

Bartels, M. (1968) In, *Pre-natal respiration*. North Holland: Amsterdam.

Biot, M. C. (1876) *Lyon Medical* **23**, 517, 561.

Byrne-Quinn, E., Sodal, I. E. and Weil, J. V. (1972) *Journal of Applied Physiology* **32**, 44.

Cheyne, J. (1818) *Dublin Hospital Report* **2**, 216.

Chiodi, H. (1957) *Journal of Applied Physiology* **10**, 81.

Dawes, G. S. (1968) In, *Foetal and neonatal physiology*. Chicago Year Book Medical Publishers.

Dowell, A. R., Buckley, C. E., Cohen, R., Whalen, R. E. and Sieker, H. O. (1971) *Archives of Internal Medicine* **127**, 712.

Edelman, N. H., Lahiri, S., Braudo, L., Cherniack, N. S. and Fishman, A. P. (1970) *New England Journal of Medicine* **282**, 405.

Editorial (1957) *Journal of American Medical Association* **165**, 1568.

Egli-Sinclair (1893) *Annales de l'Observatoire Météorologique du Mont Blanc* p. 118. Paris.

Gill, M. B. and Pugh, L. G. C. E. (1964) *Journal of Applied Physiology* **19**, 949.

Hunter, J. (1781) *Original Case Reports*. Library of Royal College of Surgeons of England.

Lahiri, S., Edelman, N. H., Cherniack, N. S. and Fishman, A. P. (1969) *Federal Proceedings. Federation of American Societies for Experimental Biology* **28**, 1289.

Lahiri, S. (1971) In, *High altitude physiology. Ed.* Porter, R. and Knight, J. Churchill Livingstone: Edinburgh and London.

Major, R. H. (1932) *Classic descriptions of disease*. Ballière Tindall and Cox: London.

Milledge, J. S. (1963) In, *Regulation of human respiration. Ed.* Cunningham, D. J. C. and Lloyd, B. B. Blackwell: Oxford.

Milledge, J. S. and Lahiri, S. (1967) *Respiration Physiology* **2**, 310.

Mosso, A. (1894) *Life of man in High Alps*. T. Fisher Unwin: London.

Pugh, L. G. C. E. (1957) *Journal of Physiology* **135**, 590.

Rahn, H. and Otis, A. B. (1947) *American Journal of Physiology* **150**, 202.

Schneider, E. C. (1932) *Yale Journal of Biological Medicine* **4**, 537.

Severinghaus, J. W., Mitchell, R. A., Richardson, B. W. and Singer, M. M. (1963) *Journal of Applied Physiology* **18**, 1155.

Severinghaus, J. W. (1971) In, *High altitude physiology*. *Ed.* Porter, R. and Knight, J. Ciba Foundation Symposium. Churchill Livingstone: Edinburgh and London.

Sorensen, S. C. and Milledge, J. S. (1971) *Journal of Applied Physiology* **31**, 28.

Tenney, S. M., Scotto, P., Ou, L. C., Bartlett, J. and Remmers, J. E. In, *High altitude physiology*. *Ed.* Porter, R. and Knight, J. Ciba Foundation Symposium. Churchill Livingstone: Edinburgh and London.

Tyndall, J. (1960) *Glaciers of the Alps and mountaineering in 1861*. Everymans Library. *Ed.* Rhys. Dent: London.

Ward, M. P. (1953) *Personal observations of Everest expedition 1953*.

Ward, M. P. (1973) *Annals of Royal College of Surgeons of England* **52**, 330.

Warren, C. B. M. (1936) In, *Everest. The unfinished adventure*. Hodder and Stoughton.

CHAPTER TWELVE

The Cardiovascular and Capillary Systems

Cardiac Output

The cardiac output is the product of the heart rate and stroke volume (the amount of blood ejected at each beat).

Heart Rate

In acute hypoxia or the exposure to high altitude of an unacclimatised person, an increase in heart rate occurs, which as the stroke volume remains little changed is considered to be the main cause for the rise in cardiac output.

Even at an altitude of 4000 ft (1219 m) in a decompression chamber an increase in rate was noted in 25 per cent of one group of individuals (Lutz and Schneider 1919).

At 10,000 ft (3048 m) and above, in unacclimatised subjects at rest, the increase in rate is gradual up to about 14,000 ft (4267 m) but then steepens with every 1000 ft (300 m) of ascent (Schneider and Truesdell 1921).

Individual variation is considerable, but in general those who are physically fit tend to have both a lower resting rate and a less steep increase in rate, than those who are not.

In an ascent by train from sea level to about 15,000 ft (4500 m), the average increase in six subjects at rest was from 65 to 76 beats/minute (McFarland 1937).

If the subject remains at altitude or the level of low Po_2 remains constant for more than an hour the pulse rate tends to slow and revert to its normal sea-level value. This adjustment seems to take place up to about 15,000 ft (4572 m). Above this level even in acclimatised man there always appears to be some increase in heart rate (Rahn and Otis 1947; Ward 1961). If the exposure to hypoxia is brief, say a matter of hours, the rate returns to normal immediately exposure is ended, or the person descends. However, if some acclimatisation has taken place the heart rate may remain lower than normal for some days after return to sea level.

Table 17. Heart rate in high-altitude visitors (Pugh *et al.* 1964; Ward 1961)

Height ft	m	Work rate kg m/min	MPW	Mean heart rate
Sea level		Rest	66	
		300		92
		600		110
		900		132
		1200		153
		1500		182
		1800–2000		187
15,300	4650	Rest	74–66	
		300		104
		600		125
		900		139
		1200		155
		1500		167
19,000	5800	Rest	80–66	
		300		106
		600		126
		900		136
		1200		143
21,000	6400	Rest	80	
		300		122
		600		139
		900		144
24,500	7440	Rest	108	
		300		130
		600		140

Acclimatised residents living at 8000 ft (2440 m) showed no increase in heart rate.

Some observers (Barcroft 1925) considered that no increase occurred up to 14,000 ft (4267 m), and Monge (Monge 1931) observed that some high-altitude residents had a bradycardia at 12,000 ft (3658 m).

A slight increase in resting heart rate was noted in Sherpas at 16,000 ft (4877 m) and above.

In high-altitude natives the resting heart rate was lower than in high-altitude visitors but showed a greater increase with work. In high-altitude visitors the resting rate was higher, but the maximal rate lower. (Pugh *et al.* 1964)

The maximum heart rate at sea level in high-altitude visitors was 189–190, whilst at 19,000 ft (5791 m) the maximum rate was 140–150. In high-altitude natives the maximum heart rate at altitude was 196.

Table 18. Resting heart rate in high-altitude resident (Sherpas) (Jackson and Davies 1960)

Height		Mean rate
ft	m	
4000	1219	65
7000	2134	67
11,700	3500	65
16,400	5000	81
17,900	5400	80
19,100	5800	93

Cardiac Output and Stroke Volume

At an altitude of about 14,000 ft (4267 m), which is equivalent to an oxygen saturation of 75 per cent, the cardiac output starts to increase (Harrison and Blalock 1927).

Investigation of two subjects at 14,000 ft (4267 m) showed that the cardiac output increased steadily over a period of 4–5 days reaching a level of nearly 50 per cent above its sea-level value. It then slowly declined to its normal level as the haemoglobin concentration was increased (Grollman 1930).

In high-altitude natives at about 15,000 ft (4572 m), a slight increase in cardiac output was initially noted (Rotta 1947), but more recently investigations using a right heart catheter have shown no change in resting cardiac output at this altitude (Rotta *et al.* 1956).

In normal subjects at simulated altitudes of 16,000–18,000 ft (4877–5486 m) the output increased by 14 per cent per beat (Starr and McMichael 1948). A similar increase was confirmed at 17,500 ft (5334 m) in unacclimatised visitors (Galdston and Steele 1950).

In high-altitude visitors at 19,000 ft (5791 m) the cardiac output at work rates of 300, 600 and 900 kg m/min was similar to that at sea level. However maximum cardiac output was less than in high-altitude natives.

When given oxygen at sea-level pressure, the heart rate for a given work rate decreased. Work capacity was restored to nearly sea-level value. The maximum cardiac output is probably increased though not to sea-level values because of the increased haematocrit.

Table 19.   Effect of work load on cardiac performance (Pugh 1964)

Work load (kg m/min)	Cardiac output (litre/min)	Heart rate (beats/min)	Stroke volume (ml/min)
High-altitude visitors (1) Sea level			
300	8·8	92	96
600	13·3	110	121
900	16·2	132	123
1200	20·8	153	137
1500	23·7	182	130
(2) 19,000 ft (5800 m)			
300	8·7	106	82
600	12·1	126	96
900	16·8	136	124
High-altitude native (Sherpa)			
19,000 ft (5800 m)			
900	19·3	162	119
1200	22·9	186	123

In high-altitude natives (Sherpas) at 19,000 ft (5791 m), at work rates of 900 kg m/min and 1200 kg m/min the cardiac output was higher than in high-altitude visitors, probably because the heart rate could be increased to near maximum sea-level values.

In addition the work rate of 1200 kg m/min was performed for five minutes, whereas high-altitude visitors could only manage two to four minutes. Endurance therefore was improved in the high-altitude native (Pugh 1964).

In high-altitude visitors at 19,000 ft (5800 m) the stroke volume was less than at sea level at all levels of exercise.

The inability of high-altitude visitors to raise their cardiac output may be due to failure of coronary blood flow to reach adequate levels, and consequent reduction in stroke volume (Alexander *et al.* 1967).

Cardiac Dilatation

Cardiac dilatation secondary to hypoxia has been reported on a number of different occasions.

Clinical examination of mountaineers after climbing to 27,000 ft (8230 m) without oxygen revealed enlarged hearts (Somervell 1925). No clinical evidence of cardiac enlargement was found at 21,000 ft (6400 m) on Everest in 1953, even after a strenuous climb (Pugh and Ward 1956) or in 1961 after many months at 19,000 ft (5791 m). Normal young men were subjected to various degrees of acute hypoxia (up to 28,000 ft (8534 m)), and x-ray measurements showed no evidence of enlargement (Keys *et al.* 1942). Studies of the change in cardiac size were made (Graybiel *et al.* 1950) during partial acclimatisation to simulated altitudes. After three weeks, subjects were able to remain at an altitude of 22,500 ft (6850 m). The heart was found to decrease in size.

Blood Pressure

Most observers are agreed that individuals in normal health who live at altitudes up to 14,000 ft (4300 m) or higher, have no elevation of the arterial blood pressure.

By contrast it has been suggested that systemic blood pressure in high-altitude natives is lower than at sea level, and this appears to be confirmed from epidemiological studies. This is probably due to vaso-dilatation and increased vascularisation, the result of chronic hypoxia and lowering of peripheral resistance.

In high-altitude visitors too after a long residence at high altitude a low blood pressure appears normal (Marticorena *et al.* 1969).

The diastolic pressure in men at high altitude appears to be similar to that at sea level. A relation between diastolic pressure and haematocrit has been observed (McDonough *et al.* 1965), and a raised diastolic pressure has been noted in cases of Monge's disease in which there is a severe degree of polycythaemia (Penaloza *et al.* 1971).

Cardiac Hypertrophy

Hypertrophy of the right ventricle in association with hypoxia was first noted in 1912 (Strohl 1912).

Gomez (Gomez 1948) working at 8000 ft (2440 m) failed to show any increase in the transverse diameter of the heart by means of tele-roentgenograms. Nor did ECG studies show any evidence of cardiac hypertrophy.

However at 12,000 ft (3600 m) Kerwin (Kerwin 1944) found an increase of 11·5 per cent in the transverse diameter and at 14,900 ft (4540 m) an increase of 21 per cent was reported (Miranda and Rotta 1944).

It is considered that the right heart is frequently involved in this hypertrophy, which is explained by a raised pulmonary artery pressure.

General agreement has been reached on the following points:

(i) During hypoxia the pulmonary artery pressure rises, but the left atrial pressure does not.
(ii) An increase in cardiac output occurs. This could contribute to the pulmonary hypertension but to what extent is uncertain.
(iii) There is evidence that hypoxia causes constriction of the pulmonary vessels, by sympathetic stimulation or by release of vaso-active agents, possibly histamine (Hauge and Staube 1969).
(iv) Whether hypoxia has a direct effect on the pulmonary vessels is undecided.

However ECG studies in a high-altitude Asian population living at 12,000–14,000 ft (3658–4267 m) in North Bhutan revealed that though some degree of right axis deviation was present there was no evidence of right ventricular hypertrophy (Jackson and Turner 1967).

Electrocardiography

The most common finding under hypoxic conditions is that the T-wave is either decreased or inverted.

During severe degrees of hypoxia there may be some slowing of the conduction rate, with lengthening of the P–R interval, and also some deformity in the QRS complex.

Changes in the R-wave can be produced by inflating the lungs, and are not associated with hypoxia but may be due to cardiac rotation (Harris and Randall 1944). The changes in the T-wave however do appear to be cardiac in origin, since they cannot be produced by inflation of the lungs.

Reduction in the height of the T-wave was observed in an individual who had been at an altitude of 16,400 ft (5000 m) for five minutes. After one month at 24,600 ft (7460 m) there was a further decrease (Holmstrom 1971).

When subjects taken to 35,000 ft (10,668 m) breathing oxygen, had their oxygen supply disconnected the ECG showed suppressed T-wave and extra-systoles (Hemmingway 1944).

The changes in the ECG noted among men taken from sea

level to 14,900 ft (4500 m) were variable though of three main types

   (i) Shifts to the right of the frontal plane Q R S axis.
  (ii) T-wave voltage increase in the limbs and right prae-
      cordial leads.
 (iii) Variations in the P-wave.

It was suggested that these changes were due to the development of pulmonary hypertension (Penaloza 1958).

The new born showed the same electrical activity of the heart
both at sea level and at 14,900 ft (4500 m). Within a few weeks
the high-altitude children showed accentuated right A Q R S
deviation. A moderate degree of right ventricular hypertrophy
was noted (Penaloza 1960).

In high-altitude natives at 14,900 ft (4500 m) changes in
ECG suggest right ventricular hypertrophy. In newcomers to
this altitude the changes were incomplete even after twelve
months (Rotta and Lopez 1959).

In high-altitude visitors and natives ascending to 19,000 ft
(5791 m) right axis shift was noted as was inversion of the
T-wave in the right praecordial leads.

Changes in the S–T segment and T-wave changes were found
in the praecordial lead in high-altitude visitors (Jackson and
Davies, 1960).

Over some months spent at 19,000 ft (5791 m), the T-wave
inversion in the right praecordial leads which was found in all
high-altitude visitors, tended to spread across the chest.

At 24,000 ft (7315 m) there was a reversion to an upright
T in chest leads, in three of five traces. One subject showed
persistent T-wave inversion in an ECG taken $3\frac{1}{2}$ months
after return to sea level, but other subjects had returned to
normal.

There were no symptoms referable to cardiac disorder.

Oxygen administration had no effect on T-wave inversion or
changes in S–T segment, but there was some change in the
amplitude of the Q R S complex (Milledge 1963).

The cause of these changes is thought to be right ventricular
hypertrophy, rather than positional, that is, hyperventilation

causing a lowering of the diaphragm and right shift of the anatomical axis of the heart.

The decrease in amplitude of the Q R S complex at high altitude and its increase with the administration of oxygen suggests that the power of the myocardium is affected by altitude, and in high-altitude visitors cardiac output is diminished.

Coronary Vessels

Anatomy

The principal arteries of the heart are, on the left, the circumflex and anterior coronary, and on the right, the circumflex. Branches arising from these may be termed secondary branches.

In high-altitude natives, born and bred at 14,500 ft (4375 m) the number of secondary branches is increased (Arias-Stella and Topilsky 1971) and there is also an increase in the number of intercoronary anastomoses and probably an increase in smaller arteries. There was also a predominance of a right type of coronary distribution (Carmelino 1970).

The number of capillaries per myocardial fibre was increased in guinea pigs maintained in a decompression chamber at simulated altitudes (Valdivia 1962), whilst a larger capillary area was noted in puppies born at 20,000 ft (6000 m) (Becker *et al*. 1955).

Coronary Blood Flow

At Sea Level
In man, the blood after passing through the cardiac capillaries contains very little oxygen and a great deal of oxygen is extracted by the myocardium from the coronary blood. During exercise the Po_2 and oxygen content of coronary venous blood remain remarkably constant. There must therefore be an increase in coronary blood flow to supply the extra oxygen, for as work increases so the oxygen uptake by the heart increases.

Hypoxia is one of the most potent factors affecting coronary blood flow which may be increased to five times the normal level. Hypoxia reduces coronary vascular resistance, which increases the blood flow and, providing myocardial oxygen consumption remains the same, reduces the $A-V_{O_2}$ content difference.

If the heart rate increases, the coronary blood flow increases, the vascular resistance diminishes, and the oxygen consumption rises.

As the heart rate increases, the period of uptake remains the same, but diastole is shortened. Since the major part of the coronary flow occurs in diastole, the coronary flow should diminish. The observed increase in flow is probably the result of arteriolar dilatation, the result of increased metabolic activity of the cardiac muscle.

The High-Altitude Native Living at 14,300 ft (4375 m)

The coronary blood flow is reduced at altitude, the decrease in flow is not compensated for by the increased haematocrit or oxygen content of the arterial blood and therefore it appears that the oxygen supply to the myocardium is decreased at high altitude (Moret 1971).

Despite this decrease in flow and oxygen supply, the oxygenation of the myocardium seems adequate.

The consumption of oxygen by the myocardium seems lower at 14,300 ft (4375 m) and the cardiac output at this altitude did not differ from sea-level values.

Above 19,000 ft (5791 m) however some limitation of myocardial efficiency appears to be present as shown by decreasing cardiac output and diminution in the amplitude of the Q R S complex on the ECG.

Heart muscle functions continuously and at a high rate. The oxidative mechanism is small, and is largely provided by myoglobin which at normal levels of P_{O_2} remains undissociated, whereas at very low levels of P_{O_2} in tissue hypoxia it releases oxygen.

Therefore to transform chemical to mechanical energy the heart (a) uses lactic and pyruvic acid, and glucose. The amount of glucose and lactate used varies reciprocally—if lactate is absent, glucose is used in greater amounts and vice versa; (b) it also uses fat, and fatty acids are used preferentially.

At high altitude the energy provided by carbohydrate, especially lactate is more important.

In spite of low arterial Po_2 there is no anaerobic metabolism, and no sign of lactate production—in fact lactate consumption is increased.

The myocardial mitchondria show an increase in internal and external surface area per unit volume of myocardium in high-altitude animals (Kearney 1971).

In patients with Monge's disease, the coronary blood flow was found to be higher than normal, and the haematocrit is raised so the oxygen supply is higher. The oxygen consumption of the myocardium is raised (Moret 1971). However despite this it does seem that the myocardium in some regions might be under-perfused.

Epidemiological studies at 13,500 ft (4100 m) have shown that the incidence of angina of effort, ECG signs of myocardial ischaemia and hypertension are lower than at sea level (Ruiz *et al.* 1969).

In 300 autopsies performed on high-altitude natives (14,300 ft (4375 m)) no cases of myocardial infarction or significant coronary artery disease was found (Ramos *et al.* 1967).

A similar inference was made from studies in North Bhutan at 12,000–14,000 ft (3658–4267 m) (Jackson and Turner 1967).

Capillary System

Anatomy

The pattern of the blood capillary system varies in different regions of the body, according to the function. The basic function is nutrition, but in certain specialised organs such as the liver and spleen this nutritive function is masked.

The basic pattern of a capillary bed concerned with nutrition is a central channel—or arterio-venular channel—and a side branch—the true capillary.

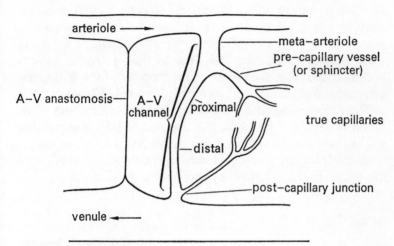

Fig. 18   Capillary bed.

Arterio-venular channels. Under normal conditions these remain open and act as a communication between arteriole and venule. They consist of four portions, the meta-arteriole, 8–15μ in diameter with discontinuous muscle cells; the proximal portion with typical muscle cells; the distal portion with no muscle cells (the arterio-venular capillary); and the venule with no muscle cells.

After it leaves the capillary bed, the venule attains muscle cells. Blood flow is continuous even in tissue at rest.

The arterio-venular channel must be distinguished from the *arterio-venous anastomosis.* This latter is a relatively short muscular vessel serving as a shunt from an artery to its corresponding vein. They vary in size, the smallest connecting a terminal arteriole to its corresponding venule.

When open, the arterio-venous anastomosis will cut off the circulation in the capillary bed. This occurs in frostbite and results in tissue gangrene.

True capillary. This is a side branch of the arterio-venular channel. The pre-capillary vessel or sphincter, gives rise to and controls the blood flow through the true capillary. The pre-capillary vessels have muscular walls and with the meta-arteriole change in calibre in response to nerve stimuli, humoral changes and local metabolites. It leads to the true capillary, whose wall is composed of a single layer of flattened endothelial cells. These present little resistance to the passage of oxygen and nutrients from the plasma. The diameter of the true capillary varies from 5–20μ and its length from 0·4–0·7 mm.

The endothelial cell has some inherent movement and when blood flow ceases the capillaries decrease in size, due possibly to the elasticity inherent in living endothelium.

Blood from the true capillaries enters the distal portion of the arterio-venular channel by post-capillary junctions.

Blood Flow

Blood flow through the true capillary is variable and depends on the alteration in calibre of the pre-capillary vessel or sphincter. The lumen of the true capillary is so narrow that the red blood cell passing in single file is squeezed out of shape as it progresses. This may facilitate passage of oxygen and carbon dioxide. The rate of flow is slower than in arteries and there is no pulsation.

The resistance to the flow of blood is determined by the internal friction, i.e. the viscosity of the blood. In cold conditions and at high altitude, this will be raised because of the high haematocrit. The velocity of flow varies directly with the arterial blood pressure.

The capillary system shows great variation in size. Normally the greater part is closed. During exercise however the capacity of the capillary bed may be increased 750-fold.

At high altitude the number of capillaries per unit area may be increased. This will result in an increase in capacity of the capillary bed and easier oxygen diffusion.

Capillary Permeability

Any factor which causes an increase in respiration causes an increase in the flow of lymph. Increased respiration produces a rise in intra-abdominal pressure during respiration and 'suction' of lymph into the thorax.

Working with dogs Maurer (Maurer 1941) found that increase in lymph production began when the arterial oxygen saturation reached 75 per cent (c. 17,000 ft (5200 m)). The greatest production took place at an arterial saturation of 52·5 per cent (20,000 ft (6100 m)). Because increased lymph flow persisted even after breathing pure oxygen, and since red cells appeared in the lymph, it was felt that the capillaries had been damaged and an increase in capillary permeability had occurred.

Henry (Henry *et al.* 1947) studied capillary permeability in human beings using a cuff technique. Four individuals were subjected to a simulated altitude between 18,000 and 20,000 ft (5485 and 6095 m). No significant difference between subjects and controls was noted.

There is apparent consensus that hypoxia within physiological limits has little if any effect on capillary permeability. Permeability to fluid and protein does not increase unless the venous Po_2 falls below 10–12 mmHg.

It is possible that the lung capillaries are somewhat more susceptible to hypoxia, although this view has been questioned.

Cutaneous Circulation at Altitude

In both visitors and natives the blood flow in the skin of the hand is lower at high altitude than at sea level. This difference however is only statistically significant when the ambient temperature is more than 24°C (i.e. when skin temperature is over 33°C) when the local blood supply is high.

In visitors to high altitude the skin blood flow to the hand is reduced immediately on arrival and then remains at a steady level. Even after one month's residence it is lower in high-altitude visitors than in high-altitude natives.

High-altitude natives have the same blood flow whether living at 12,300 or 17,060 ft (3750 or 5200 m), whereas in high-altitude visitors there is a further reduction at the higher altitude.

As the mean arterial pressure is no different at sea level and altitude, and as there was no major alteration in venous pressure, the reduction in skin blood may be considered to be due to arteriolar vasoconstriction.

There is a decrease in skin blood volume in both high-altitude visitors and natives. This decrease in distensibility in visitors appeared immediately after arriving at altitude and grew more pronounced with time. Even after one month this decrease was greater in visitors than in natives. When high-altitude natives descended to sea level and then returned to high altitude the reduction in the distensibility of skin vessels was most marked. By this mechanism about 2·5 ml of blood per 100 ml of hand volume is mobilized, which is about half the blood present in the skin of the hand at a room temperature of 24°C. This represents 300 ml for the whole skin area.

This blood may be diverted to the pulmonary blood volume and be a factor in the incidence of high-altitude pulmonary oedema. However some workers have found a decrease in pulmonary blood volume at altitude. Alternatively it could go to increase the splanchnic blood volume (Durand and Martineaud 1971).

Venoconstriction on acute exposure is sustained for at least 24 hours following arrival and appears to precede changes in plasma volume. Administration of oxygen to an equivalent altitude does not cause venoconstriction if hypocapnia is prevented but does if hypoxia and hypocapnia are associated. However hypoxia of a greater severity than 14,000 ft (4300 m) produces venoconstriction in the absence of hypocapnia (Weil *et al.* 1969). These factors may contribute to the incidence of frostbite at high altitude.

References

Alexander, J. K., Hartley, L. H., Modelski, M. and Grover, R. F. (1967) *Journal of Applied Physiology* **23**, 849.

Arias-Stella, J. and Topilsky, M. (1971) Anatomy of coronary circulation at high altitude. In, *High altitude physiology*. *Ed*. Porter, R. and Knight, J. Ciba Foundation Symposium. Churchill Livingstone: Edinburgh and London.

Barcroft, J. (1925) Respiratory function of the blood. In, *Lessons from high altitudes*. Cambridge University Press.

Becker, E. L., Cooper, R. G. and Hataway, G. D. (1955) *Journal of Applied Physiology* **8**, 166.

Carmelino, M. (1970) Tesis de Bachiller. Universidad Peruana Cayetano Heredia. Lima.

Durand, J. and Martineaud, J. P. (1971) In, *High altitude physiology*. *Ed*. Porter, R. and Knight, J. Ciba Foundation Symposium. Churchill Livingstone: Edinburgh and London.

Galdston, M. and Steele, J. M. (1950) *Journal of Applied Physiology* **3**, 229.

Gomez, G. E. (1948) *Journal of the American Medical Association* **137**, 1297.

Graybiel, A., Patterson, J. L. and Houston, C. S. (1960) *Circulation* **1**, 991.

Grollman, A. (1930) *American Journal of Physiology* **93**, 19.

Harris, A. S. and Randall, W. C. (1944) *American Journal of Physiology* **142**, 452.

Harrison, T. R. and Blalock, A. (1927) *American Journal of Physiology* **80**, 169.

Hauge, A. and Staube, N. C. (1969) *Journal of Applied Physiology* **26**, 693.

Hemingway, A. (1944) *Journal of Aviation Medicine* **15**, 298.

Henry, J., Goodman, J. and Meehan, J. (1947) *Journal of Clinical Investigation* **26**, 1119.

Holmstrom, F. M. G. (1971) In, *Aerospace medicine*. *Ed*. Randel, H. W. Williams and Wilkins: Baltimore.

Jackson, F. S. and Davies, H. (1960) *British Heart Journal* **22**, 671.

Jackson, F. S. and Turner, R. W. D. (1967) In, *Report of IBP party to North Bhutan. Ed.* Ward, M. P., Jackson, F. S. and Turner, R. W. D.

Kearney, M. (1971) Discussion. In, *High altitude physiology Ed.* Porter, R. and Knight, J. Ciba Foundation Symposium. Churchill Livingstone: Edinburgh and London.

Kerwin, A. J. (1944) *American Heart Journal* **28**, 69.

Keys, A., Stapp, J. P. and Violante, A. (1942) *American Journal of Physiology* **138**, 763.

Lutz, B. R. and Schneider, E. C. (1919) *American Journal of Physiology* **50**, 280.

McDonough, J., Hames, C. G., Garrison, G. E., Stulb, S. C., Lichtman, M. A. and Hefelfinger, D. C. (1965) *Journal of Chronic Diseases* **18**, 243.

McFarland, R. A. (1937) *Journal of Comparative Psychology* **23**, 181.

Marticorena, E., Ruiz, L., Severino, J., Galvez, J. and Penaloza, D. (1969) *American Journal of Cardiology* **23**, 364.

Maurer, F. W. (1941) *American Journal of Physiology* **131**, 331.

Milledge, J. S. (1963) *British Heart Journal* **25**, 291.

Miranda, A. and Rotta, A. (1944) *Anales de la Facultad Medicina (Lima)* **26**, 49.

Monge, C. M. (1931) *Anales de la Facultad de Medicina (Lima)* **17**, 727.

Moret, P. R. (1971) Coronary flow and myocardial metabolism. In, *High altitude physiology. Ed.* Porter, R. and Knight, J. Ciba Foundation Symposium. Churchill Livingstone: Edinburgh and London.

Penaloza, D., Echevarria, M., Marticorena, E. and Gamboa, R. (1958) *American Heart Journal* **56**, 493.

Penaloza, D., Gamboa, R., Dyer, J., Echevarria, M. and Marticorena, E. (1960) *American Heart Journal* **59**, 111.

Penaloza, D., Sime, F. and Ruiz, L. (1971) In, *High altitude physiology. Ed.* Porter, R. and Knight, J. Ciba Foundation Symposium. Churchill Livingstone: Edinburgh and London.

Pugh, L. G. C. E. (1964) *Journal of Applied Physiology* **19**, 441.

Pugh, L. G. C. E., Gill M. B., Lahiri, S., Milledge, J. S., Ward, M. P. and West, J. B. (1964) *Journal of Applied Physiology* **19**, 431.

Pugh, L. G. C. E. and Ward, M. P. (1956) *Lancet* **271**, 1115.

Rahn, H. and Otis, A. B. (1947) *American Journal of Physiology* **150**, 202.

Ramos, A., Kruger, H., Muro, M. and Arias-Stella, J. (1967) *Boln. of Sanit Pan-Am* **62**, 496.

Rotta, A. (1947) *American Heart Journal* **33**, 669.

Rotta, A., Canepa, A., Hurtado, A., Velasquez, T. and Chavez, R. (1956) *Journal of Applied Physiology* **9**, 328.

Rotta, A. and Lopez, A. (1959) *Circulation* **19**, 719.

Ruiz, L., Figueroa, M., Horna, C. and Penaloza, D. (1969) *Archivos del Instituto de Cardiologia de Mexico* **39**, 474.

Schneider, E. C. and Truesdell, D. (1921) *American Journal of Physiology* **55**, 223.

Somervell, T. H. (1925) *Journal of Physiology* **60**, 282.

Starr, I. and McMichael, M. (1948) *Journal of Applied Physiology* **1**, 430.

Strohl, J. (1912) *Atti dei Laboratori scientifici A. Mosso, Torino.*

Valdevellano, J. (1951) *Anales de la Facultad de Medicina (University San Marcos, Lima)* **34**, 572.

Valdivia, E. (1962) *Federation Proceedings. Federation of American Societies for Experimental Biology* **21**, 221.

Ward, M. P. (1961) Personal observation.

Weil, J. V., Battock, D. J., Grover, R. F. and Chidsey, C. A. (1969) *Federation Proceedings. Federation of American Societies for Experimental Biology* **28**, 1160.

CHAPTER THIRTEEN

Exercise at High Altitudes

One of the most important factors that limits muscular activity is the rate at which the muscles can be supplied with oxygenated blood. This depends on circulation and respiration.

Circulation

Active muscles show marked vasodilatation and an increase in blood flow. The mechanism involved is thought to be due to local metabolites acting directly on capillaries, and, via an axon reflex, on the arterioles.

The effect of vasodilatation alone would be to lower arterial blood pressure but as associated changes include vasoconstriction in viscera and skin and an increase in cardiac output, caused by increase in stroke volume and heart rate, from 3-4 litres/min up to 20-25 litres/min, the normal result is to increase blood pressure.

In athletes the heart rate may remain relatively low and the cardiac output is raised by an increase in stroke volume. As the diastolic volume does not increase the only possible conclusion is that the ventricles empty more completely during systole. This may be brought about by increased discharge of sympathetic stimuli combined with an increase in secretion of catecholamines from the adrenal medulla.

In severe exercise in sea-level man the maximum heart rate rarely exceeds 180/min while the cardiac output may increase up to 25 litres/min. As the stroke volume at rest is about 70 ml, it must increase to about 140 ml on severe exercise. In milder exercise the cardiac output is increased largely by the increase in heart rate, with a relatively small increase in stroke volume (up to 50 per cent).

Respiration

In order to increase oxygen intake, pulmonary ventilation is increased, both in rate and depth. When breathing air at normal barometric pressure about 24 litres of ventilation are needed for each litre of oxygen consumed, or in other words the lung can extract only about one fifth of the oxygen presented to it.

The pulmonary ventilation is fairly accurately proportional to the oxygen uptake. During severe exercise the pulmonary ventilation may rise above 100 litres/min.

Even greater rates are possible during voluntary hyperventilation, and this suggests that the limit of oxygen absorption during exercise is not set by the ability to circulate air in the lung, but rather by the rate of diffusion from alveoli to blood, and possibly by the limited time that the blood and alveolar air are in contact.

Tissues

At the start of exercise, circulatory adaptation falls behind increasing tissue consumption. After fifteen seconds of work the mixed venous P_{O_2}, which at rest is 35 mmHg, falls to 22 mmHg. After five minutes it rises to 25 mmHg. Oxygen consumption at the start of exercise is therefore carried out at the expense of the oxygen stored in haemoglobin and myoglobin.

After a delay of thirty seconds at the start of exertion the mixed venous P_{CO_2} started to rise from a resting figure of 45 mmHg to a maximum of 61·5 mmHg after five minutes. This delayed rise suggests an enlarged storage capacity for carbon dioxide in the tissues (Edwards *et al.* 1972(a)).

In man the extra oxygen obtained from the increased reduction of the haemoglobin of venous blood is about 100 ml, and from myoglobin about 500 ml. As the amount of oxygen needed is much greater these sources are soon exhausted and energy is obtained from hydrolysis of ATP (adenosine triphosphate) and CP (creatine phosphate) and the glycolysis of glycogen to lactate.

$$\text{ATP} \rightleftharpoons \text{ADP} + \text{P} + \text{energy}$$

Anaerobic:

$$\text{CP} \rightleftharpoons \text{C} + \text{P} + \text{energy}$$

Aerobic: food $+ O_2 \longrightarrow CO_2 + H_2O + \text{energy}$

Anaerobic: glycogen $\rightleftharpoons$ lactic acid $+$ energy

work

Under normal circumstances oxidative metabolism restarts and proceeds at the same time and ATP, CP and carbohydrate are reformed at high speed. The limiting factors are the rate at which oxygen can be supplied by the blood stream, and the rate at which the cytochrome system can use oxygen.

Breakdown of carbohydrate follows the same path in aerobic and anaerobic conditions.

In aerobic conditions the primary end product is pyruvic acid.

The pyruvic acid passes into the tricarboxylic acid cycle and is degraded to carbon dioxide, and H^+ ions are transferred to the cytochrome system. Fatty acids may also be utilised in the same way. About 90 per cent of the carbohydrates follow this route.

In anaerobic conditions lactic acid accumulates. In the intact mammal lactic acid is removed by the circulating blood and either oxidised or taken to the liver and reformed to glycogen. As lactic acid is not on the normal aerobic pathway it does not appear in the circulating blood unless the level of exercise exceeds the oxygen supply to the muscles or the ability of the cytochrome system to process oxygen is impaired.

For exercise of a longer duration oxygen must be supplied and carbon dioxide removed by the circulatory blood so that the continued oxidation of carbohydrates and fatty acids occurs. Protein is not directly broken down and there is no increase in the excretion of nitrogen products during exercise.

When exercise begins oxygen consumption rises rapidly but not immediately. It continues at a raised level when exercise is over.

During very strenuous exercise of a short duration like a 100 yards sprint only a minute proportion of the work performed is accounted for by the current oxygen uptake. The level of exercise that can be maintained for more than five minutes is dependent on the maximum rate at which oxygen can be taken in. In a fully trained athlete this may be 5 litres/min.

The extra oxygen consumed after exercise, the oxygen debt, is to repay the muscles which became hypoxic in the initial stages.

At sea level in man exercising at a steady state no appreciable quantity of lactic acid is produced unless the energy requirement for oxygen is greater than can be met by oxygen intake. Under hypoxic conditions, the maximum oxygen intake falls, and lactic acid formation takes place at a correspondingly lower level of work (Piiper *et al.* 1966).

In all conditions therefore lactic acid production only reaches appreciable levels when the work load increases above maximum oxygen intake.

However blood lactic acid levels have been observed to increase during submaximal work. Essentially the level increases during the initial stage of work, but ceases to increase and usually falls once oxygen consumption has become adequate and the subject performs a steady rate of work (Saiki *et al.* 1967).

During submaximal work at sea level it is therefore well established that there is an increased production of lactic acid. This is possibly due to a delay in adequate oxygen delivery at the onset of work.

After physical training there is a lowering of blood lactate concentration at the same submaximal work load. This difference is more marked when comparing non-athletes with athletes.

The intracellular concentration of pyruvate may influence production of lactic acid (Huckabee 1958) and further it has been shown that regardless of sufficient oxygen supply there is an increased lactate concentration in the venous blood draining the muscle when the mean capillary Po_2 is below 50 mmHg (Carlsson and Pernow 1961).

Intermittent exercise, with work periods of ten seconds, are associated with lower perceived grades of exertion than when work periods were longer, i.e. 30–120 seconds.

However, oxygen uptake, ventilation, heart rate and blood lactate are all significantly higher for intermittent exercise than for continuous exercise with the same average power output (Edwards *et al.* 1972(b)).

Oxygen Uptake at High Altitude

At rest the body needs about 250 ml of oxygen each minute, and even at very great altitude, the oxygen transport system is adequate to provide this amount.

On the first ascent of Mt Everest 29,002 ft (8888 m) Hillary removed his oxygen mask for about ten minutes, before symptoms occurred. On the second ascent, Swiss mountaineers remained on the summit intermittently without oxygen for about two hours.

Four Americans have bivouacked without oxygen at 28,500 ft (8680 m) for about six hours, and two British mountaineers spent three nights without oxygen at 27,400 ft (8280 m) in 1933.

A temporarily acclimatised visitor was kept for thirty minutes at 30,000 ft (9120 m) simulated altitude. His resting ventilation (BTPS) averaged 47 litre/min (five times the basal level). The Palv.o_2 levelled off at 31 mmHg and Palv.co_2 at 11 mmHg. He remained fully conscious. A further lowering to 33,000 ft (10,030 m) brought the Palv.o_2 to 24 mmHg and Palv.co_2 to 10 mmHg. No hypocapnoeic symptoms nor cerebral vasoconstriction occurred.

A high-altitude native at 32,000 ft (9730 m) simulated altitude, only needed to breath at three times the normal resting level to keep the PAlv.O_2 above the critical level of 22 mmHg. A high-altitude visitor on the other hand had to ventilate at eight times the resting level to keep PAlv.O_2 above a critical level of 28 mmHg. (His PAlv.CO_2 was 10 mmHg.) This suggests considerable adaptation (Balke 1972).

At lower levels, it is only during muscular exercise that the whole oxygen transport system is fully extended and its limitation reached.

Oxygen uptake is related directly to work rate at all altitudes, and is independent of altitude. In other words, at whatever altitude, a certain rate of work demands a certain oxygen uptake. This appears to be true in both high-altitude natives and high-altitude visitors.

However in trained athletes, middle distance runners, at 7450 ft (2270 m) though maximum oxygen uptake was persistently reduced, work rate exceeded sea-level values due to increased overall efficiency (Pugh 1964).

The maximal oxygen uptake falls progressively from sea level upwards.

Table 20.   Oxygen uptake and altitude (Pugh *et al.* 1964)

| Altitude | | Max. oxygen uptake |
ft	m	litres/min
Sea level		3·5–4·0
15,000	4572	2·5–2·7
19,000	5791	2·0–2·5
21,000	6401	1·85–1·90
24,500	7465	1·3–1·5

If one considers those figures in graphic form, plotting oxygen uptake at maximal and normal climbing rate in ml/kg/min against altitude, it can be seen that as the 25,000 ft (7620 m) level is approached, so maximal oxygen uptake and normal climbing rate tend to coincide—or to maintain a normal climbing rate (2–3 litres of oxygen/min) maximal work has to be performed.

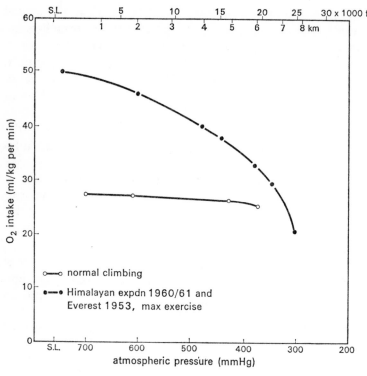

Fig. 19   Maximum oxygen intake at various altitudes and oxygen intake of men walking uphill at their habitual pace (Pugh 1965).

Up to about 20,000 ft (6100 m), after adequate acclimatisation it is possible to proceed at a normal Alpine climbing pace—a fact noted by many pre-war Everest mountaineers. It is also possible to exert oneself to the almost Alpine levels necessary to accomplish the physically difficult routes that are now being completed at higher altitudes.

Working nearer to their maximum capacity however mountaineers are unable to continue for as long at 20,000 ft (6100 m) and above as at lower altitudes. The number of hours a day spent climbing tends to decrease and whereas an individual may be capable of spending 10–14 hours a day for many days on end in the European Alps (10–15,000 ft) (3050–4500 m), at 21,000 ft

(6400 m) he will only be able to climb for say five to eight hours a day over a long period.

Above 25,000 ft (7620 m) it is not possible to climb continuously without oxygen at a normal climbing rate, because the oxygen uptake necessary for this is higher than the maximum. As a result climbing becomes intermittent, with periodic rests, rather than continuous. Anaerobic working occurs during climbing and the oxygen debt is repaid whilst at rest. At 27,000 ft (8230 m) and above Somervell describes how when climbing without oxygen he had to take seven to ten complete respirations for each step. Even so he had to rest for a minute or more every twenty yards. In one hour he and his companion had ascended only 80 feet over relatively easy ground.

With acclimatisation there appears to be a smaller fall in maximum oxygen uptake with increasing altitude.

In unacclimatised man the maximum Vo_2 is reduced by about 3 per cent for every 1000 ft (300 m) of altitude, whereas in the better acclimatised the decrease was 2 per cent.

According to some, the reduction in maximum oxygen uptake improves with increased stay at altitude; others find no improvement.

On return to sea level an increased maximum Vo_2 has been reported by some workers after long residence at altitude.

During maximum work at altitude, aching in the respiratory muscles occurs, which may be due to build up of lactate.

The reasons given for stopping maximum work are tabulated below. At extreme altitude overwhelming shortness of breath is the principal factor in halting exercise, probably due to the high oxygen cost of ventilation.

Table 21. Reasons for stopping maximum work (Consolazio *et al.* 1966)

Reasons	5500 ft 1600 m %	11,500 ft 3475 m %	14,100 ft 4300 m %
Legs gave out	72	52	38
General fatigue	14	20 ⎫	21
Cramps	7	6 ⎭	
Breathlessness	7	22	41

The working capacity of the high-altitude visitor is limited by dyspnoea, whereas the high-altitude native can work equally hard without dyspnoea due to his blunted ventilatory response (Lahiri *et al.* 1972).

Sea-level studies have demonstrated that intermittent working enables men to work for an hour or more with an oxygen uptake that would cause exhaustion after ten minutes if carried out continuously (Astrand *et al.* 1960). However intermittent work has been reported to lead to higher lactic acid formation and a higher maximum oxygen uptake for given work, than continuous exercise (Edwards *et al.* 1972(b)).

Sherpa porters, who can carry loads exceeding half their body weight up to and above 21,000 ft (6400 m) use the intermittent method even at low altitudes. As height increases, the periods of work become shorter but the rate of work (i.e. the speed at which they climb) seems to remain remarkably high.

Sea-level visitors tend to climb at a steady slow pace with fewer rests. It is noticeable that the intermittent method seems remarkably efficient and relatively less fatiguing for the high-altitude native, and also for the high-altitude visitor when carrying loads approximating to his own body weight.

Ventilation and Cardiovascular System

During muscular work at altitude, ventilation (BTPS) increases progressively with the altitude and the amount of work.

Not only does the minute volume increase with altitude, but also the change in ventilation rate for a given increase in work. At extreme altitude the rate of ventilation is extremely high and any increase in work rate, whether due to steeper ground, or change from hard to soft snow, results in an increase in respiration and may well cause excessive panting and halt the mountaineer.

In high-altitude visitors maximum ventilation during work is higher than at sea level, but no significant difference between values at 15,000 and 21,000 ft (4572 and 6400 m) was noted. At 24,000 ft (7315 m) maximum ventilation seemed to be impaired, but for climatic reasons a maximum rate was maintained for five minutes only (Pugh *et al.* 1964).

At 19,000 ft (5791 m) and over, maximum ventilation reached values of more than 200 litre/min. These extreme rates resulted in alveolar P_{CO_2} reaching very low levels, and pH levels were as high as 7·55.

At 19,000 ft (5791 m) the diffusing capacity of the lung in high-altitude visitors is similar to or slightly lower than that at sea level.

As it is possible to maintain remarkably high levels of exercise at this altitude, the body must be willing to accept a considerable degree of arterial hypoxaemia during heavy work.

At rest at 19,000 ft (5791 m) the mean arterial oxygen saturation is 67 per cent, during moderate exercise it is 56 per cent and in severe exercise it is 50 per cent.

As exercise levels increase alveolar P_{O_2} rises, because alveolar ventilation rises faster than oxygen consumption, but arterial oxygen saturation falls. This suggests that diffusion becomes a factor limiting exercise.

At an alveolar P_{O_2} of 50 mmHg (equivalent to 19 000 ft (5791 m)) and with a reasonable diffusing capacity (say 60 ml/mmHg) the arterial oxygen saturation will be maintained up to an oxygen consumption of 1–2 litres/min. If this work level is exceeded the arterial saturation falls unless the diffusing capacity is increased.

The main limiting factors of exercise at high altitude seem to be both diffusing capacity and cardiac output and of these the diffusing capacity appears to be the more important.

Effect of Age

In 1953, a man of 44 was found to have maximum ventilation and maximum oxygen intake at sea level and at 20,000 ft (6100 m) similar to that of a man twenty years younger. By 1961 at age 51 there was a fall in all values.

Table 22.   Effect of age on respiratory performance (Pugh *et al.* 1964)

Age	Max. oxygen intake, litres/min		Max. ventilation litres/min (BTPS)
	Sea level	20,000 ft (6100 m)	
44	3·88	2·09	137
51	3·43	1·68	110

The maximum oxygen uptake declines with age, both at sea level and at high altitude. Inevitably there is considerable individual variation.

In general, responses in older individuals were similar to those of younger subjects, namely, an initial decrease in maximum oxygen uptake followed by a progressive increase with stay at altitude. However, adaptation is slower (Dill *et al.* 1964).

Effect of Oxygen

In high-altitude visitors whilst living at altitude, oxygen at sea-level pressures resulted in a fall of ventilation (BTPS) for a given work rate. At higher work rates the reduction was greater. At 19,000 ft (5791 m) the heart rate also fell to sea-level values for given work. The maximum heart rate increased to the maximum value observed during exercise at sea level. The stroke volume and the maximum cardiac output therefore increased, though probably not to sea-level values because of the increased viscosity of the blood.

The alveolar Po_2 was raised and the blood pH decreased (Pugh *et al.* 1964).

In high-altitude natives (Sherpas), whilst living at altitude, oxygen at sea-level pressures made little difference to pulmonary ventilation, and therefore little difference to alveolar Pco_2 and blood pH.

The heart rate, at all levels of work from moderate to maximum, was decreased (Lahiri and Milledge 1966).

Lactic Acid Production

When submaximal work is carried out after acute exposure to altitude up to 13,000 ft (4000 m) the blood lactate is progressively increased. At lower work loads the blood pH remained unchanged, but at 8000 ft (2300 m) it started to fall with a work load equivalent to 3·0 litres/min and at 13,000 ft (4000 m) with a work load equivalent to 2·5 litres/min. Acute hypoxia then does not seem to impair the mechanism for the formation of lactic acid during severe exercise, and an increase in blood lactate is found (Hermansen and Saltin 1967).

With chronic hypoxia however a reduced formation of lactate occurs during severe exercise (Edwards 1936) and this is not influenced by giving oxygen. The higher the altitude, the smaller the increase in blood lactate after exhausting exercise. Essentially if excessive lactate production occurred the blood pH would fall below pH 7·0, which is incompatible with life.

It appears then that the blood pH is a limiting factor in lactic acid production, and possibly a feedback mechanism operates with a lethal acidosis being avoided by blocking part of the pathway for glycolysis (Cerretelli 1967).

In high-altitude natives the accumulation of blood lactate during exercise is in general lower than in sea-level controls and the differences become larger as work load increases. Not only does the individual at sea level accumulate more lactic acid during exercise than the high-altitude native, but its rate of disappearance is slower.

In high-altitude visitors after submaximal exercise, lactic acid production also appears to be greater than in the high-altitude native (Lahiri and Milledge 1966).

At sea level, if a given quantity of work has to be carried out in a set time, a lower rise in blood lactate concentration occurs if the work is performed at a continuous low rate than if performed intermittently with a higher work load (Edwards *et al.* 1971).

Distribution of Blood

During exercise on a bicycle ergometer at a simulated altitude of 13,100 ft (4000 m) the arterial Po_2 fell to 40 mmHg. Although the blood flow to the femoral region increased, it remained in about the same proportion to the increase in cardiac output. There was no indication therefore that the distribution of blood flow was altered by this degree of hypoxia (Hartley *et al.* 1973).

At high altitude there is a relative reduction in cutaneous circulation at rest and during exercise, and this reduction is probably responsible for skin cooling. Despite this, there is the same flow of heat from the core to the skin because the difference in temperature between core and skin is larger (Varene *et al.* 1973).

Physical Efficiency

Oxygen consumption during a steady state of exercise does not vary whether the exercise is at high altitude or at sea level. However, the total amount of oxygen used during exercise and recovery from exercise appears to be greater at high altitude than at sea level. This is due to the higher oxygen cost of ventilation.

Calculations of mechanical efficiency in subjects at high altitude for twelve days have shown that in the young to middle aged there was a decrease in efficiency. In an older group (51–77 years) there was no change, possibly due to a training effect. On return to sea level all had improved their efficiency over control values (Horvath 1972).

Whilst it is well recognised that both acute and chronic hypoxia result in a diminution of the performance of exercise, high-altitude natives have greater endurance, higher aerobic capacity, higher maximal and submaximal heart rate, lower ventilation and greater mechanical efficiency than sea-level visitors at high altitudes.

High-altitude visitors have to spend many years in residence before they reach the same capacity for work, if in fact it is ever possible for them to do so.

As far as muscular work is concerned the sea-level visitor appears from clinical observation to acclimatise best at altitudes between 12,000 and 16,000 ft (3658 and 4877 m) where a high exercise performance can be carried out without profound exhaustion. Above 17,500 ft (5334 m) this becomes progressively less possible.

References

Astrand, I., Astrand, P. O., Christiansen, E. H. and Hedman, R. (1960) *Acta physiologica scandinavica* **48**, 448.

Balke, B. (1972) Physiology of respiration at altitude. In, *Physiological adaptation. Desert and mountain. Ed.* Yousef, M. K., Horvath, S. M. and Bullard, R. W. Academic Press: New York and London.

Carlson, L. A. and Pernow, B. (1961) *Acta physiologica scandinavica* **52**, 328.

Cerretelli, P. (1967) Lactacid oxygen debt in acute and chronic hypoxia. In, *Exercise at altitude. Ed.* Margaria, R. Excerpta Medica Foundation: Amsterdam.

Consolazio, C. F., Matoush, L. O. and Nelson, P. A. (1966) *Federation Proceedings. Federation of American Societies for Experimental Biology* **25**, 1380.

Dill, D. B., Forbes, W. H., Newton, J. L. and Terman, J. W. (1964) Respiratory adaptation to altitude as related to age. In, *Relations of development and ageing. Ed.* Birren, J. E. Thomas: Springfield, Illinois.

Edwards, P. H. T., Melcher, A., Hesser, C. M. and Wigeritz, O. (1971) In, *Muscle metabolism during exercise. Ed.* Pernow, B., Saltin, B. Plenum Press.

Edwards, H. T. (1936) *American Journal of Physiology* **116**, 367.

Edwards, R. H. T., Denison, D. M., Jones, G., Davies, C. T. M. and Campbell, E. J. M. (1972(a)) *Journal of Applied Physiology* **32**, 165.

Edwards, R. H. T., Melcher, A., Hesser, C. M., Wigertz, O. and Ekelund, L. G. (1972(b)) *European Journal of Clinical Investigation* **2**, 108.

Hartley, L. H., Vogel, J. A. and Landowne, M. (1973) *Journal of Applied Physiology* **34**, 87.

Hermansen, L. and Saltin, B. (1967) Blood lactate concentration during exercise at acute exposure to altitude. In, *Exercise at altitude. Ed.* Margaria, R. Excerpta Medica Foundation: Amsterdam.

Horvath, S. M. (1972) Physiology of work at altitude. In, *Physiological adaptation. Desert and mountain. Ed.* Yousef, M.K., Horvath, M. and Bullard, R.W. Academic Press: New York and London.

Huckabee, W. E. (1958) *Journal of Clinical Investigation* **37**, 255.

Lahiri, S. and Milledge, J. S. (1966) *Federation Proceedings. Federation of American Societies for Experimental Biology* **25**, 1392.

Lahiri, S., Milledge, J. S. and Sorensen, S. C. (1972) *Journal of Applied Physiology* **32**, 766.

Piiper, J., Cerretelli, P., Cuttica, F. and Mangili, F. (1966) *Journal of Applied Physiology* **21**, 1143.

Pugh, L. G. C. E., Gill, M. B., Lahiri, S., Milledge, J. S., Ward, M. P. and West, J. B. (1964) *Journal of Applied Physiology* **19**, 431.

Pugh, L. G. C. E. (1964) *Journal of Physiology* **192**, 619.

Pugh, L. G. C. E. (1965) High altitude. In, *Physiology of human survival. Ed.* Edholm, O. and Bacharach, A. L. Academic Press: New York and London.

Saiki, M., Margaria, R. and Cuttica, F. (1967) Lactic acid production in sub-maximal muscular exercise. In, *Exercise at altitude. Ed.* Margaria, R. Excerpta Medica Foundation: Amsterdam.

Varene, P., Jacquemin, C., Durand, J. and Raynaud, J. (1973) *Journal of Applied Physiology* **34**, 633.

CHAPTER FOURTEEN

Temperature Regulation

Every living organism produces heat and this heat is either lost to the environment or stored in the body. If the heat content of the body increases, the body temperature rises and as a result the transfer of heat to the environment is increased. Thus any animal tends to reach a steady state of heat exchange with the environment.

Normal temperature implies the temperature of the body core expected in a healthy individual who is not currently nor has recently been subjected to any thermal stress.

Normal rectal temperature is commonly taken as 37·0°C (98·6°F) and oral temperature as 36·7°C (98·1°F) but the liver may be 1–2°C higher than the rectal temperature. Variations of 0·5°C from a mean temperature can be expected in healthy individuals under controlled circumstances.

Much larger normal deviation may occur; and diurnal and other fluctuations associated with ovulation may be 1°C or more.

Heat Exchange

The avenues of heat exchange available between body and environment are convection, radiation, conduction and evaporation.

Convection

This is the transfer of heat by bulk movement, either of heated fluids rising, or of cooled fluids falling.

Heat loss by convection depends on the existence of a temperature gradient between the body surface and the ambient air. If the body surface and air are the same temperature (i.e. no temperature gradient) there is no heat transfer by convection. If the air is warmer, then the body gains heat by convection.

The rate of heat exchange by convection depends upon the amount of exposed surface area of the body.

Posture

The exposed surface area of the body is almost always less than the total surface area of the body, as some regions such as the axilla, perineum and inner surface of the thighs do not contribute to exchange by convection. It also depends on posture. Curling up tends to reduce this area, and thus conserve body heat, while extending the legs and arms and separating them tends to increase the exposed area.

Heat loss from a warm surface to air occurs when the air is brought into contact with the surface either by forced air currents (e.g. wind) or air currents due to thermal gradient. The air takes up the heat from the surface and carries it away.

Wind

An important influence on the rate of heat exchange by convection is the rate at which convective air currents bring air to the body surface, and this is especially important in windy conditions. Heat loss by convection is much increased by air movement (wind) and it is probably the major avenue of heat loss in mountain country.

The insulating value of clothes depends entirely on the trapped still air. Still air is an efficient insulator but as soon as it is allowed to circulate the heat given to it by the body is lost.

Convection Currents

Trapped still air that is warmed tends to rise, then cool and descend, setting up convection currents. This effect produces the feeling of a draught on the neck as warmed air rises and leaves the body around the collar and descends again.

Bellows Effect

These currents are minimised by stopping the areas where warm air can escape, e.g. the neck. The 'bellows' effect by which air is displaced by body action is also reduced by the close fit of garments.

Despite the use of 'wind proof' outer clothing some wind penetration does occur and increases heat loss considerably.

Radiation

The other main method of heat loss from a warm surface is by radiation. This is the emission of discrete packets of electro-magnetic energy, photons, from a warm surface and would take place even if the air was replaced by a vacuum. Radiation penetrates for long distances in air but is eventually absorbed by the air with a resulting rise in air temperature. Heat loss or gain by radiation is independent of air movement (wind).

The average energy of the photons and their rate of emission increase as the temperature of the body surface is raised. Dense objects in the environment also emit photons some of which are absorbed by the surface of the body. The greatest source of radiation is the sun. In the clear air of the polar regions, or on high mountains with snow forming a reflector the radiation effect is enhanced. The overcast sky in certain other regions diminishes this effect. At night the earth loses heat by radiation to the black sky, clear nights being colder than nights when cloud cover acts as a blanket. The heat received by the body in full sunshine can amount to two or three times that generated by the normal metabolic processes.

Solar heat is absorbed on the surface of the clothing, and the amount absorbed depends on (a) the posture of the individual— i.e. the cross-sectional area presented by the body normally to the rays of the sun, (b) the reflecting power for radiation of the surface of the clothing, (c) the absorption of radiation by moisture and dust in the air and clouds, (d) the scattered radiation from all directions and (e) the diffuse reflection from the ground.

Heat Gain from Solar Radiation in Polar Regions and at High Altitude

In a clear sky the average amount of solar radiation to which man is exposed at sea level amounts to about 230 kcal/m²/hr.

The gain in heat will vary with the degree of cloudiness (less with overcast sky) and clothing. Black clothing will absorb 88 per cent solar radiation, khaki 57 per cent and white 20 per cent, the remainder being reflected.

For khaki clothing in a clear sky the amount of solar radiation absorbed will be of the order of 130 kcal/m²/hr or the equivalent to the heat output of a man during moderate exercise.

Because of the clear air, the intensity of solar radiation in Antarctica reaches levels which, in temperate latitudes, are found only at high altitude.

Table 23.   Solar heat gain (approximate) in Antarctica (coastal plain)

Solar altitude	Heat gain kcal/m²/hour		Total
	Direct	Reflected	
Clear sky			
0	80	0	80
10°	150	50	200
20°	150	100	250
30°	150	150	300
40°	150	200	350
Overcast sky			
0			0
10°			50
20°			100
30°			200
40°			250

At high altitude and in Polar areas the high albedo (reflectivity of solar radiation) of snow due to its whiteness is an important factor. This may vary from 75 to 90 per cent. In ground not under snow, the albedo does not usually exceed 25 per cent.

In Antarctica at the height of summer, the heat gain from the sun may be two to four times greater than in desert. Because of the high albedo this gain continues to rise with the increase in the altitude of the sun in the sky. In the desert the gain remains constant at a solar altitude of 30°.

On the Polar plateau, 7000–9000 ft (2134–2743 m), where conditions are more favourable, the heat gain would be higher.

At high altitudes, levels of heat gain from solar radiation are comparable with sea level in Antarctica.

At 19,000 ft (5791 m) in January when the solar altitude was about 40° in clear weather the solar heat gain to the surface of a clothed human body has been estimated to be about 350 kcal/m²/hour (Chrenko and Pugh 1961; Pugh 1963).

Conduction

This is heat transfer by direct contact.

It is the power to transport heat from one molecule to another by their collision, in which kinetic energy is exchanged. The temperature of a gas is the measure of this energy. Although in general heat exchange by air conduction is of little importance, under certain circumstances it does play a considerable part.

As water is a good conductor of heat, if clothes are wet, the result of external wetting by rain or internal wetting by sweat, they will lose much of their insulating value. It follows that loss of heat by conduction can be controlled by keeping clothes dry.

Drinking hot water will transfer heat to the body—as will a hot bath.

Contact between good conductors such as metals and the bare hand or snow and the gluteal region causes heat loss. Therefore if an accident occurs or a bivouac is necessary, direct contact with the snow should if possible be avoided.

Evaporation

This is heat transfer resulting from the energy required to change a liquid to a vapour. The thermal energy required when this process occurs at a constant temperature is called the latent heat of vaporisation.

Of the total heat loss in man, about 20 per cent is by the evaporation of moisture from the skin and respiratory tract.

In normal physiological ranges of temperature the latent heat of water is 580 kcal/litre of liquid vaporised. This large amount of heat necessary for the evaporation of water can be an important factor in heat exchange.

As the epidermis is only slightly permeable to water the rate of loss by passive diffusion through the skin is small.

Expired air, even at high ventilation rates is almost completely saturated with water. The water comes from the mucous cells lining the upper respiratory tract, and the heat loss at normal ventilation is about 200 kcal/day. At higher ventilation rates it is more.

The heat is supplied by the blood and very little heat loss occurs under normal circumstances when the respiratory tract temperature is near to that of arterial blood.

Practically all the evaporation from the respiratory tract occurs from the upper-respiratory tract and not from the lungs. Thus at high altitude the increased respiration of cold dry air should theoretically dry the naso-pharynx. In fact this has occurred—and so severe has this drying been in one man that the mucosa sloughed, nearly causing suffocation. It may also be the cause of the constant 'dry' cough which is so irritating a feature of high altitudes.

The total heat loss in a normal environment by passive skin diffusion and from expired air accounts for about 15–20 per cent of the total.

In twenty-four hours at sea level, about one third (300 ml of water) 174 kcal is lost from the respiratory tract and two thirds (600 ml) 348 kcal from the skin, making 900 ml, 522 kcal in all.

Perspiration
This is an active thermoregulatory mechanism involving the extrusion of water from the sweat glands. Relatively large

amounts of fluid may be lost by sweating, and on severe exercise or in a hot environment over a litre of sweat may be lost in an hour.

The quantity lost depends on the rate of fluid secretion and the capacity of the environment to remove water vapour.

If the ambient air is dry and windy the heat loss by evaporation is limited only by the rate of secretion of sweat.

If the ambient air is moist and stagnant the evaporative heat loss is limited by the ability of the ambient air to remove water from the skin.

Muscular exercise brings about sweating even in very cold conditions, and sweating due to overheating may result in water recondensing on outer clothing, which may then freeze. It can then evaporate again causing heat loss from the body.

About 500 times as much heat is required to evaporate a given quantity of water without raising its temperature, as is required to raise its temperature by 1°C.

Thus increased sweating results in both water loss and heat loss.

If clothes are wet, in order to evaporate the water (i.e. to dry the clothes) a very large amount of heat is required. Thus heat loss from wet clothes can be a serious factor for survival in a cold–wet situation. These facts emphasise the importance of keeping clothes as dry as possible at all times.

Mechanism of Temperature Regulation

The temperature of the body is regulated almost entirely by a nervous feedback mechanism, and this operates through the temperature-regulating centre in the hypothalamus. For this mechanism to function temperature detectors (receptors) must exist which determine whether the body temperature becomes too hot or too cold.

Receptors sensitive to temperature are located as follows

    (i) In the pre-optic area of the anterior hypothalamus, where many special heat sensitive neurones are found.

(ii) Cold sensitive neurones are found in different parts of the hypothalamus and the reticular substance of the mid-brain.

(iii) Peripheral temperature receptors—including both 'heat and cold receptors' are found in the skin. These transmit nerve impulses to the spinal cord and thence to the hypothalamus.

(iv) Deep temperature receptors are thought to exist in some internal organs.

A thermostatic centre is situated in the pre-optic and adjacent regions of the hypothalamus. This controls body temperature by altering the rate of heat production and the rate of heat loss.

The hypothalamic centres seem essential for effective temperature control in man as observations have shown that an anencephalic infant, without a hypothalamus and with a disorganised mid-brain, could not maintain its body temperature or increase oxygen consumption in the cold (Cross *et al.* 1966).

In patients too with high spinal lesions cooling of one limb can cause vasoconstriction in the other, but these spinal reflexes are insufficient to maintain body temperature except under the mildest conditions (Guttman *et al.* 1958).

The cold receptors of the skin increase their rate of discharge when cooled, but extreme cooling causes this rate to decline. The maximal discharge rate occurs in facial skin at about 27°C.

Warm receptors are less frequently found. It is likely therefore that the mechanism whereby heat is lost is brought into action largely by deep rather than skin temperature receptors.

Skin receptors play an important part in the response to cold. Sudden exposure to a cold wind can produce a burst of shivering within seconds and only a cutaneous reflex can account for this.

The stimulation of deep receptors produced little increase in oxygen consumption when the skin was cooled as well.

It appears therefore that although the stimulation of the skin receptors is necessary for any large metabolic response to cold, the degree of the response is greatly increased by stimulation of the deep receptors.

When the temperature of the thermostatic centre rises above

37°C the rate of heat loss is increased by stimulation of the sweat glands which causes loss of heat by evaporation and removing the vasoconstriction tone to the cutaneous blood vessels. This is done by inhibiting sympathetic centres in the hypothalamus. Vasodilatation occurs and heat loss, mainly by convection, results.

When the temperature falls below 37°C, conservation of heat occurs and heat production is increased.

Increased heat production is carried out by two mechanisms.

Stimulation of the motor centre for shivering, which is found in the hypothalamus, does not cause muscular shaking but increases skeletal muscle tone. This increases muscle metabolism and the rate of heat production may rise by as much as 50 per cent, even before shivering occurs. Once the tone rises above a critical level, shivering occurs. Heat production can then rise to two to four times the normal figure.

An increase in the rate of metabolism can occur as a result of circulatory noradrenaline or sympathetic stimulation. This is believed to be due to the ability of adrenaline and noradrenaline to increase oxidative phosphorylation and increased oxidation of food occurs to produce 'high-energy' compounds such as ATP.

Increased heat conservation occurs through three routes. Vasoconstriction of the skin vessels prevents heat transferred by blood vessels from the central core being lost except by conduction through the superficial layers.

Erection of hairs is unimportant in humans as there is little hair cover to the body, but in animals, erect hairs will entrap air—providing a good insulating layer.

Sweating is abolished by cooling the pre-optic area to below 37°C. This reduces heat loss by evaporation.

Heat Production

Food is the sole source of fuel for the production of heat.

When one litre of oxygen is inhaled the release of energy from each of the three main constituents of food is about the same—5 kcal.

(i) *At rest*. The expenditure of energy is at the basal rate of metabolism. In a 35 year old man, weight 75 kg and height 170 cm this is 1·2 kcal/min of which muscle produces about 20–30 per cent. Most of this is from the use of respiratory muscles. At rest most heat is produced centrally.

(ii) *On exercise*. The metabolic rate and the rate of heat production increases greatly—sometimes up to ten or more times the basal level.

Very high rates of heat production may be found, e.g. uphill skiing, 18·6 kcal/min or long distance swimming, 11·4 kcal/min.

Average outdoor heat output under polar conditions, which probably involved walking on rocky ground, was 7·0 kcal/min. The energy cost of walking on snow at 4–5·0 km/hour or skiing was 9·0 kcal/min (Brotherhood 1972).

All heat that is not stored has to be removed. If this is not possible, efficiency will be impaired.

Of the total heat produced by exercise, 80 per cent is generated in peripheral muscles and being close to the skin the heat is removed easily.

Table 24. Heat production in 75 kg man at rest

	Heat production per cent	kcal/hr	Fraction of bodyweight per cent
Brain	18	13	2
Heart	11	8 ⎤	
Kidney	7	5 ⎬	6
Hepatic portal	20	14·5 ⎦	
Muscle	20	14·5 ⎤	
Skin	5	3·5 ⎦	52
Other	19	13·5	40
Total	100	72·0 (1·2 kcal/min)	100

All warm blooded animals have a *critical temperature*. This can be defined as the environmental temperature below which the metabolic rate, and therefore heat production increases. Man's critical temperature equals that of a tropical animal and is between 26 and 27°C in air, and 33°C in water.

Shivering

Man can maintain a rate of heat production at least three times the resting value by shivering.

Shivering is a coordinated movement of voluntary skeletal muscle under involuntary nervous control. It can proceed without the cerebral cortex being present but after transection of the spinal cord is absent in those muscles innervated below the lesion.

Both flexors and extensors are stimulated, and the heat produced is all gained by the body as no external work is carried out.

Below 25°C the nude body at rest begins to lose more heat than it produces. This results in a rise in heat production due to increase in muscle tone which proceeds to shivering.

Increase in oxygen consumption in the cold can be abolished by voluntary relaxation of muscle, as well as by paralysis due to *d*-tubocurarine. Clinical observation suggests that shivering can also be diminished by the oxygen lack of high altitude.

This has also been observed in experimental animals and man under laboratory conditions and suggests that heat production might be inhibited and heat loss increased under hypoxic conditions.

Non-Shivering Thermogenesis

There is evidence that rodents possess a non-muscular mechanism for producing heat in cold conditions.

Cold-acclimatised rats whose muscles were paralysed by curare could increase their oxygen consumption in the cold, whilst animals acclimatised to warm conditions were unable to do so. It has been suggested that brown-fat found in rats and marmots was the site of this heat production. Many new-born animals are capable of non-muscular heat production without being acclimatised to cold.

This form of thermogenesis is under the control of noradrenaline released from sympathetic nerves. Fatty acids are oxidised locally but the glycerol of the fat is not, and appears in the blood. As this must be metabolised somewhere it may be responsible for the small increase in heat production reported in the liver and skeletal muscle of rats. Non-shivering thermogenesis is not an important means of increasing heat production in man, although there is some evidence that it exists in a rudimentary form. Following acclimatisation to cold man may possess some capacity for thermogenesis from brown-fat but it is small compared to that of small rodents and compared to his capacity for heat production from shivering.

The reliance in man on shivering as a method for increasing heat production frees him from the burden of carrying a seldom used specialised 'organ' such as brown-fat.

Shivering is also associated with heat *loss*, for by increasing blood flow, tissue insulation is decreased. However, shivering takes place mainly in muscles situated in the proximal parts of the limbs, and the trunk. These are covered by a relatively thick layer of fat and the heat loss is minimised.

Metabolic Rate

Thyroid hormones increase basal heat production in mammals. Recent evidence suggests however that the heat production of the body is not varied to any great extent in response to changes in the environment.

Exposure to cold does however increase the rate of release of thyroid-stimulating hormone and the uptake of ^{131}I and the output of thyroid hormones by the thyroid gland. However an increase in thyroid activity does not seem to be accompanied by any great increase in circulatory level of the thyroid hormones.

During prolonged exposure to cold most studies of basal metabolic rate are against an increase in level of active thyroid hormone in the circulation.

After observations on the most intense and prolonged exposure to cold found to be tolerable to European volunteers living for months in the Canadian Arctic and wearing light clothing, and on another group exposed for $7\frac{1}{2}$ hours a day for 19 days to air at 5–7°C, wearing shorts and footwear, no evidence of any increase in metabolic rate was noted.

However reports of an increase in metabolic rate was found in indigenous people living in Korea and Japan, and in Eskimos, during the winter. The serum PBI of the Eskimos and Japanese was reported to be higher in winter than summer. Doubt has been cast on the raised basal metabolic rate in Eskimos as it is considered that this could be due to a high protein intake. Increase in basal metabolic rate was always small compared to the increase in heat production by shivering.

High-altitude residents in Central Asia (Sherpas) and South America appear to have a small increase (21 per cent) in basal metabolic rate.

High-altitude visitors who have spent a long period (three months) at 19,000 ft (5791 m) also had an increase though this was a smaller percentage (10 per cent).

Because of the association of cold stress, and other factors, measurements of basal oxygen consumption at altitude give varied results.

Fat
Fat men increase heat production less than thin men on prolonged exposure to cold, so the rate of heat loss depends on subcutaneous fat.

An unusually thick layer of subcutaneous fat has been found in cross-channel swimmers who spend long periods in cold water. Subcutaneous fat was by far the most important factor in determining the degree of fall in body temperature in these people.

Obesity is rare in indigenous people in cold climate, such as Eskimos or mountain dwellers. Presumably therefore fat is used as a method of storing food, rather than for insulation.

Old Age
Some impairment of the central thermoregulatory mechanism

has been demonstrated in old age. Gross defects are rare but lesser degrees may be common.

In a recent survey (Fox *et al.* 1973) of elderly people the deep body temperature seemed to be 'set' at a lower level than in younger individuals. A decrease in hand temperature with age seemed to show that efforts were being made to conserve body heat.

It was found that when subjects who had already suffered one episode of spontaneous hypothermia were exposed to cold air, they suffered larger falls of rectal temperature with smaller increases in metabolic rate than control subjects of the same age.

Lack of subcutaneous fat may play a part in the abnormally large falls in rectal temperature and increases in oxygen consumption that occurred when individuals between the ages of 57 and 91 were exposed to cold.

These facts may help to explain why elderly people feel the cold more easily and do not survive as well when exposed to hypothermic conditions, for instance, to shipwreck.

Alcohol

In moderate doses alcohol causes peripheral vasodilatation in cold air.

However in moderate amounts it seems to have surprisingly little effect on heat loss in cold water. After drinking 75 ml of absolute alcohol in 200 ml of water ten naval ratings maintained higher blood flows during 30 minutes immersion in water at 15°C than did controls without alcohol, but the effect of the alcohol was considered to be trivial in comparison with the effect of fat thickness in each subject.

References

Brotherhood, J. R. (1972) *Study of the energy expenditure in the Antarctic.* Symposium of Human Biology and Medicine in the Antarctic. Scott Polar Research Institute: Cambridge.

Chrenko, F. A. and Pugh, L. G. C. E. (1961) *Proceedings of the Royal Society. Series B.* **154**, 243.

Cross, K. W., Gustavson, J., Hull, J. R. and Robinson, D. C. (1966) *Clinical Science* **31**, 449.

Fox, R. H., Woodward, P. M., Exton-Smith, A. N., Green, M. F., Donnison, D. V. and Wicks, M. H. (1973) *British Medical Journal* **1**, 200.

Guttman, L., Silver, J. and Wyndham, C. H. (1958) *Journal o Physiology* **142**, 406.

Pugh, L. G. C. E. (1963) *Journal of Applied Physiology* **18**, 1234.

CHAPTER FIFTEEN

Insulation

The clo is the practical unit of thermal insulation introduced in 1941 for describing heat exchange in man. 1 clo of thermal insulation will maintain a resting, sitting man, whose metabolic rate is 50 kcal/m²/hour comfortable indefinitely in an environment of 21°C (70°F), relative humidity less than 50 per cent and air movement 20 ft/min (10 cm/sec) (Burton and Edholm 1955).

It is equivalent to the insulation afforded by ordinary business clothing and underwear for a sedentary worker in comfortable indoor surroundings.

Insulating Value of Tissue, Air and Clothes

The relative importance of the insulating value of the tissues, clothing and the air can be inferred from the following figures. Tissues (I_T), 0·15–0·8 clo; Clothes (I_C), 0–5·0 clo; and Air (I_A), 0·8–0·2 clo.

In extremely cold conditions when the total insulation needed is many clo the physiological control of tissue insulation over a range of 0·7 clo does not seem very important. However, on the face, when no mask is used, and on the hands, the surface factor is important and this control assumes greater significance. In addition practical considerations or emergency conditions may result in clothing being reduced to a minimum.

Where insulation is just enough to provide heat balance the value of I_T will alter the tolerance time from a long period if vasoconstriction is present to a shorter period if vasodilatation occurs. Vasoconstriction can reduce but not prevent a fall in body temperature. Only an increase in heat production can do this.

Tissue Insulation

Internal Temperature Distribution

The detailed pattern of temperature distribution in the tissues is complex but certain general characteristics are present. At rest, most of the metabolic heat is produced by the deeper organs, such as the heart, viscera and brain, which are in general warmer than the superficial tissues. For this heat to be lost these organs must be warmer than the perfusing blood or surrounding tissues.

A useful but oversimplified concept is to imagine the body as consisting of (a) a central core at a relatively uniform temperature of 37°C and (b) a surrounding insulating shell with a temperature of about 33°C.

The central core consists of those tissues perfused with blood with a temperature within a few tenths of a degree of rectal temperature. Thus the core consists of almost the whole body when cutaneous vasodilatation is maximal. The shell in this instance provides only the superficial part of the epidermis.

In cold conditions, when heat is to be conserved, peripheral vasoconstriction occurs and reduces the circulation to the peripheral tissue; the thickness of the 'shell' increases and the 'central core' becomes smaller. The heat transfer to the skin surface is reduced and because the surface temperature is less, heat loss from the skin surface to the environment is also lowered. In extreme cold therefore the temperature of the central organs is maintained at the expense of the more peripheral tissues, especially in the extremities.

The skin temperature varies with ambient temperature, clothing and site.

The head is the warmest part, due presumably to its excellent blood supply, followed by the trunk, hands and feet.

Thus the thermal gradient from the head to the ambient air is the steepest and in cold conditions unless there is adequate protection more heat is lost from the head than elsewhere.

The fingers have a larger surface, per unit volume, than the arms, and the arms have more surface relative to their volume than the trunk. This is because the surface to volume ratio of a cylindrical object is inversely proportional to its diameter.

Large surface area is an advantage in losing heat to the environment but a disadvantage when heat has to be conserved in cold conditions.

Despite complete cutaneous vasoconstriction, the insulation of the tissues surrounding the central larger vessels of the limbs is not sufficient to prevent cooling of blood. However counter-current heat exchange permits the development of large longitudinal temperature gradients along the vessels and limbs. The result is that the entire distal portion of the extremity becomes part of the shell, and under extremely cold conditions the fingers, toes and distal parts of the hands and feet may be severely cooled. This preserves those organs of the 'central core' which are essential to life at a constant temperature at the expense of the 'peripheral' expendable structures.

Heat Transfer Within the Body

Heat lost to the environment is transferred from the site of production to the body surface or the epithelium lining of the airways by a combination of conduction, and convection by the circulation.

Conduction

Heat tends to flow down a temperature gradient by transfer of thermal energy between adjacent atoms. This process, conduction, results in heat transfer through material, in contrast to convection which involves the movement of material. The ratio of the temperature gradient to the heat flow is termed the volume conductivity.

The tissues of the body are not good conductors of heat and if the heat exchange within the body were solely due to conduction, large internal temperature gradients would be necessary to conduct metabolic heat away. It would also be difficult to compensate for the changing internal and external thermal stresses, as the conduction of heat for any given tissue remains constant.

Circulation

In the body, heat transfer by convection occurs through the bulk movement of the blood, that is, through the circulation, and is of great importance. The range of blood flow in the skin is immense ranging from 1 ml/min/100 gm of tissue to 100 ml/min/100 gm tissue.

The circulation modifies heat distribution in three ways.

(i) Minimising temperature differences within the body
Circulation cools some tissues and warms others. This maintains the body mass temperature at an almost uniform level.

In tissues with a high metabolic rate and perfusion, metabolic heat is removed by the circulating blood with only a slight increase in blood temperature. In tissues cooler than blood, heat is supplied by the blood.

In well-perfused tissues the distances over which heat must be transferred by conduction is small because of the profuse distribution of capillaries.

(ii) Controlling body insulation
Systemic capillaries do not extend to the superficial part of the epidermis; heat is therefore transferred from the capillaries to the skin surface by conduction only. If skin capillaries are dilated, the blood flows close to the surface and heat transfer rates are adequate. If skin capillaries are constricted, heat

transfer can only take place by conduction over larger distances and may be inadequate. Thus the ease of heat transfer is altered by changes in cutaneous capillaries. In effect these changes alter the thickness of the 'body shell' which separates the deeper 'core' from the environment.

(iii) Counter-current heat exchange between major blood vessels

Arterial blood perfusing the extremities loses heat in the surface capillaries and returns to cool the body by mixing with the warm venous blood from the splanchnic bed. The heat lost in this manner can be reduced if the arteries and veins exchange heat through their walls. Thus blood reaching the superficial skin is pre-cooled to a certain extent and the temperature gradient between capillary and skin surface is reduced. Consequently, less heat is lost from the blood while the venous blood is partially warmed. As the main arteries and veins tend to run for long distances together, the tendency is for heat to be conserved.

The thermal insulation of tissues varies from vasodilatation (0·15 clo) to vasoconstriction (0·9 clo). Another important factor is the distribution of blood to those areas where the curvature effect alters the effective insulation, e.g. the fingers. As the effective insulation of the air is less for the fingers, a shift in blood flow to the fingers will result in increased heat loss. Thus the gradient in temperature down the length of a limb may be more important in the control of insulation than the gradient from the deep organs to the skin.

Insulation by Air

Temperature

In a colder environment, as the air density increases, the loss of heat by radiation decreases. This is almost completely compensated for by an increase in loss by convection. Thus although the relative importance of radiation and convection loss varies greatly at differing temperatures, the total loss of heat remains the same.

Wind

Heat loss also varies with the wind velocity. At very low air speeds any small increase of air movement increases the heat loss a great deal, whilst there is little difference in I_A at 10 mph (4·47 m/s) and in a hurricane (Table 25).

In practice however, because of the effect of a hurricane in penetrating clothing and reducing the insulation by disturbing the trapped still air, the heat loss in a clothed man is much greater at 60 mph (26·8 m/s) than at 10 mph.

Altitude

Because of the decrease in air density at altitude, the I_A increases. If the I_A at ground level in still conditions was 0·8 clo, at 20,000 ft (6096 m) it would be 1·1 clo.

Table 25.   Standard values of air insulation I_A in wind

I_A clo	Air movement ft/min	cm/sec	mph
0·1	4500	2280	51
0·15	2000	1015	22·7
0·2	1050	534	11·9
0·4	210	107	2·4
0·6	75	39	0·85
0·8	35	18	0·4
1·0	10	5	0·1

Wind Chill

The concept of wind chill is an attempt to correlate the thermal effects of air movement with those of temperature and present them in a simplified form.

In the field it does provide an index which corresponds well with experience of the degree of discomfort and tolerance by man in cold and windy conditions. However the degree of air movement affects only the insulation afforded by air, and the total insulation in man is made up of the sum of the insulation afforded by clothes, air and tissues.

In effect, under field conditions the tolerance of man to cold and wind is determined to a great extent by those parts that are often unprotected—the hands and face. Wind is much less tolerable when one is forcing one's way into it, which exposes the face, than walking or climbing at an angle which protects the face.

The chilling power of wind can produce an almost super-cooling effect on exposed skin. This is shown by its effect at low temperatures on the nose and cheeks, where in the absence of any protection frostbite is very common.

Because of the decreased density of the air at high altitude the wind chill factor for a given temperature and wind velocity may be less than at sea level.

Table 26. Wind chill effect: equivalent effective temperature

Wind speed mph	Actual air temperature (°F)											
	50	40	30	20	10	0	−10	−20	−30	−40	−50	−60
5	48	36	27	17	−5	−5	−15	−25	−35	−46	−56	−66
10	40	29	18	5	−8	−20	−30	−43	−55	−68	−80	−93
15	35	23	10	−5	−18	−29	−42	−55	−70	−83	−97	−112
20	32	18	4	−10	−23	−34	−50	−64	−79	−94	−108	−121
25	30	15	−1	−15	−28	−38	−55	−72	−88	−105	−118	−130
30	28	13	−5	−18	−33	−44	−60	−76	−92	−109	−124	−134
35	27	11	−6	−20	−35	−48	−65	−80	−96	−113	−130	−137
40	26	10	−7	−21	−37	−52	−68	−83	−100	−117	−135	−140
45	25	9	−8	−22	−39	−54	−70	−86	−103	−120	−139	−143
50	25	8	−9	−23	−40	−55	−72	−88	−105	−123	−142	−145

Thermal Insulation by Clothing

This subject has been discussed by Adam and Goldsmith (Adam and Goldsmith 1965).

The insulating properties of a fabric are due not to the fibres of the fabric itself, but to the air trapped within the fabric. It is important to realise that the thermal insulation of clothing is proportional to the thickness of the dead space air trapped within the clothing.

Air enclosed in a narrow space is greatly superior as thermal insulation to still air in an unconfined space, because air currents are prevented. The thermal insulation per inch of trapped still air is 4·7 clo which is the best thermal insulation of clothing and approximates to the best insulating fur of animals.

To prevent leaks, the trapped air must be as immobile as possible. This prevents setting up currents of air which result in loss by convection. A windproof outer layer is necessary to prevent penetration by external air.

To maintain insulation a maximum thickness of trapped air must be maintained. This means choosing materials so that the thickness is maintained when compressed or wet.

The actual bulk of the materials used must be low so as to prevent loss of heat by conduction.

The necessity for freedom of movement of the arms and legs and other practical considerations means that the thermal insulation of clothing which is practical is different in different parts of the body. Thus the face is very often left unprotected unless conditions are extremely severe.

Curvature Effect

The effect of the curvature of a surface on its heat loss is important. Heat loss from the curved surface of a small cylinder is greater than from that of a large curved cylinder. Thus the total insulation (clothing plus air or $I_C + I_A$) is reduced in a cylinder of small diameter.

As the diameter decreases up to $\frac{1}{4}$ inch (6·5 mm) any increase in thickness of insulation material makes little or no difference to the total insulation.

This is an important factor in the insulation of the fingers, which is necessarily severely limited even if a mitt is used for the whole hand.

The theoretically ideal insulation value for clothing specially designed against cold is 4·7 clo per inch thickness of dead air. In fact a value of 4·0 clo is usually achieved for overall insulation.

The factors responsible for the failure to achieve the ideal figures are the effect of curvature in decreasing the effective insulating power of the extremities, and the presence of air spaces inbetween the layers of clothing. Here the air is not immobilised, and heat loss occurs by convection.

A value of more than 4 clo i.e. up to 5 clo, can be provided by very bulky materials such as eiderdown but these may well interfere with the individual's mobility.

However at rest bulky garments are acceptable.

Bulky garments too are more acceptable on the trunk than on the extremities. Therefore it is more difficult to insulate the extremities than the trunk.

Metabolic Cost

There is an increase of approximately 16 per cent in the metabolic cost of working with multilayered arctic clothing over the corresponding cost of just carrying this weight of clothing. This can be attributed to *friction drag*—the frictional resistance as one layer of clothing slides over another during movement, and the *hobbling effect*—the interference with movement at the joints of the body which is produced by bulk (Tettlebaum and Goldman 1972).

Effect of Wind and Movement

External Wind
If air penetrates clothing the trapped dead air is moved and insulation will diminish. The effects may be considerable. Thus in still air (under 2 mph (0·9 m/s)) a clothing assembly had an insulating value of 3·5 clo whilst at 24 mph (10·7 m/s) this fell to 2·5 clo.

The magnitude of the effect of external wind depends on the degree of wind resistance of the outer wind proof covering, and the efficiency of the 'seals' at neck, wrist and ankle.

Internal Wind
This refers to the currents of air set up by the movements of the

individual. These can lower clothing insulation to half its 'resting' value.

Overheating when exercising in the cold with loss of insulation associated with the production of sweat, and thus of damp clothing, is a well recognised hazard. However it might be argued that as the automatic decrease in insulation is of the order of 50 per cent while the increase in heat production is three times the resting value, the decrease is not as great as desired.

Clothing

The function of clothing is to protect the body from the environment, but it is essential that it interferes as little as possible with body movements. This is especially true when mountaineering.

Basic Principles

Insulation is the most important function and is provided by the trapped still air in the garment. It must be possible to vary combinations of clothing so that the degree of insulation is adjusted to meet varying amounts of heat produced by the body.

This is made very difficult if only one material, such as fur, is used for insulation. It is easier to vary insulation by being able to vary the number of layers, which can be put on and taken off at will. Rapid changes can therefore be made both to changing conditions of the environment and also the changes in heat production from the body.

Adequate ventilation, which is easily adjustable, improves this adaptability. One consequence of the multi-layer principle is that clothing must fit correctly without causing constriction or pressure on underlying tissues.

Clothes may be soaked by water from outside or from within. In a wet–cold climate, rain must be prevented from soaking underlying clothes and in this way decreasing their capacity to insulate.

Clothes can also be soaked by water from inside (perspiration). 500 ml of water each day is produced by man at rest, and much more when exercising. If a completely water-proof outer garment is worn, the moisture produced by the body will condense on the inner surface of the water-proof covering and the clothing will become soaked or frozen.

Outer layers should therefore be (a) permeable to water-vapour and allow this vapour to escape before condensing, (b) water resistant to retard water entry and (c) windproof to prevent excessive air movement in the garments of the trapped still air which provides the warm insulation.

In cold conditions heat loss is controlled by the clothing. Lapps and Eskimos in the Polar regions have fur clothing which gives them insulation equivalent to a tropical environment immediately next to the skin.

The clothing of Polar travellers may make them uncomfortably hot during dog sledging expeditions and the same applies to mountaineers who even under winter conditions may become very hot when actually climbing, yet get very cold when at rest.

For this reason mountaineers use the layer principle, removing clothes when moving and putting them on when at rest. The duvet or eiderdown jacket is often worn as an outer garment especially in winter mountaineering for this reason.

The choice of materials for clothes varies with the individual. Natural fibres are popular, especially wool and cotton. Fur was the first choice in polar regions as it was available locally. Synthetic fibres can imitate most of the characteristics of natural fibre and are tough, wear well and are easily maintained.

Trunk
Insulation of the trunk is relatively easy.

Upper trunk. On expeditions it may be difficult to wash clothing. A non-irritant garment next to the skin will absorb the skin debris that is shed. When dirty it can be replaced. A 'string-vest' which traps large amounts of air can provide considerable insulation. It must be worn next to the skin and covered by a closely woven garment to prevent air movement.

Shirts and pullovers, their size graduated so that they fit one over the other, are usual.

A scarf round the neck, draw strings for waist or hips and draught-excluding bands around the wrist prevent heat loss by the bellows effect.

'Down' jackets are extremely warm, light and comfortable and are now almost standard wear. However they are bulky and if they become wet are extremely difficult to dry. They are best used in cold–dry climates. The jacket should overlap the trousers by a large margin.

Lower trunk and legs. Insulation is influenced by the amount of movement at the hip and knee joints and the close proximity of the skin of the inner thighs which can cause severe chafing if the garments are badly fitted.

Long underpants of a soft weave wool are preferable. These should fit well especially around the ankle to prevent heat loss due to the bellows action.

Down-trousers should not be so thick so as to prevent easy leg movement. Breeches or trousers should be of hard wearing material which does not tear. The fly opening should be easily operated. The lower end of the legs should be closed at the ankles to prevent heat loss by the bellows effect. Garters, and puttees are often used. These also prevent snow from entering the top of the boot. Many methods of closure are available but it is essential to have a second method of closure especially if zip fasteners, which may break, are used. All should be easy to handle, whatever the conditions.

The survival and morale value of bright clothing is important and it is preferable, despite the fact that it may reflect the sun's rays and thus reduce heat gain by radiation. One-piece suits ('cat-suits') were used in 1961 and in 1972 on Everest and proved extremely efficient as the gap between trousers and jacket was avoided.

Feet
The feet tend to remain covered all day. This means that they are not inspected as easily as, for instance, the fingers, and injury

such as blisters or early frostbite may remain hidden for a long period. On many occasions men have slept in their boots at high camps.

The design of footwear depends on whether the conditions to be met are wet–cold or dry–cold. Unfortunately the mountaineer moves rapidly from one set of conditions to the other. Most mountaineering boots are designed basically for wet–cold conditions, except those used at very high altitude or for winter conditions in Europe. In cold–wet conditions the boot should be as water-proof as possible, as once the foot becomes wet its temperature falls.

Boots should fit well with no unnecessary pressure points. Frostbite most often affects the tips of the toes and one factor is pressure interfering with the blood supply in small vessels. All mountaineering boots should have a rigid sole.

Socks should fit well. Insoles are useful. An overboot is worn in very cold conditions. However if one *is* worn crampons have to be worn as well and as a result rockclimbing for long periods may be difficult.

Vapour barrier boots are not often used in the mountains. The basic principle here is that heat gain from condensation is made use of in the design.

The usual model of boot is one in which the insulating layer is sealed between an outer covering and an inner covering of rubber. It is worn with two pairs of socks and an insole under the most extreme conditions. Extra care however must be devoted to the skin of the feet and to drying socks, because water vapour remains, condenses in the boot and cannot escape. One therefore walks in a pool of warm water.

Whatever the footgear, care of the feet is most important. A spare pair of socks should always be taken (they can 'double' as a mitt for the hand).

When bivouacking, changing to dry socks may prevent frostbite. Under continuous cold–wet conditions it is apparent that those who take care of their feet regularly (i.e. dry them, and have clean socks) suffer far less from conditions such as immersion foot, than those who are less meticulous.

Hands
The multi-layer principle is probably best.

Gloves are often fingerless, i.e. all fingers in one compartment and the thumb separate—a mitten.

The glove must conform to the normal 'position of function' which is the physiological position of the unused hand.

The outer layer must be windproof, water-resistant, permeable to water vapour and robust. Whether it is a separate layer or incorporated in the layer containing trapped insulating air is a matter of design.

If it is necessary to use the fingers for fine work it will be necessary to wear 'contact' gloves, with individual fingers.

Their function is to provide protection from the wind and to prevent skin contact with metals, e.g. the axe head. In very cold conditions, as metals are good conductors of heat, if the finger comes in contact with a metal, heat is rapidly conducted away from the finger, causing a 'cold burn'. If the hand is damp with perspiration, the water will freeze, and the finger will stick to the metal.

Headgear
The head is an important avenue of heat loss, and some form of headgear will prevent this. The most likely areas to freeze are the ears, the nose and cheeks.

The ears are easy to protect and a painful ear is a warning of incipient cold injury. The nose and cheek are less easy, as face masks are uncomfortable and therefore unpopular.

A well designed anorak hood is essential both for protecting the face from the wind and from driven ice and snow particles. It should project well forward from the face and have a stiff but malleable wire in its 'leading edge'. This enables the hood to be arranged so that it protects the face, from whatever angle the wind comes. If necessary only a minute hole can be left through which the individual can see.

The use of goggles incorporating one frame of tinted glass provides more protection for the face than the dark glasses which are often used in mountaineering.

If oxygen is being used the mask and dark glasses can be

incorporated into a visor which provides protection for the whole face.

Care of Clothing

Wind proofs must be tough and durable. They should be kept as clean as possible. Holes and tears must be mended.

Woollen garments tend to shrink on washing. In the Korean War frostbite of the feet was caused by shrunken woollen socks.

Skin debris will cause matting of clothes, reduce the air content and so reduce the insulation value. Clothes must be washable and kept clean.

Holes in down clothing are best repaired with sticking plaster or sellotape to prevent escape of down.

Clothing Assemblies

Everest 1924
Norton at 28,000 ft (8524 m) (Norton 1925).

Body
Thick wool vest and drawers
Thick flannel shirt
3 sweaters
Lightish knickerbocker suit of wind proof gabardine.
Knickers lined with flannel.

Feet
A pair of 20 ft (6 m) elastic kashmir puttees.
A pair of boots of felt bound and soled with leather and lightly nailed with the usual Alpine nails.
Overall a very light pyjama suit of Burberry's 'Shackleton' windproof gabardine.

Hands
Long fingerless woollen mitts inside a similar pair made of gabardine.

Head
Fur lined leather motor cycling helmet.
'Pair of goggles which were sewn into a leather mask that came over the nose and covered every part of my face not naturally protected by my beard.'
'A large woollen muffler completed my costume.'

Everest 1933 (Ruttledge 1934)
   1 Shetland wool vest
   6 Shetland wool pullovers
   2 pairs Shetland wool drawers
   1 pair flannel trousers
   Socks—not recorded
   Boots—not recorded but probably leather with a few light nails. Weight 6 lb (?)
   1 silk-lined Grenfell suit
   1 Balaclava helmet
   1 pair woollen mitts
   1 pair Grenfell-cloth mitts
Total weight, 16–18 lb (7–8 kg)

Everest 1953 (Hunt 1954)
   1 string vest
   1 woollen shirt
   1 Shetland wool pullover
   1 pair long woollen drawers
   2 pairs socks
   Boots (High altitude (5 lb))
   Down jacket with hood
   Down trousers
   Windproof smock with hood
   Windproof trousers
   Woollen ear warmer or Balaclava helmet (wool)
   1 pair silk gloves
   1 pair woollen mitts
   1 pair windproof mitts
Total weight, 17 lb (7–8 kg)

Winter 1960–1. Everest Region
A similar clothing assembly to that of Everest 1953 was worn
when climbing at 22,000 ft (6706 m) in January to February.

An improvement was the incorporation of a windproof outer
lining to the down jacket. This enabled the down jacket to be
removed when actually moving, and replaced when at rest.

The duvets however contained more eiderdown and were
larger—a smaller, shorter eiderdown jacket consisting of eiderdown over the body with wool lined sleeves was sometimes
worn under the larger duvet.

'Cat-suits'—like a one-piece boiler suit—were also worn.

Annapurna (South Face) 1971 (Bonington 1971)
Head
  Crash hat
  Balaclava
  Face mask

Body
  Outer layer
    Wind proof
  Inner layer
    Suit of underwear next to skin
    Light wool sweater
    Borg fur jacket and breeches
    Down jacket
    Down breeches

Feet
  Galibier-Hivernale boots
  Neoprene overboots
  Proof nylon overboots

Hands
  Dachstein mitts—2 pairs

Everest South-West Face November 1972 at Camp 6, 27,000 ft
(8230 m) (Bonington 1972).

Head
  Oxygen mask
  Wool hat

Body
  Upper: Darmart artificial fibre underwear
          Roll neck sweater, nylon wool mix
          Thick ski sweater, wool.
  Lower: Long wool drawers
          Ski warm-up trousers padded
          Down jacket and trousers, one piece
          Windproof one-piece overall

Feet
  1 pair socks
  Galibier-Hivernale leather boots
  2 overboots

Hands
  1 pair silk gloves
  1 pair Dachstein mitts
  Outer gloves of Darmart

Temperature: $-35°C$ at 25,000 ft (7620 m) late afternoon; Wind: All India Radio: possibly gusting to 200 kph at 30,000 ft (9144 m).

Shelter

Whilst it is possible to go for weeks without food, and days without water, it is only possible to survive for a few hours at low temperatures without shelter.

Tents
Tents should be easily erected and stable in wind.
  The insulating effect of a single skin tent is small. Its main function is protection from wind. The fabric should be waterproofed if used in a wet–cold climate. When no rain is to be

encountered it should be permeable to water vapour. A double-skinned tent offers better insulation but is often time-consuming to put up and heavy to carry. A sewn-in ground sheet is essential as otherwise wind may get under the tent and collapse it. In addition, the weight of the occupants will prevent the tent being blown away if the poles are broken. Heat loss would also occur in the space between the tent walls and the separate ground sheet. A fly sheet, as a protection against rain, is necessary in very wet conditions.

The ability to join tents by their entrances so that a long 'tunnel' is formed may be useful.

Box Tents

The development of a box structure to take two or more people is an advance for mountaineers in dry–cold conditions. It is easier to erect and more stable than a tent. The flat roof allows snow to be melted on the roof by the sun. An inner skin can be used for added insulation.

Ventilation is most important. Carbon monoxide is given off by cooking stoves and if all entrances and ventilating vents are closed the inhabitants may suffer from a mild degree of carbon monoxide poisoning. At high altitude this can be serious as carbon monoxide competes more effectively than oxygen for haemoglobin and serious hypoxia may result. It is likely that the cause of a number of unaccountably late starts and poor performances especially by Sherpas who slept with little or no ventilation on early Everest expeditions was due to this cause.

Igloos

Igloos are domed shelters made from slabs of snow. The thermal insulation is good by virtue of the entrapped air cells in the snow. The outer layer of the snow slabs becomes polished ice and thus impermeable to the wind. In effect there is a windproof outer layer and an insulating inner layer.

A sleeping platform is built at a higher level than the entrance, which is by a tunnel below the surface of the snow. At the lower level lamps are placed to heat air which rises to the level of the sleeping platform and emerges through a ventilation hole in the roof.

The level of the sleeping platform is very warm and clothes are almost completely removed and placed in the tunnel, where they remain frozen which prevents them from thawing and becoming sodden.

Insulation and Oxygen Consumption

The relative importance of the insulation of tissue, air and clothes has already been stressed.

The value of I_T is of importance in the face and hands, as protection is inconvenient and the total insulation is restricted by the curvature factor.

The importance of the insulating value of clothes is paramount (Pugh 1966).

The value of I_C will vary with (a) the type of clothing; (b) whether it is wet or dry; (c) whether exercise is being taken (the bellows effect). The value of I_A will vary with wind velocity.

The following Table gives some indication of those changes in varying climatic conditions. The standard clothing assembly has an insulation of 1·5 clo when dry.

Table 27.   Activity, weather and clothing effectiveness

Activity	Conditions	Wind	I_A	I_C	$I_A + I_C$
rest	dry	still	1 clo	1·5 clo	2·5 clo
work	dry	still	0·4 clo	0·6 clo	1·0 clo[a]
work	dry	9 mph[c]	0·2 clo	0·5 clo	0·7 clo
rest	wet	still	0·3 clo	0·2 clo	0·5 clo
work	wet	9 mph	0·2 clo	0·3 clo	0·5 clo
work	wet	9 mph	0·2 clo	0·65 clo	0·85 clo[b]

[a] The low clo value for $I_A + I_C$ is thought to be due to the bellows effect in displacing static warmed air from clothing.

[b] Protective outer garments to keep clothing dry.

[c] 9 mph ≡ 4 m/s.

The relations between body temperature, ambient temperature, total thermal insulation and metabolic rate (or oxygen consumption) are shown in Fig. 20.

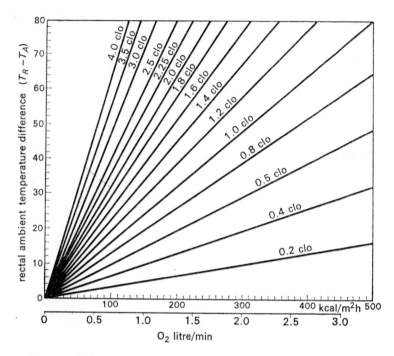

Fig. 20 Chart for predicting final body temperature (R) under conditions of ambient temperature, total thermal insulation and metabolism. Ordinate shows difference between rectal and ambient air temperature ($T_R - T_A$) in °C, abscissa shows metabolism in kcal/m^2 surface area/h and oxygen consumption for an average man of 75 kg weight and 2 m^2 surface area. The values of total insulation (ΣI) are given in units $\Sigma I = I_A + I_C + I_T$. (Pugh 1966.)

At sea level (wet–cold)

(i) Assume a standard clothing assembly of $I_C = 1 \cdot 0 - 1 \cdot 5$ clo at rest in dry, still conditions.

Whilst walking in the wet and in a 9 mph (4 m/s) wind this will fall to 0·3 clo.

In gale force winds (over 50 mph (22 m/s)) I_A will fall to 0·10 clo.

The tissue insulation during exercise is 0·5 clo. Thus the total body insulation or $\Sigma I = 0 \cdot 9$ clo.

If the ambient temperature is freezing (0°C) and the subject is walking at less than average uphill pace the oxygen consumption may be of the order of 1·5 litres/min.

The rectal–ambient temperature difference will be 28·5°C. Therefore the individual will inevitably become hypothermic.

If however, he walks faster and consumes say 2·0 litres oxygen per minute, the rectal ambient difference will be 38·0°C and he will be normothermic.

(ii) If a person wearing the same clothing assembly is wet through yet sheltering from the wind at an ambient temperature of 0°C, at sea level, then $I_C = 0.5$ clo, $I_T = 0.8$ clo and $I_A = 0.40$ clo. The total body insulation or ΣI is 1·70 clo.

To maintain a normal rectal temperature, or at 0°C ambient a rectal–ambient temperature difference of 37°C, the oxygen uptake must be of the order of 1 litre/min, or he must be able to produce 150 kcal/hour.

If he is exhausted or ill he will not be able to manage this for a long period, but if he is fit he will be able to do so.

(iii) If the same person has dry clothing, or he has waterproof overgarments, and he is sheltering from the wind at an ambient temperature of 0°C, then his $I_C = 1.5$ clo, $I_T = 0.8$ clo and $I_A = 0.4$ clo. Total body insulation or $\Sigma I = 2.7$ clo. Then to maintain a rectal–ambient temperature difference of 37°C, his oxygen uptake need only be 0·50 litres/min ($= 75$ kcal/hour) or twice the normal resting level (0·25 litres/min).

The graph also brings out the fact that at low insulation levels i.e. below about 1·5 clo it is necessary to increase the oxygen uptake very considerably to maintain thermal balance. Thus a small increase in insulation—such as extra clothing or an increase in subcutaneous fat—will lower oxygen consumption or, in other words, lower the need to work so hard to maintain body temperature.

At high altitude (dry–cold)

At high altitude where loss of subcutaneous fat due to a lowered food intake is common and the effort to maintain a reasonable oxygen consumption disproportionately difficult, a tendency towards hypothermia is more marked. The insulating value of clothing becomes vital and supplementary oxygen will aid tissue metabolism and thereby heat production—a fact noted clinically in the field.

At 25,000 ft (7620 m) without supplementary oxygen at maximum working capacity, an oxygen uptake of the order of 1·5 litre/min has been observed. On walking uphill oxygen consumption would be of the order of 1·0 litre/min, and on descent 0·75 litre/min or less.

Assuming an ambient temperature of −20°C the rectal-ambient temperature difference for thermal equilibrium would be about 55°C and with a clo value of between 3·5 and 4·0 for total body insulation (which might be the figure for pre-war Everest expeditions), then, with an oxygen uptake of 0·75 litre/min a mountaineer might just be normothermic. Hence the comment made by Smythe on the 1933 Everest expedition that he always felt cold at rest.

It also explains why despite being fully clothed a man might

Table 28.   Sea-level oxygen consumption

Mountaineers at natural pace	Average oxygen uptake at sea level litre/min
Ascent	2·5
Horizontal	2·0
Descent	1·5
Resting	0·25
Maximum	4·0

Table 29.   Maximum oxygen uptake at varying altitudes

Altitude		Maximum oxygen uptake
ft	m	litre/min
25,000	7400	1·46
21,000	6400	1·90
19,000	5800	2·30
15,000	4650	2·70
Sea level		4·0

tend towards hypothermia with resultant peripheral vaso-constriction and frostbite, whilst walking uphill.

At 4 clo total body insulation and at $-20°C$ ambient temperature oxygen consumption must be over 0·5 litre/min for thermal equilibrium. If the mountaineer at 25,000 ft (7400 m) is ill and can move only slowly—or is immobile—he may not be able to maintain even this level of oxygen consumption. He will become gradually hypothermic. This has been recorded clinically.

References

Adam, J. M. and Goldsmith, R. (1965) Cold climates. In, *Exploration medicine. Ed.* Edholm, O. G., Bacharach, A. L. Wright: Bristol.

Bonington, C. (1971) *Annapurna. South face.* Cassell: London.

Bonington, C. (1972) Personal communication.

Burton, A. C. and Edholm, O. G. (1955) *Man in a cold environment.* Arnold: London.

Hunt, J. (1954) *The ascent of Everest.* Hodder and Stoughton: London.

Norton, E. F. (1925) *The fight for Everest.* Arnold: London.

Pugh, L. G. C. E. (1966) *Nature* **209**, 1281.

Ruttledge, M. (1934) *Everest 1933.* Hodder and Stoughton: London.

Tettlebaum, A. and Goldman, R. F. (1972) *Journal of Applied Physiology* **32**, 743.

CHAPTER SIXTEEN

Man's Reaction to Cold

Essentially, man reacts to a cold environment by the use of clothing and the development of adequate shelter, rather than by physiological adaptation. By this manufacture of satisfactory microclimates the Eskimo is able to live at temperatures as low as − 70°C, and the mountaineers are able to survive in similar conditions at altitudes up to 28,000 ft (8500 m).

Evidence of general acclimatisation to cold is found neither in mountaineers nor Polar travellers. This is because the amount of time spent exposed to cold is so short.

In static Polar bases men may be out of doors for only 10 per cent, and in a sledging base for only 15 per cent, of the total elapsed time.

Probably longer periods are spent exposed to cold conditions by mountaineers because they live in unheated tents.

There is evidence that some degree of cold adaptation does occur in the hands and feet (Goldsmith 1960; Edholm and Lewis 1964).

In any event protective clothing is now so effective that as the microclimate is as warm as a temperate zone, men out of doors do not get cold except in the extremities. Indeed, some degree of heat acclimatisation may occur (Wilkins 1972).

However, reports suggest that those who spend long periods permanently under cold conditions do become tolerant to the cold. This tolerance may be estimated by measuring the time elapsing after exposure to a given temperature before shivering starts, or before the subject complains of discomfort of varying degrees. The evidence is that those who are used to working out of doors can work longer with bare hands than newcomers, are less liable to frostbite, and after an initial period when all clothing was worn, as the temperature dropped they used no additional clothing (Butson 1949).

General Acclimatisation

Essentially there are three ways in which general adaptation may occur: body temperature may be allowed to drop, insulation may be increased or heat production increased.

Body Temperature

This may fall in hibernating animals. In man, groups who have been chronically exposed to cold are able to sleep in the cold, some by shivering with a subsequently raised metabolism, others by allowing body and skin temperatures to fall.

The aboriginal Bushman can sleep naked at an ambient temperature of 0°C, with a foot skin temperature of 12–15°C, without shivering.

White controls shivered and moved about and produced a corresponding rise in heat production. The acclimatised white men shivered in their sleep, thus maintaining a higher peripheral temperature enabling them to sleep. Essentially, the aboriginal Bushman allows his body temperature to fall—and this is presumably a feature of cold adaptation (Scholander *et al.* 1958).

Insulation

Animals living in a cold climate develop an increase in insulation by an increase in the depth of fur. In man it has been noted that the hair grew faster during the Arctic winter.

An increase in skin-fold thickness is frequently observed in Polar regions with an increase in fat thickness from 1 to 2 mm.

Though this may be biologically significant the physiological value is probably slight.

There may also be a difference in the physical composition of the fat in the tissues in those who have been chronically exposed to cold (Schmidt-Nielsen 1946).

Some vascular changes, notably an early, larger cold induced vasodilatation has also been observed.

Heat Production

In laboratory animals an increase in heat production has been observed. In man the evidence is more equivocal.

The basal metabolic rate has a negative correlation with the average climatic temperature, that is, if the average temperature is high, the rate is low (Roberts 1952).

In Eskimos, a seasonal effect has been shown to be present, with a basal metabolic rate high in winter, low in summer. Values of +31·4 per cent on July 13th dropped to 23·7 per cent on August 24th (Brown 1950). Most of the evidence favours an increased metabolic rate in Eskimos, but the question of diet has been raised, in that a high protein diet rather than cold may be the cause (Rodahl 1952).

An avidity for a fatty diet has been often noted on Polar expeditions, and appetite tends to increase in cold conditions.

A high carbohydrate diet was more effective than a high protein diet for maintaining thermal balance. However, a high fat diet is even better than a high carbohydrate diet in preventing heat loss.

Increased metabolism in the cold may be largely explained by increased muscular activity both voluntary and involuntary. The weight and clumsiness of cold weather clothing also increase the metabolic cost of work.

Local Acclimatisation

The mechanism for local acclimatisation probably has an essentially vascular basis.

Both skin temperature and blood flow in the hands of eight

Eskimos at a temperature of 20°C were higher than in controls. When immersed in cold water the blood flow did not decline so abruptly in the acclimatised as in the control group (Brown and Page 1952).

Measurement of tactile discrimination of the finger tips both before and after exposure to cold shows that this decreased after exposure. However the numbness was less in those used to outdoor work.

After a period of four weeks in a cold room being exposed to temperatures of 15°C for two hours a day for five days a week, it was found that loss of tactile discrimination became gradually less—or in other words the finger tips had become acclimatised (Mackworth 1953).

Exposure to heat however can prevent this adaptation.

The man acclimatised to cold seems to maintain a smaller 'central core', so that under conditions of cold stress he has a smaller proportion of his body to maintain at a constant maximum temperature and can therefore store up more heat during periods of activity when there is no cold stress. This extra heat is used when cold stress occurs. Under continued cold stress the thicker 'outer shell' allows the acclimatised man to lose more stored heat than the nonacclimatised before his metabolism has to increase.

The acclimatised man gains the following advantages by reducing his central core: he can endure cold stress for longer periods; he can drop the total heat load to a lower level before he must start shivering, or put on warmer clothing; and the level of exercise which he must take to keep him from shivering will be lower. As a result he will be able to maintain circulation in the extremities longer with consequent protection against frostbite.

Observations have been made in the field on a Nepalese pilgrim who survived four days of exposure at 15,000–17,000 ft (4550–5300 m), in the Himalaya during mid-winter. Temperatures fell to − 13°C at night, when he slept in the snow wearing only light clothing (1·5 clo) and no gloves or shoes.

He maintained a relatively high metabolic level, possibly 50 per cent greater than basal, without shivering. With further cooling he maintained a continuous light shivering, rather than the violent intermittent shivering more usually encountered. His metabolic rate was probably twice normal. The surface temperature of his hands never fell below 10–12°C. His feet were in contact with snow or the bare ground at temperatures between 0°C and − 5°C. The skin temperature of the toes fell to 8°C. Neither in his hands nor his feet did he complain of any pain or numbness; and as the skin temperature did not drop to freezing point he did not suffer from frostbite.

Essentially he was able to maintain a high metabolic rate without discomfort or shivering, and possibly some local tissue adaptation to cold occurred. It appeared that subcutaneous fat thickness was not an important factor (Pugh 1963).

Vascular Effects of Exposure to Cold

Immersion in cold water above 10°C causes a reduction in the blood flow through the forearms. This reduction is due to (a) vasoconstriction, which affects the vessels in both the muscles and the skin, and (b) an increase in viscosity of the blood due to an increase in haematocrit.

As a similar effect has been observed in patients with a sympathectomy, the effect of cold is clearly due at least in part to a direct action on the blood vessels, as well as by sympathetic vasoconstriction (Barcroft and Edholm 1943).

Immersion of the extremities in water at temperatures between 0°C and 8°C, or exposure to air between 0°C and 15°C, initially produces vasoconstriction and decreased blood flow, but this is followed by vasodilatation and increased blood flow. The vasodilatation is often periodic in nature and although usually demonstrated in the fingers it has also been shown to occur in the toes and nose (Lewis 1930).

If the hands alone are cooled a heat loss of as much as 40 kcal/hour has been demonstrated, and a fall in rectal temperature can occur.

The explanation of the vasodilatator effect is that cold causes a paralysis of the smooth muscle which normally causes vasoconstriction.

Experiments on strips from mammalian arteries demonstrated that severe cooling reduced their response to vasoconstrictor agents. Although cooling caused an immediate loss of power to respond to adrenaline it did not abolish the contraction which had already been induced. It halted contraction but did not cause immediate relaxation. The results in smaller arteries that control blood flow were similar.

Low temperature causes only a relatively minor degree of vasodilatation in already chilled subjects. The likely explanation is that the larger proximal arteries are still reacting to noradrenaline—i.e. they are not cooled enough for their vasoconstrictor mechanisms to be paralysed (Keatinge 1957).

Various racial variations have been observed. Eskimos are found to develop cold dilatation to a greater degree, and Negros to a lesser degree than Europeans (Meehan 1955). The reason for this is not clear.

The main factor causing cold paralysis is not yet clear, but there is some evidence to suggest that the actomyosin system of arteries could contract almost as well though more slowly at 5°C as at 35°C.

Habitual exposure to cold may give blood vessels the ability to respond to noradrenaline at low temperatures, and Glover (Glover *et al.* 1968) demonstrated that rabbit-ear arteries, which are habitually exposed to lower temperatures than femoral arteries, lose their ability to respond to noradrenaline when cooled to 7°C whilst the femoral arteries lost their ability to respond at 12°C.

It is possible that the failure of the smooth muscle of the blood vessels to function at 0°C has developed either as a result of cells becoming adapted to function at 37°C, or because cold vasodilatation has a positive value for survival in cold conditions.

Any mechanism that increases blood flow and temperature at the extremity, near 0°C, is useful in avoiding frostbite. However the delay in onset and intermittent nature of the cold vasodilatation can allow the finger to freeze either before vasodilatation occurs or during a periodic wave of vasoconstriction. Vasodilatation also causes loss of heat from the body with resultant liability to hypothermia.

On balance the effect of cold vasodilatation seems to be adverse and it seems likely that the failure of arteries to respond to noradrenaline at temperatures near freezing is simply a result of their adaptation to function at 37°C.

Pain Due to Cold

Immersion of a finger in cold water produces pain. The initial pain comes on gradually, builds up, and then fades as cold-induced vasodilatation occurs. Pain is associated with vasoconstriction and relief with vasodilatation, so it is related to blood flow.

Cold Diuresis

On exposure to cold there is an increased output of urine, which is independent of water loss from the skin. There is also a gradual fall in plasma volume in the first few days.

Diuresis is markedly increased on lying down, and reduced in the upright position (Adolph and Molnar 1946).

The increased urinary output is probably due to diminished tubular re-adsorption, and was regulated by the posterior pituitary rather than renal blood flow (Bader *et al.* 1952).

This diuretic response to cold was diminished during the Polar winter (Wyatt 1962) after a year in Antarctica.

On ascent to high altitude cold may be intense and in any event the temperature falls 3°F for every 1000 ft (1°C every 150 m) of ascent and the fall in plasma volume due to cold diuresis will be in addition to that normally occurring on exposure to altitude.

References

Adolph, E. F. and Molnar, G. W. (1946) *American Journal of Physiology* **146**, 507.

Bader, R. A., Eliot, J. W. and Bass, D. E. (1952) *Journal of Applied Physiology* **4**, 649.

Barcroft, H. and Edholm, O. G. (1943) *Journal of Physiology* **102**, 5.

Brown, J. M. and Page, J. (1952) *Journal of Applied Physiology* **5**, 221.

Brown, M. (1950) *Report on Queens University, Kingston, Ontario, expedition.*

Butson, A. R. C. (1949) *Nature* **163**, 132.

Edholm, O. G. and Lewis, H. E. (1964) Terrestrial animals in cold: Man in Polar regions. In, *Handbook of Physiology.* Section 4. *Adaptation to environment. Ed.* Dill, D. B., Adolph, E. F. and Wilber, C. G. American Physiological Society: Washington, D. C.

Glover, W. E., Strangeways, D. H. and Wallace, W. F. M. (1968) *Journal of Physiology* **194**, 78.

Goldsmith, R. (1960) *Journal of Applied Physiology* **15**, 776.

Keatinge, W. R. (1957) *Journal of Physiology* **139**, 497.

Lewis, T. (1930) *Heart* **15**, 177.

Mackworth, N. H. (1953) *Journal of Applied Physiology* **5**, 533.

Meehan, J. P. (1955) *Military Medicine* **116**, 330.

Pugh, L. G. C. E. (1963) *Journal of Applied Physiology* **18**, 1234.

Roberts, D. F. (1952) *Journal of the Royal Anthropological Institute* **82**, 169.

Rodahl, K. (1952) *Journal of Nutrition* **48**, 359.

Schmidt-Nielsen, K. (1946) *Acta physiologica scandinavica* **12**, 110; *ibid.* **12**, 123.

Scholander, P. F., Hammel, H. T., Hart, J. S., Le Mesurier, D. H. and Steen, J. (1958) *Journal of Applied Physiology* **13**, 211.

Wilkins, D. C. (1972) *Heat acclimatisation in the Antarctic.* Symposium of Human Biology and Medicine in the Antarctic. Scott Polar Research Institute: Cambridge.

Wyatt, H. (1962) *Some observations on the physiology of men during sledging expeditions.* M.D. thesis. University of London.

CHAPTER SEVENTEEN

Acclimatisation and Deterioration at Altitude

There is great individual variation in the rate and degree of acclimatisation.

The ability to acclimatise appears to improve with each successive visit. The newcomer, however fit, is more affected than those who have paid previous visits, some of whom may have no symptoms until 20,000 ft (6096 m). The rate of acclimatisation has no bearing on ultimate performance and slow acclimatisers may eventually become extremely fit.

The rate and degree of acclimatisation seem to be improved by exercise below 15,000 ft (4572 m), and possibly by a high carbohydrate diet. There is no correlation between blood values and physical performance. Age seems not to be an important factor and in 1953 the Sherpas who went to the South Col 26,000 ft (7925 m) varied from 17 to 47 years. In general the early thirties appears to be the best age for very high altitudes. Women appear to acclimatise as well as men.

Although acclimatisation occurs up to about 23,000 ft (7010 m), the effects of deterioration become more marked for every thousand feet over 17,500 ft (5334 m). At altitudes less than 17,500 ft very long periods appear to be necessary for high-altitude visitors to approach the physical performance of high-altitude natives. Even after eight months at 14,000 ft (4267 m), sea-level performance was not obtained in visitors.

Complete acclimatisation to 17,500 ft (5334 m) must take a long time, if it ever occurs. Even after months at this height men were impressed by the striking feeling of well-being and energy on descent.

Acclimatisation does not persist long after return from high altitude and climbers have suffered from acute mountain sickness in the European Alps up to 16,000 ft (4877 m) within two months of returning from long periods in the Himalaya.

High Altitude Deterioration (Over 17,500 ft (5334 m))

The greatest altitude at which men are known to live permanently appears to be at about 17,500 ft (5334 m). A mining settlement, Auconquilcha, is situated at this altitude, in the Andes. Attempts to induce miners to live at a higher altitude, 19,000 ft (5791 m), to be close to their work failed because they developed the symptoms of mountain sickness and were unable to live and work at this level for long periods.

It is on this basis that the height 17,500 ft (5334 m) has been considered to represent the critical level for acclimatisation. Above this, high-altitude deterioration occurs.

The term 'high-altitude deterioration' was first used by members of early Everest expeditions, to denote a deterioration in men's mental and physical condition as a result of prolonged stay at great altitude.

Somervell (Bruce 1923) was the first to emphasise the existence of this condition, whilst the performance of Odell (Norton 1925) who twice went to 27,000 ft (8230 m) without oxygen and showed relatively slight side-effects suggested that deterioration varied considerably in severity with the individual.

Poor living conditions, with exposure to winds gusting to 100 mph and temperature of $-40°C$, associated with monotonous and often insufficient food and a low fluid intake resulting in dehydration, would result in some degrees of mental and physical deterioration, whether or not chronic hypoxia was present.

However despite excellent protection from the environment,

good living conditions and adequate food and fluid intake, prolonged stay at 19,000 ft (5791 m) in 1960–1 led to high-altitude deterioration, as shown by loss of weight and loss of appetite. Although a fall in work output was not observed and mental capacity appeared normal at this altitude there was a proneness to intercurrent infection, and a general lack of robustness. Mental and physical capacity appeared to be diminishing and none considered that they could live at this height indefinitely.

Table 30. Maximum periods spent at varying altitudes without oxygen

| Height | | Period | Expedition |
ft	m	days	
Over 17,500	5334	30–40	Various expeditions
at 19,000	5791	90–100	Makalu 1960–1
22,000–24,000	6706–7315	11	Everest 1953
23,000	7010	11	Everest 1924
24,500	7467	8	Makalu 1961
25,700	7850	5	Everest 1953
26,000	7925	4	Everest 1953
27,400	8382	3	Everest 1933
27,800	8450	1 night	Everest 1953

At greater altitudes deterioration becomes more marked, and although many expeditions have spent periods of up to six weeks or more at altitudes exceeding 20,000 ft (6096 m), almost all have reported loss of weight, mental and physical lassitude and impairment of work capacity.

In some men acclimatisation appears to occur up to 23,000 ft (7010 m), but above this altitude deterioration becomes more rapid.

The maximum periods for which men have lived at varying altitudes is given in Table 30 (Ward 1954; Ward 1968).

Age

In general men over the age of 40 do not acclimatise as well as younger men, yet men over 40 have ascended to 28,000 ft

(8534 m) without oxygen (Norton 1925). Pugh on successive visits to 19,000 ft (5791 m) and above in 1953 (aged 44) and 1961 (aged 52) tended to deteriorate faster on the second occasion. However Odell reached 23,000 ft (7010 m) on Everest at the age of 47.

Below the age of 40 successive visits to altitude appear to improve performance and diminish deterioration. Some exceptional performances have been made, e.g. Odell (Norton 1925) spent 11 days above 23,000 ft (7010 m) without oxygen, twice climbing to 27,000 ft (8230 m).

Studies carried out in 1962, on six members of the International High Altitude Expedition of 1935, that is 27 years later, revealed that in general adaptation to 17,500 ft (5334 m) was slower. At rest, the minute volume increased about as rapidly and to the same extent as in younger men. On easy exercise work was performed with the same minute volume as in 1935 but the oxygen consumption on peak performance was less in 1962. Haemoglobin seemed to increase at a slower rate (Dill *et al.* 1964).

In laboratory animals too, the older animals acclimatised less well than the younger (Altland and Highman 1964).

Sex

Women have ascended to 25,000 ft (7620 m) (Dyhrenfurth 1955), but information about their physical and mental performance at high altitude is lacking. However a women's expedition to Mt Everest is projected for 1976. Certainly their resistance to cold is better than in the male and they appear less liable to frostbite.

It has been noted too in some laboratory animals that the female has a greater tolerance to altitude, and is able to exercise better than the male (Altland and Highman 1964).

Blood Values

No change in blood values occurred over three months at 19,000 ft (5791 m) even when individuals showed clinical evidence of high-altitude deterioration.

Physical Performance

Over three months spent at 19,000 ft (5791 m) work rates attained a level of 1200 kg m/min and did not diminish. Subjectively however towards the end of this period maximum work rates appeared to take more out of the individual than initially.

At higher altitudes physical performance appears to deteriorate over a period of time though valid measurements are difficult to obtain.

Maximum work rates fell with altitude from 2000 kg m/min at sea level to 600 kg m/min at 24,500 ft (7467 m).

The cardiac output of one individual who spent five days at 25,000 ft (7620 m) appeared to be considerably lower than that of a comparably built companion; and his general condition at the end of this period was very poor.

Oxygen Cost of Ventilation

The oxygen cost of ventilation during maximal work rises steeply above 19,000 ft (5791 m). At about 24,500 ft (7467 m) it has been estimated that a critical level is reached when a further increase in ventilation will make no more oxygen available to the muscles without lowering Po_2.

Fatigue of the respiratory muscles results and oxygen intake will fall with resulting tendency to cold injury.

Heart Rate

Maximum heart rate for high-altitude visitors fell. At sea level it was about 187 whereas at 24,500 ft (7467 m) it was 140.

In high-altitude natives heart rate at altitude more nearly approaches maximal sea-level values.

This argues that cardiac output is better.

Loss of Appetite and Weight

Some loss of appetite and weight seems inevitable after prolonged stay at altitude, and this was evident over a period of twelve weeks in good living conditions at 19,000 ft (5791 m).

A desire for carbohydrate seems to be associated with prolonged stay.

One of the simplest indications of adequate acclimatisation is the possession of an appetite capable of maintaining normal weight. In general the higher the altitude and the longer the stay the greater the weight loss.

This suggests some degree of intestinal maladsorption.

Milledge (Milledge 1972) studied the adsorption of xylose from the small intestine in patients with arterial oxygen desaturation associated with chronic lung disease and cyanotic heart disease. The more serious the desaturation the less xylose was adsorbed. In cases where hypoxia was relieved by surgery or oxygen administration the xylose adsorption increased to within normal limits.

Resistent intestinal disorders not responding to antibiotic treatment have been recorded on one or two occasions. Although these cases are most likely to be due to gastro-intestinal infection, fat maladsorption has been considered a possibility.

It is interesting that oxygen administration at altitude does tend to increase general well-being including appetite, and in three of Milledge's respiratory cases oxygen administration (for 8 hours) was sufficient to increase xylose adsorption. This suggests that the effect of hypoxia on the intestinal mucosa may be of a biochemical nature.

Endocrine

The possibility that extreme exhaustion at altitude may be associated with adrenal cortical deficiency has been considered but not proved.

However, abnormally high urine levels of 17-hydroxycortico-steroids have been found with exposure to extreme altitude, 27,000 ft (8230 m) and above. Extreme exertion at those heights can lead to a shock-like state as observed clinically. The individual may take a long period to recover.

Some reduction in adrenal cortical activity has been observed after months at 19,000 ft (5791 m) though the adrenal gland was not exhausted and seemed capable of responding to stress (Pugh 1962; Ward 1968).

Mental Performance

Diminution in mental performance occurs at extreme altitude.

Memory

An increasing impairment of memory occurs with altitude; some is apparent at 8000–10,000 ft (2438–3048 m) but the decline is more rapid above 12,000 ft (3658 m).

For this reason all observations should be noted down immediately rather than carried in the memory.

The inability to remember names and numbers has often been noted.

Mental Ability

After three months at 19,000 ft (5791 m) on the Himalayan Scientific Expedition 1960–1 mental fatigue was the rule. Subjectively, mental performance seemed little impaired though mistakes in calculation were commoner and all mental activity required a greater effort to initiate and carry through, than at sea level.

Statistically significant change in mental performance is shown by the falling off in efficiency of card-sorting which was recorded after three weeks at 19,000 ft (5791 m) (Gill *et al*. 1964).

Behaviour amongst members of the 1960–1 party did not deteriorate to any significant extent despite relatively cramped quarters.

Sleep may become fitful and accompanied by unpleasant dreams and nightmares. This tends to enhance deterioration.

Prolonged stay at very high altitude leads to a decreased intellectual efficiency for a period after return to sea level. The intensity and persistence of these changes seem to be related to the heights attained and the length of stay. Unusual mental tiredness may persist for several weeks after returning to sea level. Some disturbance of memory is common but tends to pass off.

Some expedition members have suffered from depression, which necessitated psychiatric consultation.

Permanent mental damage has not been reported and of eight individuals who have been to 28,000 ft (8534 m) without oxygen, none has shown any degree of mental deterioration, all have had distinguished careers—three being Fellows of the Royal Society.

There is a relation between arterial oxygen saturation and altitude with mental performance tests in unacclimatised subjects. Breakdown in performance occurs at an altitude of 18,000 ft (5486 m) or arterial oxygen saturation between 70 and 75 per cent. With acclimatised subjects adequate mental performance might persist to higher altitudes.

Special Senses

Visual Ability

At 16,000 ft (4877 m) the ability to see may be reduced to 50 per cent of sea-level performance. In other words, twice as much light would be required for the perception of a given stimulus.

At 18,000 ft (5486 m) at high illuminations there is little or no decrease in the ability to resolve a given target. At low illumination some decrease occurs at about 8000 ft (2438 m).

Presumably both light sensitivity and visual acuity might become more impaired with prolonged stay at altitude.

Auditory Sensitivity

Some impairment occurs at about 17,500 ft (5334 m).

Disease

Above 17,500 ft (5334 m) mountaineers rarely experience more than mild attacks of mountain sickness. Because their endurance and capacity for work is greatly reduced, difference in altitude between camps of 1000–2000 ft (300–600 m) only are normal. Thus they are not exposed to large differences in barometric pressure. However Longstaff (Longstaff 1950) ascended from a camp at 17,500 ft (5334 m) to 23,000 ft (7010 m) in one day and returned, without symptoms.

Pulmonary oedema has been reported at 24,000 ft (7315 m), and it is likely that the higher the altitude the greater the mortality.

Thrombotic episodes also seem to occur at higher rather than lower altitude, possibly because of the additional factors of inactivity and dehydration.

It is an impression too that cold injury is commoner at high altitude than at comparable temperature at lower levels. Hypothermia and frostbite occurred in one man suffering from high-altitude deterioration after five days, at 25,000 ft (7620 m) and above. He became exhausted after ascending to about 25,800 ft (7823 m) and fell repeatedly on an easy descent to camp at 25,000 ft. Before losing consciousness for 24 hours, he had a rigor. This suggests that his core temperature had fallen to about 33°C, despite his being fully clothed.

Muscular fatigue and the high oxygen cost of ventilation probably contributed to lower oxygen consumption. In addition, the diminished ability to shiver which may occur at high altitude may have decreased heat production.

Certainly many mountaineers have observed how often they feel cold above 23,000 ft (7010 m), and frostbite has occurred in fully clothed men on occasion.

References

Altland, P. D. and Highman, B. (1964) In, *The physiological effects of high altitudes. Ed.* Weihe, W. H. Pergamon Press: Oxford.

Bruce, C. G. (1923) *The assault on Mt Everest.* Arnold: London.

Dill, D. B., Forbes, W. H., Newton, J. L. and Terman, J. W. (1964) Respiratory adaptation to altitudes as related to age.

In, *Relations of development and ageing. Ed.* Birren, J. E. Thomas: Springfield, Illinois.

Dyrenfurth, G. O. (1955) *To the Third Pole.* Werner Laurie: London.

Gill, M. B., Poulton, E. C., Carpenter, A., Woodhead, M. M. and Gregory, M. H. P. (1964) *Nature* **203**, 436.

Longstaff, T. G. (1950) *This my voyage.* Murray: London.

Milledge, J. S. (1972) *British Medical Journal* **3**, 557.

Norton, E. F. (1925) *The fight for Everest.* Arnold: London.

Pugh, L. G. C. E. (1962) *British Medical Journal* **2**, 621.

Ward, M. P. (1968) *Diseases occurring at altitudes exceeding 17,500 ft.* Thesis for M.D. University of Cambridge.

Ward, M. P. (1954) *Proceedings of the Royal Society* Series B **143**, 40.

CHAPTER EIGHTEEN

Clinical Effects of High Altitude

The clinical effects of high altitude differ with each individual, the rate at which he is exposed to low barometric pressure, the period that he spends at each altitude, and the height which he attains.

In the majority of people successive ascents are associated with less disturbance and most acclimatise well. At about 17,500 ft (5334 m) the converse process, high altitude deterioration, starts and this becomes progressively more rapid with altitude.

Table 31. High-altitude visitors. Approximate climbing rates

Height		No oxygen		Open circuit oxygen	
ft	m	ft/hr	m/hr	ft/hr	m/hr
0–12,000	0–3658	2500	765		
19,000	5791	1500	460		
21–22,000	6401–6706	1000	305	1000	305
22–24,000	6706–7315	up to 700	up to 210	600	180
24–26,000	7315–7925	up to 500	up to 152	600	180
26–27,000	7925–8230	300	91	350	106
27–28,000	8230–8534	200	61	300	91
28–29,000	8534–8839			200	61
26–28,500	7925–8684			600[a]	180[a]

[a] Closed circuit oxygen

The two processes, acclimatisation and deterioration, go hand in hand and are influenced by a number of factors.

Up to 12,000 ft (3658 m)

In the majority of those ascending on foot the fully developed features of acute mountain sickness are uncommon. Few however escape some acute symptoms, and about half have symptoms if they stay more than twelve hours.

Climbing rates of 2000–2500 ft (610–750 m) per hour can be maintained on long ascents, but some undue increase in pulse rate has been noted, as has hyperpnoea. Resting pulse rate was not raised however.

Cheyne-Stokes (periodic) breathing during sleep has been noted as low as 9000 ft (2743 m) and a slight headache, light-headedness and irritability are not uncommon.

All these effects however soon wear off.

Up to 18,000 ft (5486 m)

Between 15,000 and 18,000 ft (4573 and 5486 m) acute symptoms are particularly liable to occur as the oxygen pressure is by this stage considerably reduced, and by the fact that at this altitude mountaineering parties move their camps up 2000–3000 ft (610–914 m) a day and thus expose themselves to relatively large falls in barometric pressure.

The majority of people suffer some ill effects and this is most marked in newcomers. Those who have been to altitude before are much less affected and some may have no symptoms until they ascend above this level.

Residents who are accustomed to living at altitudes up to 16,000 ft (4877 m) appear to suffer no ill effects. Sherpas can carry loads of 60 lb all day without signs of fatigue. The physical performance in newcomers is still inferior even after a long period, although this is not always appreciated.

Symptoms consist mainly of dyspnoea, muscular weakness, and lassitude with reduced endurance.

Film sequences taken on Everest in 1953 at this level showed men cutting steps with precision and climbing with apparently normal rhythm and balance. Climbing however required more effort.

Severe headaches, loss of appetite, nausea and vomiting were not uncommon. Appetite tended to remain poor and under the tented condition on Everest in 1953, the average loss of weight was 11 lb in 26 days. Men developed cravings for certain foods, such as tinned salmon and pineapple cubes, and they preferred to go without rather than eat distasteful food. The appetite for sweet foods was much increased, and the consumption of sugar doubled from 6 oz per man per day on the approach-march to 12 oz per man per day. As physical performance improved so did appetite and tolerance to a bulky diet.

Individuals became very conscious of hyperpnoea, especially at work. Periodic breathing was observed particularly whilst asleep. Cycles usually consisted of six respirations followed by a pause of about ten seconds. However a note made at 18,000 ft (5486 m) records observations on two men. In one the respiratory cycle consisted of two respirations, each lasting three seconds, followed by a ten second pause; in the other there were three respirations with a ten second pause.

Cyanosis became apparent and observers have commented on the absence of normal conversation at meals, with a reduction in casual activity and customary gaiety.

Initially there is a marked disinclination to make any mental effort—but this passed off after 14 days. Complicated mental work could be done accurately though more slowly and with more effort than at sea level.

Men slept 10–12 hours at night, though whether as well as at sea level is open to question. Occasional attacks of paroxysmal nocturnal dyspnoea were noted. In general if the individuals remained free from illness, symptoms seemed to last up to two weeks, gradually diminishing in severity.

The resting pulse ranged from 80–88 as compared with 50–70 in the same men at sea level. At work, sustained pulse rates of 120–140 were normal.

The blood pressure seemed unaffected although slight diastolic rise was noted in some men.

At 19,000 ft (5791 m)

Acclimatisation can occur to a marked degree as illustrated by the fact that ascents over steep and difficult ground can be carried out at a speed similar to that attained in the European Alps (up to 16,000 ft (4877 m)). Heavy loads can be carried and extreme exertion is possible but exhaustion after these efforts can be profound and men may take up to 48 hours to recover. Physical endurance whilst mountaineering was decreased and a six-hour day was normal average compared with a ten-hour day in Europe.

Objective evidence of acclimatisation is provided by work on a bicycle ergometer. After 20 days, work at 600 kg m/min was maximal, whereas after 40 days 1200 kg m/min was possible.

Concentration and memory seemed to improve after a period.

Subjectively however, permanent residence at this altitude, even under ideal conditions, was not considered possible and gradually increasing lethargy occurred.

Diminution of appetite and loss of weight occurred even under ideal conditions. Over a period of three months, a weight loss of up to 10 lb was noted in individuals weighing 155–175 lb at sea level. One man lost 8 lb in ten days and had to descend. Episodes of 'deterioration' can occur and cause men to become ill within a few hours. This process is reversed even after a small descent, to 15,000 ft (4572 m). Proneness to intercurrent infection has also been noted.

Blood values remain constant at this altitude. Haemoglobin estimates and red blood cell counts showed no change and remained static over a period of three months. No evidence of a change occurred even in men with evidence of deterioration.

Psychometric tests involving card sorting showed a definite increase in the percentage of delayed responses after nine weeks at this altitude.

Resting pulse is initially raised, but returns over a period of weeks to normal sea-level values.

From 20,000–22,000 ft (6096–6706 m)

Individual tolerance to altitude becomes more marked, and there is wide variation in performance and well-being from day to day, or even within the day.

Undue muscular fatigue can be caused by going for long periods without food—or by making too great a muscular effort for too long without rest. The beneficial effects from an easily assimilated carbohydrate (sugar) are more striking than at lower levels.

The more acute symptoms of oxygen lack may not be obvious for two reasons: time has already been spent acclimatising, and the reduction in capacity for work may prevent men placing camps too far apart. The curve relating height to barometric pressure is beginning to flatten out and the change of pressure within this range of altitude is less.

Mental activity is not severely impaired. The *Times* crossword puzzle was completed in normal sea-level time by one observer and gas analysis could be carried out for six hours a day by another, with relatively few mistakes in the calculations. Prose and poetry, subsequently published, have also been composed at this height.

Acclimatisation can still occur at 21,000 ft (6401 m) as observed by Somervell on Everest. On three successive occasions, 13, 17 and 19 May 1922, he climbed from 21,000 to 23,000 ft (6401 to 7010 m). On the first occasion 'each step was a hardship and every foot a fight', whilst on May 19th, 'the ascent occasioned no more discomfort than that produced by breathlessness'.

Confirmation is provided by Ward, who in 1953 twice ascended from 21,000 to about 24,000 ft (6401 to 7315 m) with an interval of three days. On the first occasion he was almost completely exhausted, whereas on the second his general condition was much improved.

Deterioration however does occur. In 1953, Lowe, after working for five days between 21,000 and 24,000 ft (6401 and 7315 m) without oxygen but with adequate shelter and food and fluid intake, suffered from loss of appetite, his general physical condition became worse, and his work output diminished. In

1961 a maximum work rate on the bicycle ergometer of 900 kg m/min was considered maximal against a sea-level value of 1800 kg m/min.

Food intake in 1953 averaged 3000–4000 kcal per day but there was an average weight loss of 4 lb in four weeks: extreme emaciation was reported by pre-war Everest parties. Oxygen had surprisingly little effect on acclimatised man at rest. During climbing there was a 20–50 per cent reduction in ventilation, though little increase in speed. There was however a feeling of increased energy and strength. Endurance was also much improved.

At 21,000 ft (6401 m) up to 50 per cent increase in resting pulse from a sea-level value of 70 to 90–100 per minute was noted.

From 22,000–26,000 ft (6706–7925 m)

Individual variation in tolerance to oxygen lack becomes more marked, as do the effects of oxygen lack.

Weakness, fatigue and shortness of breath become more marked. On Everest in 1953 two newcomers to these altitudes became exhausted.

Film shows feeble strokes with the ice-axe and considerable unsteadiness on the feet—but the climbers were unaware of the extent of their incapacity.

There is considerable impairment of mental performance. Routine jobs are done successfully, but those which require initiative take much longer and require more effort.

Some recovery from fatigue does occur. Thus Ward, though initially very fatigued, improved over a period of several days.

Lowe in 1953 at the end of nine days without oxygen within this altitude range said that only at the end of this time was he beginning to deteriorate.

Greene on Everest in 1933 remarked that deterioration started above 23,000 ft (7010 m) and that climbers ascended progressively more slowly on each ascent to 25,000 ft (7620 m).

Although the appetite of the mountaineers was good, considerable weight loss occurred.

Deterioration became more marked at 24,000 ft (7315 m) and in 1961 both West and Ward, who spent six and eight days respectively at this height, became increasingly nauseated.

Considerable mental impairment occurred and neither individual was able to appreciate his own or his companion's poor condition.

It is doubtful if any acclimatisation occurs at or above this height.

Oxygen increased general awareness and enjoyment of surroundings. It also increased endurance and decreased fatigue. Whilst some slept well without its use, most observers felt that it enhanced both the depth and the revivifying effect of sleep. It restored warmth to cold extremities.

Resting pulse-rates were raised.

At 25,000 ft (7620 m) the resting pulse in Ward was 108 as compared to a sea-level value of 66.

Oxygen uptake during maximal work in two individuals of the same build and acclimatisation were 1·6 litre/min and 2·0 litre/min. The lower uptake may represent evidence of deterioration as this individual became ill after five days at this altitude.

26,000–28,000 ft (7925–8534 m)

The effects of oxygen lack became most marked at these altitudes. However after acclimatisation at least six men have climbed to just above 28,000 ft (8534 m) on Everest without oxygen.

Some extracts from these accounts are recorded.

Norton in 1924 said that at 27,500 ft (8382 m) he began to see double. This was thought at the time to be due to oxygen lack, but was more probably due to incipient snow-blindness.

He records that

> Our pace was wretched. My ambition was to do 20 consecutive paces up hill without a pause to rest and pant: yet I never remember achieving it—thirteen was nearer the mark. The process of breathing in the intensely cold dry air, which caught the back of the larynx had a disastrous effect on poor Somervell's already

very bad sore throat and he had constantly to stop and cough. Every five or ten minutes we had to sit down for a minute or two and we must have looked a sorry couple.

He reached 28,000 ft (8534 m).

His climbing rate was from 26,800 to 28,100 ft (8200 to 8564 m) in six hours, that is, 200 ft (60 m)/hour.

Somervell in 1924 records that he took 7–10 complete respirations for each step upwards, and he had to rest for a minute every 20–30 yards (20–30 m).

Both he and Norton suffered severely from thirst, and when met on their return to a lower camp he commented 'we don't want the damned oxygen, we want drink.' He also comments that their appetite was very poor, that they ate from a sense of duty, and that it was impossible to take enough food.

Odell spent 11 days in 1924 at a level above 23,000 ft (7010 m) climbing on two occasions to 27,000 ft (8230 m). On each occasion he tried oxygen using an open circuit set, and reported that it had not benefited him in any way. In fact he climbed as well carrying the set but not using the oxygen, as he did using it. He was remarkably little fatigued by these ascents—was able to make geological observations (by profession he is a Professor of Geology) and suffered very little from thirst.

Climbing rates: From 23,000–25,300 ft (7010–7720 m) in three hours = approx 700 ft (213 m)/hour.
From 25,300–27,000 ft (7720–8230 m) in six hours = 300 ft (100 m)/hour.

Wager in 1933 noted on leaving his tent at 27,400 ft (8382 m) that excessive panting resulted in rapid loss of body heat.

Smythe in 1932 remarked that seldom did he feel warm on Everest.

He reached his highest point, 28,100 ft (8564 m) and comments on two curious phenomena.

All the time that I was climbing above I had a strange feeling that I was accompanied by a second person. I stopped to try to eat some mint cake; I carefully divided it and turned round with one half in my hand. It was almost a shock to find no-one to whom to give it.

When at 27,000 ft (8390 m)

> I saw two curious looking objects floating in the sky. They strongly resembled kite-balloons in shape but one possessed what appeared to be squat under-developed wings and the other a protuberance suggestive of a beak. They hovered motionless, but began slowly to pulsate, a pulsation incidentally much slower than my own heart beats. The two objects were very dark in colour, and were silhouetted sharply against the sky, or possibly a background of cloud.

He spent that night alone at 27,400 ft (8380 m), 'I woke after the best night I had yet had above the North Col'.

Whilst the first episode has been noted by other observers at sea level, the second was almost certainly due to hypoxia.

Shipton, his companion, describes climbing at this height as being 'like a sick man walking in a dream'.

The main features noted in this altitude range were those of physical and mental depression. Both thought and action were retarded, and insight was impaired.

An example of retardation is shown by Bourdillon on Everest in 1953 taking $1\frac{1}{2}$ hours to go through a procedure for detecting faults in a closed circuit oxygen apparatus, which at 21,000 ft (6401 m) took him 20 minutes.

Routine procedure can be carried out normally, but the increase in effort required to initiate thought or action was considerable.

Impairment of insight and judgement also occurred. After three days on the South Col at 26,000 ft (7925 m) Hunt's condition had deteriorated a great deal and despite a reeling and drunken gait he considered he was quite fit to lead the party on the descent. Hunt in his diaries seems not to have been fully aware of his condition.

A similar episode occurred to the author who on Mt Makalu in 1961 after eight days at and above 24,500 ft (7473 m) became unconscious, probably due to the effects of hypoxia and hypothermia. At no time did he have full insight into his condition, despite being a doctor.

The use of oxygen emphasised the previous blunting of mental faculties and enabled climbers to take an active interest in their surroundings. At rest, oxygen brought an immediate feeling of warmth, greatly improved recovery from fatigue and induced sound sleep. Whilst climbing, although giving no definite feeling of a 'boost', oxygen increased endurance, decreased fatigue, decreased the rate of breathing and greatly improved the climbing rate.

Evans and Bourdillon, using closed circuit oxygen, climbed from 26,000 to 27,500 ft (7925 to 8382 m) at a rate of 930 ft (300 m)/hour carrying loads of 43 lb. This is an Alpine rate of climb.

Hillary and Tensing using open circuit oxygen at 4 litre/min over much the same ground, climbed at a rate of 620 ft (183 m)/hour. No ill effects were noted on turning off the oxygen, provided the mountaineer rested. Sudden failure of oxygen during climbing caused acute dyspnoea, dizziness and weakness, and incontinence of urine. Slow failure passed unnoticed until increasing fatigue and breathlessness brought the climber to a halt.

Some degree of dehydration and weight loss seems inevitable at this altitude, as neither fluid nor calorie intake is sufficient.

28,000–29,000 ft (8534–8839 m)

Climbers have always used oxygen to ascend to the summit of Mt Everest.

In 1953 on Everest, Hillary and Tensing spent a night at about 28,000 ft (8534 m). They used sleeping oxygen for about four hours. From the final camp to the summit took five hours, a rate of climb of 200 ft (60 m)/hour.

In 1963 after climbing Everest by two different routes, four American mountaineers bivouacked without shelter at 28,400 ft (8650 m). Fortuitously it was not a particularly windy night and all survived. Two sustained serious frostbite and lost all their toes, and one man lost the tips of each little finger. The other two were less severely affected and lost no tissue. Each man however was so hypoxic and exhausted that he had difficulty in recalling details of the night.

Periods of up to an hour have been spent at rest on the top

of Everest without oxygen. Hillary spent ten minutes without it, before he became a little 'muzzy in the head'.

Some dehydration occurred in both Hillary and Tensing and both passed urine infrequently during the summit day and the day after. In addition both lost weight during this period (Hillary 4 lb in three days), possibly a combination of dehydration and tissue loss.

One Sherpa, Gompu, has climbed to the summit of Everest on two occasions. On the second occasion he removed his oxygen set for about 25 minutes. At rest he suffered no symptoms but when moving he became light-headed. Towards the end of the period he noted paraesthesiae in his legs which started in the calf and moved upwards to the thighs. He did not consider that he could remain indefinitely on the summit without oxygen.

An 18 year old boy, a stowaway on an aircraft, spent about five hours without oxygen at 29,000 ft (8839 m) and above at a temperature between $-4°C$ and $-6°C$. Although unconscious for most of this period he survived without any untoward sequelae (Pajares and Merayo 1970).

Reference

Pajares, C. and Merayo, F. (1970) *Aerospace Medicine* **41**, 1416.

CHAPTER NINETEEN

Mountain Sickness

Introduction

Illness due to the hypoxia of altitude is the result of an abnormal response to physiological stress rather than a separate disease entity.

Thus although a number of different disease patterns are described, the main aetiological factor is essentially the same.

Initially the term 'mountain sickness' was used to denote any physical or mental incapacity that occurred as a result of ascending to high altitude. The existence of these conditions has been known to travellers for centuries.

The early mountaineers were quick to note and describe any abnormality in physical or mental well being. Although to some it assumed an overwhelming importance others either ignored the symptoms or suffered little. This discrepancy may be explained by individual variation, fatigue, physical training, nutrition, and rate of ascent.

It has been suggested that geographical location influenced the severity of symptoms and that the height at which mountain sickness occurred varied with location. Barometric pressure levels for equivalent altitudes appear to be the same although there are variations with latitude, season and weather.

The term '*acute mountain sickness*' is used to denote an acute clinical condition characterised by symptoms of a general nature, which include headache, lassitude, weakness, nausea and vomiting, and which occurs within a few hours of ascending to altitude.

Sudden exposure to great altitude may cause death, and fatalities occurred on early balloon flights when insufficient oxygen was available.

The first comprehensive description of acute mountain sickness to appear in the Western literature was that of Father Joseph d'Acosta who gives the following account of crossing a pass of 14,000 ft (4267 m) in the Andes in 1570 (De Acosta 1850).

> I was surprised with such pangs of straining and casting as I thought to cast up my soul too; for having cast up meat, phlegm, and choller, both yellow and greene, in the end I cast up blood with the straining of my stomach.

He considered that this was due to 'the elements of aire (which is there so subtle and delicate as it is not proportionable with the breathing of man which requires more grosse and temperate aire)'.

Edward Whymper (Whymper 1879) was one of the first to attempt to investigate mountain sickness. He mounted an expedition to the Bolivian Andes, specifically for this purpose. He gives a good description of the condition, and comments that the clinical features did not immediately occur on ascending to altitude but took a few hours to develop. He distinguished between an acute transitory and a permanent form, and put forward a theory that the acute, temporary, condition was due to equalisation of the internal and external pressure of the body.

Joseph Barcroft (Barcroft 1925) gives a more detailed clinical description of acute mountain sickness or 'Seroche' as it is called in South America, occurring in individuals making an ascent by train from near sea level to 16,000 ft (4877 m). The clinical features either subsided after a few days or persisted to a lesser degree throughout the individual's stay at high altitude. Four of the eight members of Barcroft's party had to stay in bed for periods of up to four days; the remainder had symptoms which were not severe enough to be disabling. After the symptoms had subsided all eight were able to work for up to ten hours each day.

Later Barcroft lived in a decompression chamber in which the partial pressure of oxygen was reduced to that corresponding to 18,000 ft (5486 m) over a period of six days. During this period he complained of the typical symptoms of mountain sickness. These disappeared on his 'descent'.

Some degree of acute mountain sickness seems to affect every person who ascends to altitudes around 10,000–12,000 ft (3048–3658 m). The symptoms may vary considerably. Individual variation is very marked, and Longstaff climbed Mt Trisul 23,000 ft (7010 m) from a camp at 17,500 ft (5334 m), in one day, a total of 5500 ft (1675 m) ascent, without any symptoms (Longstaff 1950). Cases too have been recorded of men flying from Kathmandu 4000 ft (1219 m) to Solakhumbu 14,000 ft (4267 m) without symptoms, even after a stay of 48 hours at the higher altitude. But individuals can be completely prostrated and on one Himalayan expedition after an attempt was made to place a base camp at 17,000 ft (5182 m) by plane, several experienced mountaineers were forced to descend in order to recuperate.

Patho-Physiology

The following changes occurred in men acutely exposed to 14,100 ft (4300 m); all had some degree of symptoms.

Ventilation

Resting ventilation rose rapidly during two days from a sea-level value of 8·3 litre/min BTPS to 12·0 litre/min BTPS by day five.

The tidal volume roughly paralleled ventilation.

The rate of respiration showed a tendency to increase at two days and then return to sea-level values. After five days therefore a deeper breathing at normal rate occurred.

Arterial Blood Gas and pH

Arterial Po_2 rapidly declined on ascent reaching a minimum value of about 40 mmHg after two days. On the third day there was some recovery, and then a steady state Po_2 of about 50 mmHg was obtained.

Oxygen saturation seemed to be in accordance with the fall in arterial Po_2. It reached a steady state value of around 90 per cent after 14 days exposure.

Measurements of Pco_2 showed an initial rapidly developing fall in the first three days of exposure. The change then proceeded more slowly reaching a new value of 20 mmHg after 14 days.

The arterial pH reflected respiratory alkalosis, but the value after 14 days was not greatly different from that at sea level. The renal excretion of bicarbonate and fixed base was increased and partially compensated for the respiratory alkalosis induced by hypoxia.

The haemoglobin and haematocrit increased so that after 14 days the oxygen content of the blood returned essentially to sea-level values despite the reduced oxygen saturation.

Within three days of exposure to altitude a marked change in the body water content of each of the body's compartments had occurred. On the average a three-litre shift of fluid from extracellular to intracellular compartments was manifest together with an early reduction in plasma volume.

During the first three days the subjects experienced the most symptoms and this was the period when the major water shift occurred. After eight days the shift was complete and symptoms nonexistent (Carson et al. 1969).

As hypoxia causes cerebral vasodilatation and increased cerebral blood flow, and since the brain and cerebrospinal fluid are not compressible, there must be a shift of CSF away from the cerebral cavity. The pressure of the CSF is apparently raised and adsorption of CSF is increased temporarily until a new equilibrium is reached.

The increase in pressure of the CSF, subclinical fluid retention and mild cerebral oedema that occur on going to high altitude almost certainly accounts for the symptoms of acute mountain sickness. In addition papilloedema has been observed in one or two cases.

The more severe symptoms of acute mountain sickness may be related to the state of hydration. The fact that symptoms occur even in the presence of dehydration suggest that changes in internal water and the redistribution of blood volume may be important factors (Aoki and Robinson 1971).

The main symptoms are associated with the central nervous system and gastrointestinal tract. Symptoms such as nausea and vomiting are well known to indicate cerebral compression, whilst those referable to the central nervous system may be due to a combination of increased cerebral blood volume, increased pressure of the cerebrospinal fluid and increased brain tissue water leading to swelling of the brain (Shenkin and Bouzarth 1970).

Hypocapnia and respiratory alkalosis which occur on exposure to high altitude may help to decrease cerebral blood flow and thus relieve brain swelling. However the diminished plasma volume and dehydration observed with the hyper-ventilation of altitude (Buhlmann *et al.* 1970) may compromise brain perfusion and lead to further cerebral hypoxia.

Deviation of the CSF pH from the expected normal may possibly mean a relative incompetence in acclimatisation. Clinical studies at sea level demonstrate an association of mental disorientation with abnormal CSF pH (Posner *et al.* 1965; Bulger *et al.* 1965).

It appears that there may be an inverse relation between the ventilatory response to hypoxia and acute mountain sickness. A large response would reduce the Po_2 gradient between inspired and alveolar air and pulmonary blood and this would lessen the hypoxic stress (King and Robinson 1972).

A high carbohydrate and low fat diet generally reduced the clinical symptoms at altitude. Men who had a high carbohydrate diet showed considerably better performance in the heaviest work at altitude and could more than double the duration of their work on a tread mill (Consolazio *et al.* 1969).

Anorexia, a common symptom, may result in a 20–25 per

cent decrease in food intake. If anorexia can be avoided by careful and slow acclimatisation in individuals who are physically fit, the many biochemical changes attributed to hypoxia may be avoided.

It seems however that some degree of dehydration occurs during the first few days of exposure to hypoxia whether or no fluid intake is inadequate (Consolazio *et al.* 1972).

Clinical Features

Onset

Symptoms occur within a few hours of exposure to an altitude of about 10,000 ft (3000 m), and are commoner if the ascent has been rapid. Ascents on foot are usually associated with less pronounced clinical features.

Previous acclimatisation does not mean that ascent will be symptom free; lack of previous altitude experience does not result necessarily in severe symptoms.

Symptoms which may vary from being mild to prostrating become manifest only after several hours exposure. They reach their maximum severity during the first and second day, and then recede over the next two to four days. By the fifth day there are essentially no symptoms.

Above 17,500 ft (5334 m) mountaineers rarely experience more than a mild attack. As their endurance and capacity to work is reduced, differences of altitude between camps are rarely more than 2000 ft (610 m), so great differences in barometric pressure are not encountered.

The clinical features of acute mountain sickness seem to represent the reactions of the body to any severe stress. The following extracts from an account of men exposed to high ambient temperatures could well be substituted for that of acute mountain sickness:

> There is a sense of overwhelming oppression...Trifling work is fatiguing...A throbbing headache may develop and reach cruel intensity...Dizziness occurs...Dyspnoea may be a problem...

Lack of coordination reduces efficiency...Outbursts of irritability ...Judgement and morale decline...(Bean 1961).

Headache is perhaps the commonest symptom but the mechanism of its production is not clear. A number of theories have been put forward:

(i) Stretching of arterial walls from increased cerebral blood flow.

(ii) Distortion of cerebral structures due to cerebral oedema and increased cerebrospinal fluid pressure (Hansen and Evans 1970; Singh *et al.* 1969).

(iii) Extracerebral arteries may be the source of pain since ergotamine, which causes vasoconstriction of scalp arteries, provides relief (Carson *et al.* 1969).

Compression of the superficial temporal artery, which had become enlarged on acute exposure, was associated with the disappearance of headache in a number of subjects.

Water Balance

Loss of potassium, which is associated with alkalosis, may contribute to the clinical features of mountain sickness. Symptoms appeared to be worse and more prolonged in those on a low potassium diet. This group also tended to retain sodium and become more oedematous (Waterlow and Bunje 1966).

It has been suggested too that some subclinical water retention occurs on acute exposure to high altitude (Williams 1966).

Acetazolimide (Diamox), which acidifies the blood by its action on carbonic anhydrase has been used to prevent symptoms of acute mountain sickness (Cain and Dunn 1966). However besides acidifying the blood, acetazolimide is a diuretic and the removal of body fluid rather than its effect on pH may be its mode of action (Forwand *et al.* 1969).

Hypocapnia

Angelo Mosso, the Italian physiologist, noted that carbon

dioxide was lost at altitude because of increased respiration. He suggested that the resulting acapnia might be the cause of mountain sickness (Mosso 1898). Attempts to reduce acapnia by various methods such as breathing carbon dioxide and ingesting ammonium chloride have not met with great success in ameliorating symptoms.

Symptoms

The first symptoms are often a feeling of light-headedness, associated with an increase in the rate and depth of respiration.

Headache, usually frontal in position and often increasing in severity is also not uncommon, and there is increasing lassitude, fatigue and weakness. This is associated with an undue breath-lessness on exertion, dizziness, palpitations and a feeling of 'other-worldliness'.

Sleeplessness at night associated with nightmares is not un-usual, and periodic breathing may be especially noticeable. Cheyne–Stokes snoring has been described. Sleep is not usually beneficial and the individual wakes up feeling tired.

The hands and feet may feel cold, there is tachycardia and often cyanosis of the lips and nails is noticed.

Some individuals become very depressed, and there may be temporary auditory and visual impairment.

Appetite is generally poor whilst nausea and vomiting are relatively common. The lack of food intake further accentuates the feeling of weakness.

In the majority, symptoms subside after two to four days and normal activity is resumed.

It must be stressed that individual variation can be very marked, and previous visits to high altitude seem to minimise the symptoms, though this is not always the case. Some people may be very ill for a short period and deaths have been recorded within six hours of reaching high altitude.

In earlier case reports epistaxis and haemoptysis were com-monly noted. However these do not appear to be a common feature of acute mountain sickness. If haemoptysis occurs then the possibility of pulmonary oedema must be considered.

Cerebral and pulmonary oedema may represent more severe manifestations of mountain sickness.

The addition of cold stress to hypoxia (11,000 ft (3353 m)) impaired critical flicker frequency, which represents the general state of the excitability of the central nervous system (Nair *et al.* 1972).

This suggests that at high altitude both hypoxia and cold are factors to be considered in assessing cerebral function, and in the causation of acute mountain sickness.

Treatment

In general those who ascend slowly on foot to high altitude are less likely to suffer from acute mountain sickness than those who ascend rapidly by transport.

Various methods have been used to try to speed acclimatisation and reduce symptoms.

Drugs

A comparison of codeine with methylamphetamine showed that at 15,000 ft (4572 m) (simulated altitude) the performance of subjects was better with codeine. At 2000 ft (610 m) (simulated altitude) amphetamine enhanced performance (Carson *et al.* 1969).

250 mg of acetazolamide were given four times daily for two days before ascent to 14,100 ft (4300 m) and for three days afterwards. The results were compared with a placebo; and acetazolamide was found to produce a small rise in arterial Po_2, a reduction in Pco_2, a smaller rise in arterial pH, and a minimal reduction in symptoms. There was no change in performance (Carson *et al.* 1969).

Acetazolamide is a mild diuretic and it may be that its benefits are due to this. However, the primary action may be to create a metabolic acidosis to offset the respiratory alkalosis of altitude. It may also act by increasing concentration of H^+ ion in the cerebrospinal fluid and allowing a greater degree of hyperventilation which results in a higher Po_2 and lower Pco_2. An additional mechanism may be the influence of a higher CSF H^+ ion concentration on cerebral blood flow. On initial exposure to altitude the increase in cerebral blood flow is antagonised by a low P_{CO_2} and low concentration of H^+ ion in the CSF. On acclimatisation or acetazolamide administration the CSF H^+ ion concentration is restored to normal and cerebral blood flow increases (Gray *et al.* 1971).

Furosemide has been suggested as a useful prophylactic (Singh *et al.* 1969) but dehydration is a problem at high altitude and furosemide would aggravate the reduction in plasma volume. Its use on a group on arrival at 17,500 ft (5334 m) gave no relief from symptoms (Gray *et al.* 1971; Aoki and Robinson 1971). However, in subjects acclimatised for three weeks at 11,000 ft (3353 m) furosemide decreased oxygen debt, increased physical work capacity and increased oxygen uptake during exercise (Nair and Gopinath 1971).

Results suggest that ergotamine ameliorates headache, but gastrointestinal upset was an almost uniform side effect (Carson *et al.* 1969).

Diet

A high carbohydrate diet at simulated altitude (11,000 ft (3353 m)) resulted in a higher alveolar and arterial oxygen pressure, and a higher arterial oxygen saturation. Thus a high carbohydrate diet increases ventilation and improves oxygenation during acute exposure (Hansen *et al.* 1972).

Oxygen

Oxygen appears to have little effect.

The severity of acute mountain sickness during abrupt exposure to altitude may be greatly reduced without drug therapy providing

  (i) Individuals are physically fit prior to exposure.
 (ii) A minimal carbohydrate consumption of 320 gram/day is undertaken.

(iii) Normal food and fluid intake is maintained, especially as a natural diuresis occurs due to cold and hypoxia, with subsequent decrease in total body and intracellular water (Consolazio *et al.* 1972).

Ideally however individuals should be exposed gradually rather than abruptly. It is probably better to be physically fit, and for some degree of exercise to be taken during exposure.

References

Aoki, V. S. and Robinson, S. M. (1971) *Journal of Applied Physiology* **31**, 363.

Barcroft, J. (1925) The respiratory function of the blood. In, *Lessons from High Altitude*. Cambridge University Press.

Bean, W. B. (1961) *Pathologic physiology*. Saunders: Philadelphia.

Buhlmann, A. A., Spiegel, M. and Straub, P. W. (1970) *Lancet* **1**, 1021.

Bulger, R. J., Schrier, R. W., Arend, W. P. and Swanson, A. G. (1965) *New England Journal of Medicine* **274**, 433.

Cain, S. M. and Dunn, J. E. (1966) *Journal of Applied Physiology* **20**, 882.

Carson, R. P., Evans, W. O., Shields, J. L. and Hannon, J. P. (1969) *Federation Proceedings. Federation of American Societies for Experimental Biology* **28**, 1085.

Consolazio, C. F., Matoush, L. O., Johnson, H. L., Krzywicki, H. J., Daw, T. A. and Isaac, G. J. (1969) *Federation Proceedings. Federation of American Societies for Experimental Biology* **28**, 937.

Consolazio, C. F., Johnson, H. L., Krzywicki, H. J. and Daws, T. A. (1972) *American Journal of Clinical Nutrition* **25**, 23.

Consolazio, C. F., Johnson, H. L. and Krzywicki, H. J. (1972) *Environmental sciences. Physiological adaptations. Desert and mountains. Ed.* Yousef, M. K., Horvath, S. M. and Bullard, R. W. Academic Press: New York and London.

De Acosta, J. (1880) *The natural and moral history of the Indes.* London.

Forwand, S. A., Landowne, M., Follansbee, J. N. and Hansen, J. E. (1968) *New England Journal of Medicine* **279**, 839.

Gray, G. W., Bryan, A. C., Frayser, R., Houston, C. S. and Rennie, I. D. B. (1971) *Aerospace Medicine* **42**, 81.

Hansen, J. E. and Evans, W. O. (1970) *Archives of Environmental Health* **21**, 666.

Hansen, J. E., Hartley, L. H. and Hogan, R. P. (1972) *Journal of Applied Physiology* **33**, 441.

King, A. B. and Robinson, S. M. (1972) *Aerospace Medicine* **43**, 419.

Longstaff, T. G. (1956) *This my voyage.* Murray: London.

Mosso, A. (1898) *Life of man on the High Alps.* T. Fisher Unwin: London.

Nair, C. S. and Gopinath, P. M. (1971) *Aerospace Medicine* **42**, 268.

Nair, C. S., Malhotra, M. S. and Gopinath, P. M. (1972) *Aerospace Medicine* **43**, 1097.

Posner, J. B., Swanson, A. G. and Plum, F. (1965) *Archives of Neurology* **12**, 479.

Shenkin, H. A. and Bouzarth, W. F. (1970) *New England Journal of Medicine* **282**, 1465.

Singh, I., Khanna, P. K., Srivastava, M. C., Lal, M., Roy, S. B. and Subramanyam, C. S. V. (1969) *New England Journal of Medicine* **280**, 175.

Waterlow, J. C. and Bunje, H. W. (1966) *Lancet* **2**, 655.

Whymper, E. (1892) *Travels amongst the Great Andes of the equator.* Murray: London.

Williams, E. S. (1966) *Proceedings of the Royal Society. Series B* **165**, 266.

CHAPTER TWENTY

'Monge's Disease'

Introduction

'Chronic mountain sickness', 'chronic seroche' and 'Monge's disease' are names that have been given to a clinical picture that appears when individuals normally acclimatised to and residing at high altitude lose their ability to adapt to the low oxygen tension at which they have been living for a long period without symptoms. On descent to lower altitudes the clinical picture is reversed.

To make a genuine diagnosis it must be established that there is no pulmonary disease; the thoracic cage must function normally; and there must be no history of mining work.

A clinical picture mimicking Monge's disease can be produced in a high-altitude native by lung diseases such as silicosis or pulmonary fibrosis, which impair oxygen diffusion. Other forms of alveolar hypoventilation secondary to obesity, kyphoscoliosis or pulmonary emphysema when occurring at high altitude may also give a clinical picture similar to Monge's disease.

It has been suggested that these conditions be termed Monge's syndrome or secondary chronic mountain sickness (Monge and Monge 1966; Arias-Stella 1971). However these terms are confusing and diminish the merit of Monge's original concept and description.

It should be realised that as Monge himself noted some people never completely acclimatise to high altitude despite months of residence.

Doubt has been expressed as to whether Monge's disease does in fact exist, or whether it is an as yet unexplained condition associated with abnormal lung function.

History

The original description of this condition was made by Monge (Monge 1928) in 1928. He distinguished a number of different clinical variations of this condition but these distinctions are no longer considered as valid.

The number of documented cases is relatively small. Arias-Stella (1971) collected 81 cases from the literature.

Of these, 62 were men and 19 women. Twenty had some pathology which could be associated with alveolar hypoventilation (obesity, kyphoscoliosis, etc).

The mortality rate was 12 per cent (7 out of 81).

All these cases were observed in South America. Despite a number of surveys carried out of high-altitude populations in Asia, mainly on the inhabitants of the high Himalayan valleys, no cases have yet been recorded from this area.

Lahiri, who has worked in both areas, records that he saw a few cases in South America, whereas he has seen none despite several years work in the Himalaya (Ward 1965; Lahiri and Milledge 1971). Climatic differences may be a factor in this incidence.

Aetiology

Evidence that has accumulated seems to suggest that in view of the clinical and physiological findings Monge's disease is a particular variety of alveolar hypoventilation with similar respiratory, haematological, cardiovascular and neuropsychiatric features.

The mechanism for hypoventilation is not clear. Some ascribe it to a decreased sensitivity of the respiratory centre to carbon dioxide (Hurtado 1960), whilst others consider that the alveolar hypoventilation may be due to an irreversible insensitivity of the peripheral chemoreceptors to hypoxic stimuli, the result of chronic exposure to hypoxia (Severinghaus et al. 1966).

The pathophysiology of the hypoventilation of Monge's disease seems to be comparable with that of primary or idio-pathic alveolar hypoventilation.

No cases of Monge's disease have had their lungs exhaustively examined so far, so some condition such as centrilobular emphysema might easily have been missed. Also minor degrees of silicosis or other lung disease associated with mining may have been overlooked (Heath 1971). However moderate changes in lung function do not generally produce alveolar hypoventilation.

Physiological Data

Patients with Monge's disease show lower values of arterial oxygen saturation, and higher figures for haemoglobin and

Table 32.   Oxygenation and blood-pressure in Monge's disease

	Monge	HA native	SL residents
Mean arterial oxygen saturation, %	69·6	81·1	95·7
Haemoglobin, g%	24·8	20·1	14·7
Haematocrit, %	79·3	59·4	44·1
		mmHg	
Mean R atrial pressure	3·9	2·9	2·6
Mean R vent pressure	29	15	9·0
Systole ⎫	64	34	22
Mean ⎬ Pulmonary arterial pressure	47	23	12
Diastole ⎭	33	13	6
Mean pulmonary wedge pressure	5·7	6·9	6·2
Systole ⎫	136	124	127
Mean ⎬ Systemic arterial pressure	105	91	94
Diastole ⎭	88	72	70

haematocrit, than those observed in normal high-altitude dwellers.

The degree of pulmonary hypertension in Monge's disease was higher than in healthy high-altitude natives.

The pulmonary wedge pressures were no different from healthy high-altitude natives.

Clinical Features

Monge's condition is generally observed at altitudes exceeding 10,000 ft (3000 m) and may develop either in high-altitude natives or high-altitude visitors, that is subjects who have ascended to and acclimatised at these altitudes.

Most cases seem to occur in young male adults, although some cases have been recorded in women.

The absence of a history of mining work, of previous pulmonary disease, of previous pulmonary dysfunction and the reversal of the clinical picture on descent to sea level are necessary criteria before a correct diagnosis can be made.

The main clinical manifestations are related to (a) severe hypoxaemia, (b) severe polycythaemia, (c) accentuated pulmonary hypertension and (d) neurological and psychic disturbance.

The diagnosis is relatively simple in the advanced case, but early cases are difficult to distinguish.

Decreasing exercise tolerance, associated with a gradually increasing fatigue were the commonest symptoms. Headache, dizziness, paraesthesia and a feeling of somnolence were frequent.

Cyanosis and clubbing of the finger were also common.

Patients with extreme cyanosis often had signs of congestive cardiac failure, whilst the pulmonary second sound was increased in most cases, and was associated with a systolic murmur in some.

The diastolic pressure was often raised, and some cases had systolic hypertension.

X-Ray Photographs

These showed a variable degree of cardiac enlargement mainly due to right ventricular and right atrial enlargement.

Hilar vascular engorgment, associated with a prominent pulmonary artery was also found.

Electrovector Cardiographic Studies

The pulmonale P-wave pattern was found in most cases.

An accentuated degree of right A QRS deviation or upward A QRS positions was frequently seen in association with the RS precordial pattern.

Tall R waves over the left precordial leads were observed in some of the more severe cases.

The ischaemic T-wave pattern was often seen over the right pre-cordial leads.

Changes on Descending to Sea Level

Clinical

The general clinical condition improved considerably. Cerebral signs disappeared rapidly, as did the feeling of fatigue and cyanosis.

Heart size progressively diminished, particularly in those who spent the longest time at sea level.

Signs of right ventricular and right atrial overload almost disappeared.

Physiological Changes

Arterial oxygen saturation became normal. Haemoglobin and haematocrit diminished—the greatest fall occurring in those who spent the longest time at sea level.

Mean pulmonary artery pressure fell, as did the pulmonary resistance and right ventricular work.

The greatest change in mean pulmonary arterial pressure occurred during the first few days of residence at sea level. This reduction increased as the time at sea level increased.

Table 33.   Physiological changes after descending to sea level in three cases of Monge's disease (Penaloza *et al.* 1971)

	Hct. %	Hb. g%	Art. O$_2$ satn. %	R Atrium mean	Blood pressure mmHg			Pulmonary wedge mean	Systemic mean
					Pulmonary artery				
					Systolic	Diastolic	Mean		
High altitude	83	27	75	5	74	43	55	7	100
Sea level for three days	80	25	95	9	42	22	34	10	103
High altitude	84	27	65·5	2	68	38	53		110
Sea level for eleven days	79	21·5	92·5	1	35	15	26		95
High altitude	86	23	67	6	78	48	62	6	100
Sea level for 60 days	50	17	98	3	37	9	24	5	87

Chest X-Ray

There was a reduction in cardiac size and the prominence of the pulmonary artery and the density of vascular markings also diminished.

Treatment

The clinical course is always unfavourable whilst the patient stays at high altitude. The definitive cure therefore is to descend to sea level. A return to high altitudes may result in a recurrence of the condition.

Some palliation may be obtained by bleeding. Sime (Sime 1971) reported results on six patients treated in this fashion. The arterial oxygen saturation improved and pulmonary hypertension decreased. The cardiac output did not vary significantly, neither did the haematocrit.

	Mean hct %	Mean art. O_2 saturation %	Mean pulmonary arterial pressure mmHg
Before bleeding	72	63·8	39
5 days after bleeding	66	73·4	30

The improved arterial oxygen saturation might be due to improved ventilation after bleeding, but in Monge's disease the primary cause is usually considered to be alveolar hypoventilation, the result of a diminished sensitivity of the respiratory centre or peripheral chemoreceptors.

The use of oxygen produces an increase in arterial oxygen saturation and this is associated with an improvement in the neuropsychiatric symptoms.

The pulmonary artery pressure decreases slightly more than in healthy high-altitude natives. This suggests that in Monge's disease there is a greater degree of arteriolar constriction.

Since Monge's disease is a chronic condition, oxygen inhalation even for several days is unlikely to result in any significant diminution in the excessive polycythaemia or in structura changes of the heart or pulmonary vessels.

By contrast acute forms of high-altitude disease, such as pulmonary oedema, often improve rapidly and even recover after a relatively short term administration of oxygen.

References

Arias-Stella, J. (1971) Chronic mountain sickness. Pathology and definition. In, *High altitude physiology. Ed.* Porter, R. and Knight, J. Ciba Foundation Symposium. Churchill Livingstone: Edinburgh and London.

Heath, D. (1971) In, *High altitude physiology. Ed.* Porter, R. and Knight, J. Ciba Foundation Symposium. Churchill Livingstone: Edinburgh and London.

Lahiri, S. and Milledge, J. S. (1971) In, *High altitude physiology. Ed.* Porter, R. and Knight, J. Ciba Foundation Symposium. Churchill Livingstone: Edinburgh and London.

Monge, M. and Monge, C. (1966) *High altitude diseases: Mechanism and management.* Thomas: Springfield, Illinois.

Monge, C. (1928) *Anales de la Facultad de medicina. University St Marcos, Lima* **11**, 1–316.

Penaloza, D., Sime, F. and Ruiz, L. (1971) Cor pulmonale in chronic mountain sickness: present concept of Monge's disease. In, *High altitude physiology. Ed.* Porter, R. and Knight, J. Ciba Foundation Symposium. Churchill Livingstone: Edinburgh and London.

Severinghaus, J. W., Bainton, C. R. and Carcelen, A. (1966) *Respiratory Physiology* **1**, 308.

Sime, F. *et al.* (1971) In, *High altitude physiology. Ed.* Porter, R. and Knight, J. Ciba Foundation Symposium. Churchill Livingstone: Edinburgh and London.

Ward, M. P. (1967) In, *Report of I.B.P. Party to North Bhutan. Ed.* Ward, M. P., Jackson, F. S. and Turner, R. W. D.

CHAPTER TWENTY-ONE

High-altitude Pulmonary Oedema

Probably the earliest recorded case of high altitude pulmonary oedema was that of Dr Jacottet, a physician of Chamonix, who died at the Vallot Hut, 14,300 ft (4347 m) after climbing Mt Blanc, 15,580 ft (4807 m).

The following is the original description as given by Angelo Mosso (Mosso 1894).

On the 1st of September, 1891, after two days rest in the Vallot Hut 14,300 ft (4347 m), during which Jacottet seemed to feel better than he did at first, he climbed to the summit (15,800 ft (4807 m)), remained there an hour and then returned to the Hut. During the night he did not sleep, and coughed much and complained at breakfast of a headache and lack of appetite. During the morning he wrote a letter to his brother at Vienna, in which he remarked that he had passed so bad a night that he would not wish the like to his worst enemy. His distress increased to such a degree that Imfeld advised him to descend to Chamonix, but he refused. He wrote another letter to one of his friends, telling him that he was suffering from mountain sickness like the others, but that he meant to study the influence of atmospheric depression, and acclimatise himself. This was, alas, his last letter. He afterwards threw himself off his bed trembling with cold.

On the 2nd September at 3.00 a.m. violent shivering fits seized him, and soon he was no longer able to carry his glass to his mouth himself; he seemed as though paralysed and began to wander. Oxygen was given to him to breathe, but without result. The respiration was very superficial (60–70 breaths per minute), the pulse irregular (between 100 and 120), the temperature 38·3°C.

Towards six o'clock in the evening he suddenly ceased to speak, became somnolent, and then the death agony began. His face grew pale, and towards 2.00 a.m., he expired in the glacier hut, a victim to his devotion to science, like a soldier on the field of battle.

The post-mortem was carried out by Dr Wizard of Chamonix. The relevant parts read as follows:

Heart: Normal, valves competent.
Lungs: Violet colour, swollen, bilateral congestion.
  Considerable oedema. Bronchial mucous membranes much infected. On cut section—frothy fluid, congestion evenly distributed.
[The diagnosis was] Capillary bronchitis, and lobular pneumonitis. The more immediate cause of death was therefore probably a suffocative catarrh accompanied by acute oedema of the lung.

The description is very suggestive. Previous to this attack Dr Jacottet had suffered from some 'indisposition' and had not been able to help some workmen out of a crevasse.

Mosso also describes another case with similar clinical features occurring in a fit 22 year-old soldier. The initial diagnosis was penumonia, and Mosso finally concluded that this case was 'inflammation of the lung arising from paralysis of the vagus nerve.'

Probably the first case recorded in the Himalaya was that of a European who developed 'pulmonary oedema' during an attempt to climb Mt Godwin-Austen, 28,523 ft (8680 m) in 1902 (Dyhrenfurth 1955). He recovered.

It seems likely that cases occurred on the pre-war expeditions to Mt Everest but they may have been misdiagnosed.

For instance in 1921 (Howard-Bury 1922) a physician, Dr A. M. Kellas, died of 'heart failure' at 17,000 ft (5182 m) on the March-In, through Tibet. During this expedition another European is described as being sent to lower levels with a similar condition.

On both the 1933 and 1936 Expeditions (Ruttledge 1934, 1937), Ongdi, a Sherpa, suffered from 'double pneumonia'. He recovered sufficiently to carry heavy loads.

In 1934 on another Himalaya peak, Nanga Parbat 26,658 ft (8100 m), a German mountaineer died of 'pneumonia with oedema of the lungs' (Bauer 1956), whilst in 1954 on Mt Godwin-Austen (K2) a fit young Italian guide died at 19,000 ft (5791 m), despite the use of oxygen (Desio 1964).

Hurtado (Hurtado 1937) was probably the first to suggest that the clinical picture of pulmonary oedema was due to high altitude alone, and not an infective process. He described the case of a Peruvian Indian who became ill after returning from Lima (sea level) to Casapalca, 13,665 ft (4140 m). On returning to sea level his condition improved.

Other observers (Lundberg 1952; Lizarraga 1955) have recorded cases in South American populations, whilst Houston (Houston 1960) emphasized the importance of this condition to those who ski and climb.

Indian observers (Singh *et al.* 1965) have recorded cases occurring in men posted to high altitude.

The existence of this condition as a clinical entity is now well established, and it seems likely that minor cases may be more frequent than expected.

Steele (Steele 1972) reported a number of cases on the International Everest Expedition, the majority of whom recovered after treatment at lower altitudes and returned to take part in the attempted ascent of the peak by the South-west Face.

Aetiology

Catheter studies have confirmed that pulmonary hypertension is present at high altitude and this is especially so during exercise (Rotta *et al.* 1956). In pulmonary oedema, pulmonary hypertension may be very marked reaching 144/104 in one case (Severinghaus 1971).

There is no evidence of left ventricular failure in recorded cases, and post mortem studies show no evidence of enlargement or dilatation of the left ventricle, nor of underlying cardiac pathology.

The main pathological features are widespread oedema of the alveoli, perivascular haemorrhage, intravascular thrombosis, dilated arterial and arteriolar bed and congested capillaries. Occasionally a hyaline membrane has been reported. This could be explained by alveolar fluid from which water had been re-adsorbed after desaturation and precipitation of proteins (Arias-Stella and Kruger 1963; Hultgren *et al.* 1962).

Catheter studies on a patient with pulmonary oedema who had a very small patent foramen ovale revealed no evidence of increased left atrial pressure (Fred *et al.* 1962).

As the perivascular spaces are the points of lowest pressure in the lung, perivascular cuffing occurs as the earliest form of pulmonary oedema. Only when these spaces are completely distended does their pressure rise above the pressure of the alveoli, and water is forced into the alveoli. In animal experiments in which hypoxic pulmonary oedema was induced by breathing 8 per cent oxygen when exercising, the oedema was mainly perivascular (Severinghaus 1971).

There is little evidence that hypoxia produces an alteration in capillary permeability. However an increase in lymph flow from the right lymphatic duct in dogs exposed to simulated altitudes up to 21,000 ft (6401 m) has been recorded. The flow diminished when pure oxygen was given (Warren and Drinker 1942).

Though the pulmonary lymphatics are dilated there is no direct evidence of obstruction (Arias-Stella and Kruger 1963).

That peripheral vasoconstriction occurs during the initial period of acclimatisation is inferred from cold hands and feet (Barcroft 1925). Blood pressure studies confirm this view (Hultgren and Spickard, 1960) and oxygen induces a feeling of warmth at great altitude (Ward 1968). Peripheral arteriolar vasoconstriction has also been noted (Durand and Martineaud 1971).

Cold also causes peripheral vasoconstriction, and this is especially so with any degree of cold injury. Immersion in cold water has been associated with pulmonary oedema and death at altitude (Horrobin and Cholmondeley 1972).

A low level of arterial P_{CO_2} causes contraction of peripheral veins (Wood and Roy 1970; Weil *et al.* 1971) and the thoracic blood volume may be increased.

Acute anoxia does not appear to immediately increase thoracic blood volume, though an increase has been noted in high-altitude natives (Monge *et al.* 1956).

Some degree of water retention may occur at altitude even when clinical oedema is absent (Williams 1966). Potassium loss with sodium- and water-retention has also been reported (Waterlow and Bunje 1966) and gravitational oedema of the eyelids when recumbent for long periods has also been observed (Ward 1968).

Diuresis on descent from altitude has been described (Sutton 1973).

Low oxygen tension may produce hypothalamic lesions, causing an increase in pulmonary blood volume and oedema (Maire and Patton, 1956).

Cold injury to the lungs may also be implicated, but this seems unlikely as temperatures much lower than those observed at high altitude have been recorded in Polar regions without pulmonary oedema.

Humoral factors such as serotonin which produces pulmonary hypertension in dogs have also been considered (Borst *et al.* 1957).

Vigorous exercise will greatly increase the blood return to the right side of the heart, and so tend to overload the pulmonary circulation.

Any respiratory infection will increase the rate of fluid secretion in the respiratory tract and may increase the permeability of the pulmonary capillaries.

A block to pulmonary blood flow may occur in some part of the lung due to embolism, thrombosis or intense vasoconstriction. Therefore another mechanism in the aetiology of high-altitude pulmonary oedema may be that the hypoxic vasoconstriction is uneven throughout the lung. Thus flow through the capillaries in less vasoconstricted areas will be torrential, producing oedema (Hultgren 1969).

A similar position may be reached by supposing that the initial vasoconstriction breaks down in certain areas (Davies 1973).

Both these explanations account for the findings of patchiness in the distribution of oedema seen at autopsy and on x-ray.

Clinical Features

Young, well muscled males seem to be more at risk than females. The late 'teens and early 20s seem to be the period when individuals are most susceptible. Rapid exposure, associated with hard exercise, are precipitating factors.

Most cases occur under 12,000–15,000 ft (3600–4500 m), though an occasional case has been reported from higher altitudes.

Thoroughly acclimatised patients returning to altitude after a stay at lower levels seem to be more at risk than those who are ascending for the first time, and the main period of risk appears to be within 12 to 72 hours after ascent. The association of physical exercise is not clear cut, yet young males are less likely to rest on ascending to altitude, especially if they are returning from lower levels.

Once established, pulmonary oedema may be aggravated by exercise and mountaineers, especially those with a restricted holiday, may be inclined to 'press on', in the face of a mild attack.

Individual susceptibility occurs and recurrent attacks in the same individual have been reported. Whether there is a familial as well as an individual susceptibility is open to question.

Occasionally fulminating cases occur in whom no form of therapy appears to influence the outcome.

Sub-clinical cases of pulmonary oedema may be commoner than generally realised. One of the most annoying features of first ascent to altitude is a chronic, irritative, nonproductive cough. Episodes of paroxysmal nocturnal dyspnoea have also been recorded, which are relieved by elevating the upper part of the body. Other symptoms such as dyspnoea at rest are not uncommon.

Symptoms

Undue fatigue and weakness followed by increasing shortness of breath and a mild cough are the commonest symptoms. A productive cough with blood-tinged sputum or a frank haemoptysis may follow.

Other symptoms include headache, nausea, vomiting and palpitations.

Most of these symptoms—other than haemoptysis—are normal on ascending to altitude and it is the degree that is important in diagnosis.

Cases may present with cerebral symptoms such as irrational behaviour. This is presumably due to impaired lung diffusion.

In the majority of cases there is no evidence of infection, the temperature is normal and chills are absent.

Signs

Tachycardia and rapid respiration are common. Cyanosis may be marked. The blood pressure is usually within normal limits.

There is no clinical evidence of heart failure, the heart sounds are normal, and there are no murmurs. Neck veins are not distended and there is no hepatic tenderness or enlargement.

Crepitations are usually found at the lung bases but they may be more widespread.

Investigations

Haemoglobin and packed cell volume in one series was lower than normal values for resident high-altitude natives, but as these patients had just returned from sea level this was to be expected.

The sedimentation rate and white cell count are normal.

ECG changes indicate right ventricular strain or hypertrophy, together with tachycardia.

After treatment, there is a decrease in heart rate, a lowering of the P wave and a decrease in the degree of right ventricular strain.

Chest X-Rays

In the acute phase there are bilateral, asymmetrical, patchy areas—though occasionally these are unilateral.

A hilar opacity with sparing of the periphery and bases is common.

Enlargement of the pulmonary vessels may be marked.

Cardiac enlargement seems very uncommon although the hilar vessels are enlarged, and the pulmonary artery is prominent. This prominence disappears on recovery.

In high-altitude natives returning to high altitudes from sea level, some measure of right ventricular enlargement may be present in any event.

Progress

Death whilst undergoing treatment has been reported both in hospital and in the field. It is possible too that death occurring in acute fulminating mountain sickness (acute seroche) may be due to the onset of acute pulmonary oedema. These cases go into a shock-like state, but show no clinical evidence of pulmonary oedema.

With adequate treatment most patients recover in a few days.

Treatment

Prevention

An increasing number of people are visiting high-altitude areas due to improved transport. In South America travel between the altiplano and coast may be undertaken many times in the year. Increasing use of aircraft also lifts travellers from low to high levels in a matter of hours.

Mountaineering and skiing have increased in popularity and with this the incidence of pulmonary oedema.

It seems possible that a considerable number of mild cases occur without full-blown symptoms.

Susceptible subjects are those who have experienced previous attacks and all previously acclimatised individuals returning to high altitude after a stay at lower levels.

Despite the prophylactic use of drugs, e.g. Furosemide, the

only real protection is gained through acclimatisation which can sometimes be a lengthy process. Adequate time should always be allowed for acclimatisation, especially in a susceptible person. On arrival at altitude a brief period of rest and relative inactivity is wise. Any undue cough, shortness of breath, mental aberration, or haemoptysis must be regarded as pulmonary oedema and treated as such.

Any person with a pulmonary infection should be forbidden to ascend to high altitude, and ascent in any event should be slow.

Curative

The patient should be rapidly removed to lower altitudes if transport facilities are available. If possible the patient should be taken to hospital where absolute bed rest and continuous oxygen are available.

Immediate treatment includes the positioning of the patient in a position where oedema is dependent—i.e. he should sit rather than lie down. Continuous oxygen, if available, should be given. The use of rotating tourniquets has been advocated. In the absence of tourniquets, handkerchiefs may be used. These are placed on three limbs at a time, as close to the trunk as possible. They should not occlude the artery—i.e. the pulse distal to the tourniquet must be palpable—but the venous return should be obstructed. Every five to ten minutes one tourniquet is removed and placed on the free limb and this is continued in an orderly manner either in a clockwise or anticlockwise direction (Sutton 1973).

This is a simple and effective method of reducing the venous return to the heart and lungs and will help to prevent overloading.

Morphia (15 mg IM), which dilates the peripheral veins (Herney *et al.* 1966) and allays fear can be used, preferably by the medically qualified.

An antidiuretic such as Lasix (Furosemide) should be injected, 80–120 mg IM immediately, followed by 40–80 mg every six to eight hours. I/V Cortisone has also been used.

Oxygen equipment for use in emergencies should always be available in parties going to altitudes over 15,000–18,000 ft (4572–5486 m).

It must be stressed that death has occurred within a few hours in fit young people despite the use of oxygen and other measures.

References

Arias-Stella, J. and Kruger, H. (1965) *Archives of Pathology* **76**, 147.

Barcroft, J. (1925) Respiratory function of the blood. In, *Lessons from high altitude*. Cambridge University Press.

Bauer, P. (1956) *The siege of Nanga Parbat*. Hart Davis: London.

Borst, H. G., Berglund, E. and McGregor, M. (1957) *Journal of Clinical Investigation* **36**, 669.

Davies, H. (1973) *Lancet* **1**, 999.

Desio, A. (1964) Personal communication.

Durand, J. and Martineaud, J. P. (1971) Resistance and capacitance vessels of the in permanent and temporary residents at high altitude. In, *High altitude physiology. Ed.* Porter, R. and Knight, J. Ciba Foundation Symposium. Churchill Livingstone: Edinburgh and London.

Dyhrenfurth, G. O. (1955) *To the third Pole*. Werner Laurie.

Fred, H. L., Schmidt, A. M., Bates, T. and Hecht, H. H. (1962) *Circulation* **25**, 929.

Herney, R. P., Vasko, J. W., Brawley, R. K., Oldham, H. N. and Morrow, A. G. (1966) *American Heart Journal* **72**, 242.

Horrobin, D. F. and Cholmondeley, H. G. (1972) *East African Medical Journal* **49**, 327.

Houston, C. S. (1960) *New England Journal of Medicine* **263**, 478.

Howard and Bury, C. K. (1922) *Mt Everest. The reconnaissance*. Arnold: London.

Hultgren, H. N. and Spickard, W. (1960) *Stanford Medical Bulletin* **18**, 76.

Hultgren, H. N., Spickard, W. and Lopez, C. (1962) *British Heart Journal* **24**, 95.

Hultgren, H. N. (1969) In, *Biomedicine of high terrestrial elevations. Ed.* Hegnauer, A. H. U.S. Army Research Institute of Environmental Medicine, Clearinghouse for Federal Scientific and Technical Information: Springfield, Va.

Hurtado, A. (1937) *Aspectos fisiologicos y patologicos de la vida en la altura.* Imp. Edit. Rimas. S.A.: Lima.

Lizarraga, L. (1955) *Anales de la Facultad de medicina. Lima* **38**, 244.

Lundberg, E. (1952) *Edema agudo del pulmon en el Seroche.* Conferencia sustentada en la Association Medica de Yauli Oraya.

Maire, F. W. and Patton, H. D. (1956) *American Journal of Physiology* **184**, 345.

Monge, C., Cazorla, A., Whittembury, C., Sakata, Y. and Rizo-Patron, C. (1956) *Anales de la Facultad de medicina. Lima* **39**, 498.

Mosso, A. (1894) *Life of man on the High Alps.* T. Fisher Unwin: London.

Rotta, A., Canepa, A., Hurtado, A., Velasquez, T. and Chavez, R. (1956) *Journal of Applied Physiology* **9**, 328.

Ruttledge, H. (1934) *Everest 1933.* Hodder and Stoughton: London.

Ruttledge, H. (1939) *Everest. The unfinished adventure.* Hodder and Stoughton: London.

Severinghaus, J. W. (1971) Trans-arterial leakage: a possible mechanism of high altitude pulmonary oedema. In, *High altitude physiology. Ed.* Porter, R. and Knight, J. Ciba Foundation Symposium. Churchill Livingstone: Edinburgh and London.

Singh, I., Kapila, C. C., Khanna, P., Nanda, R. B. and Rao, B. D. P. (1965) *Lancet* **1**, 229.

Steele, P. (1972) *Doctor on Everest.* Hodder and Stoughton.

Sutton, J. (1973) *Alpine Journal* **78**, 153.

Ward, M. P. (1968) *Diseases occurring at altitudes exceeding 17,500 ft.* M.D. Thesis. University of Cambridge.

Warren, M. F. and Drinker, C. K. (1942) *American Journal of Physiology* **136**, 207.

Waterlow, J. C. and Bunje, H. W. (1966) *Lancet* **2**, 655.

Weil, J. V., Byrne-Quinn, E., Battock, D. J., Grover, R. F. and Chidsey, C. A. (1971) *Clinical Science* **40**, 235.

Williams, E. S. (1966) *Proceedings of the Royal Society. Series B* **165**, 266.

Wood, J. E. and Roy, S. B. (1970) *American Journal of Medical Science* **259**, 56.

CHAPTER TWENTY-TWO

Thrombosis

History

A number of major and minor episodes attributed to thrombosis have been recorded at high altitude.

In 1895, whilst exploring the Amne Machin range of mountains in Eastern Tibet, the Russian traveller Roborovsky recorded that whilst crossing the Mangur Pass, 14,000 ft (4300 m), he 'had a stroke of paralysis which attacked all the right part of my body from head to the toes of my right foot; my tongue hardly obeyed my will. I lay in a disgusting and unbearable state for eight days'. He gradually recovered from this episode (Roborovsky 1896).

Two further cases of hemiplegia on each of the 1924 and 1938 expeditions to Mt Everest are recorded. No detailed information is available but one of the men, a Ghurkha, died, whilst the other, a Sherpa, recovered (Norton 1925; Tilman 1948). A further fatal case was recorded of a Sherpa who suffered from hemiplegia on Mt Kangchenjunga (Evans 1956). These three cases were fit young men who had spent a considerable time over 20,000 ft (6096 m).

In 1954 an American mountaineer, Gilkey, aged 24, spent five nights stormbound in a tent at 24,500 ft (7465 m) on Mt Godwin-Austen, 28,523 ft (8680 m). He was confined more or less completely to his sleeping bag and his food and fluid intake was considerably restricted. After two days he developed thrombophlebitis of the calf and two days later began coughing up bloody sputum. A diagnosis of pulmonary embolus was made and the patient was evacuated. Unfortunately in the descent the party was involved in an avalanche and Gilkey was swept off (Houston and Bates 1955).

In 1961, an episode of pulmonary thrombosis occurred in a fit New Zealand mountaineer aged 32. Whilst climbing without oxygen at 27,400 ft (8382 m) he complained of a pain in his chest and began to cough up blood-stained sputum. Becoming more and more shocked, and developing generalised hypothermia and frostbite, he was eventually evacuated to 15,000 ft (4572 m) after spending five days above 25,000 ft (7620 m) and a further four above 15,000 ft (4572 m) after the episode. His lung complications included a bronchopleural fistula and an empyema from which he finally recovered. He also had to have both legs amputated below the knee.

A further case of transient hemiplegia, associated with dysphasia, also occurred on this expedition. The paralysis lasted about 36 hours, and the difficulty with speech about three days (Ward 1968).

Transient dysphasia, associated with an extremely severe headache has also been reported at 21,000 ft (6400 m). As this patient also suffered from migraine it is difficult to be certain as to the exact cause of this episode (Shipton 1943).

A number of cases of thrombophlebitis occurring mainly in the legs have been recorded on Himalayan expeditions.

It is not without interest that post mortem studies showed that 10 out of 24 cattle with high mountain disease had pulmonary artery thrombosis (Alexander and Jensen 1963).

Aetiology

The increase in haemoglobin and red cell count noted at high altitude leads to an increase in blood viscosity (Dill 1938).

In perfusion experiments, when haematocrits exceeded 45–50

per cent the apparent viscosity increased steeply. In addition a fall in arterial pressure below 50 mmHg also increased viscosity slightly (Whittaker and Winton 1933). Further perfusion experiments indicated that blood viscosity increased when vasoconstriction occurred (Pappenheimer and Maes 1942).

Both hypoxia and cold lead to peripheral vasoconstriction, thus decreasing blood flow. Cold is also associated with a raised haematocrit.

At high altitude further factors which may increase the likelihood of thrombosis are extreme dehydration due to increased respiration, especially over 23,000 ft (7010 m), and curtailment of physical activity, especially when stormbound.

Treatment

Adequate hydration and exercise are obviously important in prevention.

In severe cases oxygen should be given, and the patient evacuated to lower levels as soon as possible.

Anticoagulants should not be started until adequate control is available.

Table 34. Serious thrombotic episodes

Condition	Height ft	m	Personal details
Hemiplegia recovery	14,000	4267	European, under 40
Hemiplegia death	20,000	6096	Sherpa, under 40
Hemiplegia death	over 20,000	6096	Sherpa, under 40
Hemiplegia recovery	over 21,000	6401	Sherpa, under 40
Hemiplegia recovery	over 19,000	5791	European, 41
Pulmonary embolus death by accident	24,500	7465	European, 23
Pulmonary infarction recovery	26,000	7925	European, 32

To prevent further episodes it is probably wise to make some sort of height barrier. A height of 14,000 ft (4267 m) though associated with polycythaemia allows the individual to take enough exercise and as his appetite and well being should be the same as at sea level the possibility of dehydration is negligible.

The mortality rate is high, three deaths resulting among seven serious cases occurring at high altitude.

References

Alexander, A. F. and Jensen, R. (1963) *American Journal of Veterinary Research* **24**, 1094.

Dill, D. B. (1938) *Life, heat, altitude.* Harvard University Press: Cambridge, Mass.

Evans, R. C. (1956) *Kangchenjunga. The untrodden peak.* Hodder and Stoughton: London.

Houston, C. S. and Bates, R. (1955) *K.2. The savage mountain.* Collins: London.

Norton, E. F. (1925) *The fight for Everest.* Arnold.

Pappenheimer, J. R. and Maes, J. P. (1942) *American Journal of Physiology* **137**, 187.

Roborovsky (1896) *Geographical Journal* **8**, 161.

Shipton, E. E. (1943) *Upon that mountain.* Hodder and Stoughton: London.

Tilman, H. W. (1948) *Mt Everest 1938.* Cambridge University Press.

Ward, M. P. (1968) *Diseases occurring at altitudes exceeding 17,500 ft.* M. D.Thesis. University of Cambridge

Whittaker, S. R. F. and Winton, F. R. (1933) *Journal of Physiology* **78**, 339.

CHAPTER TWENTY-THREE

Cold Injury. Introduction

Types of Cold Injury

In general cold injury, or hypothermia, the individual is said to be suffering from exposure.

Local cold injury may be classified under three heads.

(i) Non-freezing
At temperatures above freezing but below 15°C, usually in wet–cold conditions but also in a dry–cold climate.

It is most often encountered when the hands or feet are kept immersed in water just above freezing point, and so is called 'immersion hand' or 'immersion foot'.

(ii) Freezing
At temperatures below freezing (dry–cold condition) the tissues freeze and crystals form in between the cells. This is termed 'frostbite'.

Local cold injury may or may not be associated with hypothermia.

(iii) Variation
When local cold injury affects the limbs the degree of cold injury may vary, as the more proximal part of the limb is warmer than the distal and the deeper tissues warmer than the superficial.

The superficial and distal tissue may cool to below freezing and become frostbitten, whilst the proximal and deeper parts may be above freezing yet still suffer damage (immersion injury).

Limbs with severe cold injury therefore show a patchy distribution of blackened tissue. The fingers and toes can be quite black whilst more proximally on the legs and arms gangrene may be patchy or absent. In the more proximal part of the limb the main damage may be to muscle and nerve, as occurs in immersion injury, rather than to the skin.

Climate

There are two distinct types of cold climate—wet–cold and dry–cold.

The wet–cold climate covers large areas of the world's so-called temperate zones, where the range of air temperature varies from between 10°C down to −5°C. Wind, rain, sleet and mud are not uncommon.

Hypothermia and immersion injury occur under these conditions.

In dry–cold regions the temperature rarely rises above freezing point so snow, ice and wind contribute to cold stress. Hypothermia, frostbite and immersion injury can occur.

The wind-chill effect is an important factor, as the cooling effect of wind and cold on exposed tissues is more dangerous than that of cold alone.

The climate of mountainous areas is particularly prone to produce cold injury. As the temperature drops about 1°C for every 180 m (3°F for every 1000 ft) of ascent and as a still day is rare, the wind-chill factor has always to be taken into account. Sudden changes in climatic conditions, with storms, rain and hail, and blizzards associated with precipitate drops in temperature, are common, especially in periods of disturbed weather.

Cases of frostbite and hypothermia occur on normal Alpine routes in mid-summer. In Great Britain cold–dry conditions are rarer but some degree of hypothermia due to a combination of rain and wind causing considerable heat loss is probably more common than realised.

In the Andes and Himalaya the added factor of high altitude must be taken into account. In winter very low temperatures of the order of -40 to $-50°C$ with winds gusting up to 100 mph are encountered. Under these conditions men are only able to move for a very short period away from the shelter of a tent or snow cave.

People at Risk

Cold injury is an uncommon condition in civilian life despite the fact that large numbers live at least for part of the year in subzero temperatures. Populations of the order of one hundred million may be at risk in Siberia, Europe, Scandinavia, Canada and Alaska. At least another ten million live at altitudes exceeding 12,000 ft (3600 m) in South America and Central Asia.

During warfare in subzero temperatures, cold injury occurs as a complication of wounds and disease. Frostbite for instance was common amongst soldiers during Napoleon's campaign in Russia, during the Second World War in the winter in Northern Europe, in the Korean Campaign, and in the fighting between Indian and Chinese troops in the Himalayas.

Air crews, especially waist-gunners in the US Air Force in the Second World War, were particularly prone to frostbite and at one time during the winter of 1943, frostbite injuries among US heavy-bomber crews were greater than all other casualties combined. Most of these occurred in aircraft flying between 24,700 ft (7500 m) and 34,500 ft (10,500 m) in temperatures between -32 and $-43°C$, the guns being operated through open waist ports into air rushing by at over 320 mph.

Polar travellers of the pre-1920 era suffered severely from frostbite but it is now uncommon except in the case of accidents. This is due to improved clothing, a better diet (there is evidence that Scott's Polar party suffered from scurvy) and improved living conditions.

Mountaineers especially are exposed to cold injury, and on

early Everest expeditions mild degrees of frostbite were accepted. However at least two Sherpa members of these expeditions appear to have died from frostbite. When attempting a peak over 20,000 ft (6000 m) the margin of safety, already narrow due to high altitude, may have to be cut drastically to complete an ascent in bad weather. However, frostbite is not inevitable at high altitude and most of the highest peaks have been climbed successfully without such injury. Everest, K2 and Kangchenjunga—the three highest—have all been climbed using oxygen and without any cold injury. Attempts without oxygen on Nanga Parbat, Annapurna and Everest appear to have been associated with a relatively high incidence of frostbite.

With care and preparation frostbite may be avoided. Bradford Washburn has taken at least one hundred people into the high peaks of Alaska with only one mild case.

Improvement in technique, equipment and clothing has resulted in an increasing popularity of winter climbing in the European Alps.

A winter spent at 19,000 ft (5791 m) in the Everest region with the ascent of a technically very difficult peak of over 22,000 ft (6706 m) in February 1961 was made possible by exceptionally good acclimatisation and equipment. The recent ascents of the South Face of Annapurna in the spring of 1971 and the attempt on the South-west Face of Everest in the autumn of 1972 indicate that the trend towards hard technical and winter mountaineering has spread to the Himalayas.

High Altitude and Cold Injury

Clinical observation suggests that cold injury may be more prevalent at high than at low altitude for comparable temperatures.

Mountaineers on pre-war Everest expeditions suffered mild frostbite of the extremities despite being fully clothed, physically fit and ascending normally. One member commented that he felt cold the whole time that he was on the mountain. In 1961, after five days at 25,000 ft (7620 m) one climber became unconscious following a severe 'rigor'. Descent 36 hours later, despite being fully clothed, was associated with frostbite of the fingers and toes. An increased tendency towards cold injury may exist at high altitude because of the following factors:

(i) Hypoxia leads to loss of concentration and forgetfulness. Thus vital items of equipment such as gloves may be lost or not worn.

Hypothermia may also be associated with some loss of mental function.

(ii) Maximum oxygen uptake falls with altitude. In one individual it was 4·0 litre/min at sea level and 1·6 litre/min at 25,000 ft (7620 m). On the summit of Everest men have rested for periods of up to an hour without oxygen. This suggests a maximum intake of 250–500 ml/min.

As the ability to work is diminished, heat production will be less at high altitude than at sea level.

(iii) With increased respiration heat loss via the lungs will be increased. This loss will be more important the greater the altitude.

At altitudes over 24,000 ft (7315 m) the oxygen cost of ventilation during maximal work is very high. Oxygen intake may fall due to fatigue of the respiratory muscles.

(iv) Loss of appetite and loss of weight are cardinal features of high altitude deterioration. Fat is lost from the subcutaneous tissue diminishing the body insulation. Later, muscle wasting occurs and this is associated with muscle weakness and inability to do work, and hence to produce heat.

In addition there is a gradually increasing distaste for fatty foods with altitude. On acute exposure to altitude, anorexia may lead to some weight loss and loss of subcutaneous depot fat. Acute exposure at −5°C also resulted in an increase in fat mobilisation (Wilson *et al.* 1969).

(v) High altitude is associated with a high haematocrit due to (a) an increase in haemoglobin content (up to 50 per cent is normal) and (b) relative dehydration, the result of increased fluid loss from the lungs and decreased fluid intake because of poor living conditions.

These two factors, together with the associated relative inactivity at altitudes over 23,000 ft (7010 m), may result in an increased tendency to thrombosis.

Cold is also associated with an increased haematocrit (up to 24 per cent at 23°C body temperature) (Fisher *et al.* 1958) and increased blood viscosity leading to a diminution in blood flow.

Thus cold and high altitude both show a tendency to produce local haemoconcentration. If damage to capillary walls occurs the chances of intravascular sludging with resulting impairment of tissue nutrition and necrosis are much increased.

A decrease in plasma volume occurs both on acute exposure to high altitude and on exposure to cold.

(vi) At normal temperatures the blood flow in the skin has been shown to be reduced at high altitude—the result of arteriolar vasoconstriction (Durand and Martineaud 1971).

(vii) Cardiac output is decreased in high-altitude visitors, and a low basal metabolic rate has also been recorded (Hartley *et al.* 1967).

(viii) The ability to shiver may be decreased. Lactic acid so produced cannot be rapidly metabolised under hypothermic conditions and the associated hypoxia of altitude may increase the production of lactic acid for given work. If shivering were allowed to proceed too rapidly the blood pH would fall to levels incompatible with life. Hence some blocking mechanism may be brought into play (Cerretelli 1967).

(ix) The oxygen dissociation curve is shifted to the left by cold, and this results in a very low partial pressure of oxygen in the tissues. The pH is lowered by both high altitude and cold and this has the effect of shifting the curve to the right, as has the effect of 2,3-DPG.

These effects appear to cancel each other.

(x) The only factor where high altitude does not appear to potentiate liability to cold injury is the wind-chill factor. Because of the relatively less dense atmosphere, this is diminished in comparison with sea-level values (Burton and Edholm 1955).

In general therefore there do appear to be physiological reasons supporting the clinical observation that individuals are more liable to cold injury at altitude than at sea level.

References

Burton, A. C. and Edholm, O. (1955) *Man in a cold environment.* Arnold: London.

Durand, J. and Martineaud, J. D. (1971) Resitance and capacitance vessels of the skin in permanent and temporary residents at high altitude. In, *High altitude physiology.* Ciba Foundation Symposium. *Ed.* Porter, R. and Knight, J. Churchill Livingstone: Edinburgh and London.

Cerretelli, P. (1967) Lactic acid oxygen debt in acute and chronic hypoxia. In, *Exercise at altitude. Ed.* Margaria, R. Excerpta Medica Foundation: Amsterdam.

Fisher, B., Fedor, E. J. and Lee, S. H. (1958) *Annals of Surgery* **148**, 32.

Hartley, L. H., Alexander, J. K., Modelski, M. and Grover, R. F. (1967) *Journal of Applied Physiology* **23**, 839.

Wilson, O., Laurell, S. and Tibbling, G. (1969) *Federation Proceedings. Federation of American Societies for Experimental Biology* **28**, 1209.

CHAPTER TWENTY-FOUR

Accidental Hypothermia. Pathophysiology

Hypothermia is defined as a lowering of the temperature of the human body below the arbitrarily chosen level of 35°C (95°F).

Exposure is not a strict medical term, but in general usage describes serious effects that result from exposure to climatic hazards. In general its use is limited to cold environments. Thus a working definition would be, serious chilling of the body surface leading to a progressive fall in body temperature with the risk of death from hypothermia.

Hypothermia may be classified according to the length of exposure into

(i) Acute, as in sudden immersion in water; less than six hours.

(ii) Sub-acute, as in fell-walkers; more than six and less than 24 hours.

(iii) Chronic, as in geriatric patients; more than 24 hours.

Experimental

The inhuman experiments carried out by German doctors at Dachau Concentration Camp during the Second World War, on individuals immersed in water at near 0°C, revealed that death occurred when rectal temperature fell to between 24·2 and 25·7°C (Alexander 1946).

As rectal temperature lagged behind the temperature of the heart when cooling was rapid, the lethal temperature for the heart will be 1–2°C below this, i.e. 23–25°C. This corresponds well with evidence from individuals recovering from accidental cooling to similar temperatures (Rees 1958; Arneil and Kerr 1963; McNichol and Smith 1964) but occasional exceptions show that this lower limit is by no means absolute. Thus a rectal temperature of 18°C was recorded in a Negro woman who collapsed after drinking alcohol. She recovered after being allowed to re-warm slowly in hospital (Laufman 1951).

Deliberate cooling to 9°C under anaesthesia has been used in the hope of curing advanced cancer. At this temperature, an ECG recording showed that the heart had stopped, and it remained in asystole for 60 minutes. Following active re-warming the patient survived, but only recovered consciousness ten hours after the body temperature was restored to normal. Although the possibility of temporary brain damage was entertained the patient was later described as pleasant and alert (Niazi and Lewis 1958).

Cerebral Activity

Some cerebral activity has been observed at very low temperatures and people have been recorded as maintaining conversation with a body temperature as low as 33–35°C. One patient with accidental hypothermia and a rectal temperature of 27°C was able to nod her head in response to questions (Laufman 1951).

However cerebration is obviously impaired and may well be a major factor in deaths in the field.

Shipwrecked survivors in cold water become delirious and confused, letting go of wreckage to which they are clinging and drifting away. Amnesia may occur, even when cooling has not been severe enough to cause confusion or unconsciousness (Currie 1798; Keatinge 1959).

Cardiovascular System

Lowering the body temperature from 37°C to 28°C increases the time that the circulation to the brain can be halted from five minutes to ten (Ross 1957).

However, the most important effect of cold is on the heart. The experiments in Dachau showed that in hypothermia, death was due to cardiac arrest, whilst respiration was still continuing.

The most obvious effect is slowing the pace-maker. The rate of beating fell as the body temperature fell until atrial activity ceased at 13°C (Niazi and Lewis 1958). An ectopic focus continued to maintain ventricular activity until the heart stopped completely at 10·5°C.

Associated with this slowing is a fall in cardiac output, the result of a fall in rate rather than stroke volume. Although in theory an artificial pace-maker might restore normal output, in practice this does not occur.

Ventricular fibrillation is a more serious complication—but it rarely develops at body temperature above 33°C. Auricular fibrillation develops below 33°C, below 28°C ventricular fibrillation may develop if the heart is mechanically irritated, whilst ventricular fibrillation may occur spontaneously below 25°C.

As is well known auricular fibrillation interferes little with cardiac function, whereas ventricular fibrillation destroys the 'pump mechanism'.

In the field, ventricular fibrillation is usually fatal as spontaneous reversal to normal rhythm is rare. In hospital, external cardiac massage and defibrillation can restore normal rhythm.

The evidence points to ventricular fibrillation being the result of insufficient oxygen supply to the cardiac muscle—especially as hypothermia results in increased blood viscosity and a fall in arterial pressure, which will reduce coronary blood flow. The use of hyperbaric oxygen might be considered in these cases.

The loss of salt and water, possibly due to impairment of renal tubular cells by cold, together with increased vascular permeability, can cause serious loss of blood volume in prolonged hypothermia. The haematocrit rises by as much as 24 per cent at a body temperature of 23°C (Fisher *et al.* 1958).

Oxygen Transport

Cooling haemoglobin diminishes the amount of oxygen that it will release at a given partial pressure. To a certain extent this is counteracted by the greater solubility of carbon dioxide at low temperature, which favours dissociation. Even allowing for this, at temperatures lower than normal, oxygen is less easily given up by haemoglobin (Barcroft and King 1905; Callaghan *et al.* 1961).

The result of the combined effect of poor oxygen dissociation and impaired coronary blood flow is that at low temperature the supply of oxygen to the cardiac muscle is barely sufficient for its needs even at rest. At high altitude however the rightward shift of the oxygen dissociation curve by 2,3-diphosphoglycerate may counteract these effects.

Disturbances of Renal Function

Exposure to cold with no fall in body temperature leads to a temporary increase in the excretion of salt and water—the so-called 'cold diuresis'. This is countered by pitressin and may be a mechanism to remove some of the 'increased' blood volume, the result of vasoconstriction.

Hypothermia causes a more serious disturbance with persistent excretion of salt and water, leading to haemo-concentration.

Acid–Base Balance

The excretion of acids is impaired by hypothermia which allows them to accumulate in the blood. This together with the greater solubility of carbon dioxide results in a relative acidosis. Lactic acid cannot be metabolised rapidly and if its rate of production is high, as in shivering, will also contribute.

Dangerous acidosis is however rare while the temperature is low but on warming severe acidosis may occur (Fairley *et al.* 1957).

A pH of 7·0 was recorded in patients rewarmed to 35–37°C. Associated with loss of consciousness and depressed respiration, it was successfully treated with I/V bicarbonate.

The relatively minor degree of acidosis that occurs during hypothermia does not appear to cause much harm though ventricular fibrillation has been reported in hypothermic dogs. The sudden reversal of acidosis can cause ventricular fibrillation, even in the absence of hypothermia. For this reason, when artificial ventilation is necessary in severe hypothermia, it should not be carried out vigorously.

Environment

Wet–cold conditions are extremely common in mountain regions. Hypothermia is more insidious, and probably commoner than normally recognised in these conditions and the subject will be discussed in relation to that context.

Many cases occur in cold–wet conditions, often at temperatures close to freezing point with gale force winds and when the individual is wet through. Hypothermia can occur in temperatures up to 10°C above freezing, if the factors of wind and wetting are present and if clothing is inadequate.

In cold–dry conditions the possibility of hypothermia is much more obvious to the individual. Thus he is mentally prepared, and is probably wearing clothing that is warm and more appropriate to the climatic conditions.

Clothing and Exercise

In wet–cold conditions clothing must protect against wetting, provide sufficient insulation and be wind proof.

It must be stressed that the insulating value of much clothing is too low, especially when sodden.

Experiments in a climatic chamber showed that the combination of exercise, wind and wetting reduced the effective thermal insulation of a typical clothing assembly to a tenth of its nominal value determined at rest in dry, still conditions.

The results also showed that when a subject was exercising at a given work rate in wet–cold conditions his oxygen uptake was 50 per cent more than at the same work rate in dry conditions.

A high work rate will increase heat output and decrease the shivering and discomfort of cold–wet conditions. Thus in one experiment under conditions of a 15 kph wind and a standard clothing assembly wetted at 17–19°C, shivering persisted and work was more tiring at a rate below 800 kg m/min; above this rate shivering decreased and discomfort diminished.

Mountaineers and hill walkers habitually operate at 2·0–2·5 litre/min oxygen uptake, or between 50 and 60 per cent of their maximum capacity. Their heat production is 450–600 kcal/hour. This means that they are walking fast enough to keep themselves warm under stress of average cold conditions. They are as a result immune from discomfort and fatigue under average wet–cold conditions.

The effect of cold stress is to increase metabolic rate, and this was approximately equal to that brought about by a 300 kg increase in work load and amounted to 15–20 per cent of the subjects' maximum uptake.

In wet clothes strong hill walkers in cold–wet conditions can maintain a fast enough pace (i.e. can approach their maximum oxygen uptake) to keep themselves warm, despite the low insulation value of these garments.

Slow walkers, or mountaineers with a lower physical working capacity, will work close to their maximum capacity (or maximum oxygen uptake) in order to keep warm. Even so they may not have a high enough heat production to combat heat loss and maintain thermal equilibrium. Over a period of hours they cool off until balance and muscle control are affected. Their pace falls, heat production falls with it, and their rate of body cooling accelerates.

If mountaineers maintain a slower pace, they will suffer an obligatory increase in oxygen uptake of up to 30 per cent due to cold stress, as well as intense discomfort (Pugh 1967).

The clothing of boys who died of hypothermia during the Four Inns Race in 1964 was examined and the clo value established. The clothing consisted of:

Anorak with hood, wool jersey, Viyella shirt, string vest, cotton underpants, jeans, 1 pair socks, shoes and gloves.

This is a fairly standard assembly with a clo value when dry of 1·5 units.

If the heat production of each boy was about 500 kcal/hour, the minimum clothing insulation for thermal balance would work out at about 0·68 clo which is the likely value for this clothing when wet through. This would mean that if the individual were unable to maintain a heat production of 500 kcal/hour he would cool down.

If his clothing remained dry (i.e. 1·5 clo) he could just keep warm with a heat production of 330 kcal/hour. This is equivalent to an oxygen consumption of 1·1 litre/min which is the oxygen consumption required for walking on the level at 3·0 mph (Pugh 1964).

Fatigue

The association between subcutaneous fat and resistance to cold has been convincingly demonstrated. Under wet–cold conditions, when clothes are wet through, the individual is in much the same position as a cross-channel swimmer. It is known that cross-channel swimmers can continue swimming with a rectal temperature as low as 34·5–35·5°C without muscle weakness. By contrast a non-adapted swimmer failed regularly with muscle weakness at a rectal temperature of 34·5°C (Pugh and Edholm 1955). However, exhaustion may come on while the rectal temperature is still above 37°C, but in this case the rectal temperature falls extremely rapidly after cessation of active exercise.

There is evidence that the metabolic response to cold passes off when rectal temperature falls below 34°C and this would greatly hasten body cooling.

Shivering usually ceases at rectal temperature of 30–33°C and is succeeded by muscular rigidity. On re-warming shivering begins again on reaching rectal temperature above 30°C.

The role of local muscle cooling in accidental hypothermia is difficult to evaluate. It is suggested that muscle temperature might fall low enough to cause serious weakness by the time rectal temperature had fallen to 34·5°C.

Low muscle temperature might also be related to other symptoms of incipient hypothermia such as stiffness, stumbling and cramp.

The combination of cold and fatigue will bring the point of exhaustion nearer, than when only one factor is involved.

In severe weather conditions, the added fatigue brought on by combating gale force winds is important.

Adolph and Molnar (Adolph and Molnar 1946) studied nude subjects at rest and performing ergometer exercises. Working at a rate they could maintain, i.e. 380 kg m/min, under severe cold stress (temperatures at 2–4°C and wind 3–7 mph) they became exhausted within 1½–2 hours. Metabolism during exercise was found to be 30 per cent higher than doing similar work under warmer conditions. They considered that these high levels of energy expenditure explained early exhaustion.

Extreme fatigue by itself unassociated with hypothermia can produce mental symptoms.

Individual variation in response to cold stress depends on a combination of factors—degree of clothing insulation, physical type and age, thickness of subcutaneous fat and sensitivity to cold.

This variation may explain the random incidence of hypothermia casualties.

If a party caught out by bad weather increases its pace to keep warm, those who can maintain the extra oxygen uptake imposed by the response to cold stress will suffer no extra fatigue, whereas those who cannot will become exhausted much sooner.

Within certain limits metabolism rises to a level necessary to maintain thermal balance and this may be achieved by increasing work rate, shivering and by other unexplained means.

In severe cold stress the metabolic demand may be so high that only very fit people can meet it over a prolonged period.

References

Adolph, F. E. and Molnar, G. W. (1946) *American Journal of Physiology* **146**, 50.

Alexander, L. (1946) Combined Intelligence Objectives Subcommittee, item No. 24 File No. 26–37.

Arneil, G. C. and Kerr, M. M. (1963) *Lancet* **2**, 756.

Barcroft, J. and King, W. O. R. (1909) *Journal of Physiology* **39**, 374.

Burton, A. C. and Edholm, O. (1955) *Man in a cold environment*. Arnold: London.

Callaghan, P. B., Lister, J., Paton, B. C. and Swan, H. (1961) *Annals of Surgery* **154**, 903.

Currie, J. (1798) *Medical reports on the effects of water, cold and warm. Appendix 2*. Cadell and Davis.

Fairley, H. B., Waddell, W. G. and Bigelow, W. G. (1957) *British Journal of Anaesthesia* **29**, 310.

Fisher, B., Fedor, E. J. and Lee, S. H. (1958) *Annals of Surgery* **148**, 32.

Keatinge, W. R. (1959) *The effect of work, clothing and adaptation on the maintenance of body temperature in water*. R.N.P.R.C. Report R.N.P. 60/97. Medical Research Council.

Laufman, H. (1951) *Journal of the American Medical Association* **147**, 1201.

McNicol, M. W. and Smith, R. (1964) *British Medical Journal* **1**, 19.

Niazi, S. A. and Lewis, F. J. (1958) *Annals of Surgery* **147**, 264.

Pugh, L. G. C. E. and Edholm, O. (1955) *Lancet* **2**, 761.

Pugh, L. G. C. E. (1964) *Lancet* **1**, 1210.

Pugh, L. G. C. E. (1967) *British Medical Journal* **2**, 333.

Rees, J. R. (1958) *Lancet* **1**, 556.

Ross, D. N. (1957) *Proceedings of the Royal Society of Medicine* **50**, 76.

CHAPTER TWENTY-FIVE

Accidental Hypothermia. Clinical Features and Treatment

The clinical features of hypothermia may be tabulated as follows.

Table 35.   Clinical features of hypothermia (Golden 1972; Laufman 1951)

Core temperature °C	
37–34	Shivering
35–34·5	Disorientation, confusion
34–33	Amnesia, apathy
33–30	Semi-conscious, cardiac arrythmias, muscular rigidity (instead of shivering)
30	Unconscious, pupils dilate, absent tendon reflex
28	Ventricular fibrillation
below 26	Death (failure to revive)
16–18	Lowest recorded with survival.

Sub-Acute Hypothermia

Clinical Features

Mild (*Core Temperature over 32·2°C*)
A normal physiological response is seen. Peripheral vaso-constriction and pallor, associated with shivering, rising in

blood pressure pulse, and diuresis. Consciousness is not impaired.

Severe (Core Temperature below 32·2°C)
There is a gradual slowing of the rate of progress, clumsiness in placing the feet, and a tendency to stumble and fall.

Complaints of undue coldness are fairly common, and some mountaineers who are aware of this condition can distinguish a feeling of 'central coldness' (especially marked at high altitude) (Ward 1961) as opposed to the more peripheral feeling normally encountered.

Unexpected and unreasonable behaviour, associated with failure to understand and respond to questions and directions and slurring of speech, may be associated with outbursts of violent language and spasms of unexpected energy.

Sudden shivering fits of great intensity are also a feature. Abnormality or failure of vision often occurs and should be treated with extreme seriousness.

Signs
There is extreme pallor, often with absence of the peripheral pulses, and associated generalised rigidity. The patient has a corpse-like appearance and a 'chill' may emanate from his body.

The skin may develop blue patches, and becomes puffy and oedematous—presumably due to the shift of fluid from plasma to interstitial spaces. The respiration may be so shallow (under 10/min) as to be barely perceptible and the patient may appear dead. However stertorous breathing, exaggerated reflexes and widely dilated pupils have also been recorded.

The pulse, if palpable, is thready and rapid.

If cooling is considerable the pulse rate falls and may become irregular with auricular fibrillation. Ventricular fibrillation is a common cause of death.

Investigations
A low reading thermometer is necessary to record the low temperature.

Rectal temperatures are easy to take. However it should be remembered that rectal temperatures respond slowly to changes in arterial temperature. Urine temperature is also an indication of core temperature.

Both haemoglobin and white cell count may be raised due to the shift of fluid from plasma to interstitial space.

X-Ray
May help in detecting respiratory infection.

ECG
Characteristically this shows J waves, bradycardia; atrial fibrillation and prolongation of the Q–T interval are also recorded.

Pulmonary function
Pulmonary function is usually inadequate and oxygenation impaired. The P_{CO_2} is usually normal but may be raised.

Prevention

Adolescents and young people are more at risk than adults for a number of reasons.

   (i) Because they are less willing to conserve energy, they tend to become exhausted more rapidly.
   (ii) Being less emotionally mature, they panic more easily, use up more energy, and become fatigued and unable to keep up their heat production. They may even forget to take the correct measures to combat hypothermia.
   (iii) Some adolescents have very little subcutaneous fat and are therefore less well insulated against the cold.

It is essential that enough warm and wind-proof clothing be available.

Both an anorak and windproof trousers are necessary. Windproof trousers are rarely taken as spare clothing, yet the legs account for 36 per cent of the total surface area of the body and heat loss is considerable.

Heat loss from the head, because of its plentiful vasculature and because it is the warmest part of the body, may be very high. Therefore some form of head covering is also essential.

Wet clothing has its insulating value reduced by 50 per cent or more. Therefore a reserve of dry clothing must be available. The insulating value of clothing depends on the stagnant air trapped in its substance, and wind and body movement cause this air to circulate and thus lose its insulating value. Outer windproof garments prevent this as does the closure of gaps at wrist, ankles, neck, etc.

Water increases the heat loss from the body so to keep the central core temperature normal, metabolism and oxygen consumption have to be increased. Fatigue and exhaustion may therefore be accelerated.

Once the central core temperature falls below a certain level, shivering ceases and is succeeded by muscular rigidity and death.

The majority of hill walkers and mountaineers take fewer calories as food on the day's outing than the number of calories that they expend during that day. The deficit is made up on return to shelter. In the event of an accident or emergency this negative energy balance will increase, which in turn will affect the ability to perform muscular exercise to keep up heat production. Very high calorie values are obtained in certain concentrated foods which are light and should always be taken as an emergency.

Adequate fluid intake is also essential especially under certain dry–cold conditions and at high altitude.

Too much should not be expected of a person who has recently had an illness. Although he may seem perfectly well and able to carry out his normal daily work effectively, the added stress of mountain conditions and continued exercise may result in an increased liability to fatigue and hypothermia.

The majority of people are urban dwellers and more or less insulated from the environment by the conditions under which they live at home and at work.

The transition to the harsh mountain environment can be a considerable psychological stress to some. This is especially important in newcomers, and although no physiological

acclimatisation occurs on a short holiday, psychological accept-
ance is important.

Careful attention to detail has resulted in no cases of cold
injury occurring in the last few years in the British Antarctic
Survey other than as the result of accident.

Curative

In the Field and Camp

The possibility that this condition may occur must always be
present in the minds of those who travel in mountain country
and under cold conditions.

It is especially important for those who organise groups of
adolescents to be aware that minor degrees of hypothermia
are commoner than realised.

It must be stressed too that hypothermia may cause death
within two hours. Even in the low hills and mountains of Great
Britain the combination of wind and rain associated with above-
freezing temperatures can cause severe cases of hypothermia.
All potential and suspected cases should be treated seriously.

In those adults who are basically fit, it may be possible to
increase heat production to such a level that they can be
'walked out of trouble'. Putting on warm dry clothes next to
the skin is also important as it decreases heat loss; having something to eat causes a temporary peripheral vasodilatation and
feeling of warmth. The enforced rest and calorie intake may en-
able greater energy to be expended thus increasing oxygen uptake and heat production. At very high altitude, supplementary
oxygen induces a feeling of warmth, presumably due to vasodilatation.

If activity proves impossible or unwise, the individual should be
placed in a spot that is sheltered from the wind. If practicable,
dry clothing must be placed next to the skin.

The patient should be insulated from the ground as well as
protected from the wind.

Gradual re-warming is preferable to rapid re-warming as it is
easier to carry out in the field or camp, safer, and rapid re-

warming may cause an 'after drop' in body temperature by the flow of cooled peripheral blood into the central circulation.

If possible the patient should be placed in a tent, polythene bag, or failing that a sleeping bag or something else relatively impermeable to heat. This diminishes heat loss and provides protection from the wind.

If the victim is still breathing, and provided carbon dioxide build up from expired air can be avoided, it is reasonable to put the face inside the bag. This will 'warm up' the bag by capturing heat loss from the expired air and the head. He should be allowed to warm up slowly by his own heat production and by heat produced from other bodies lying either in the same bag, or beside him.

If he is conscious he should be given warm fluids and easily digested food such as sugar or glucose. However, warm fluids by mouth may cause peripheral vasodilatation and subsequent drop in central core temperature.

If he is unconscious and without a pulse, mouth to mouth respiration and continuous closed cardiac massage should be started. Even those who are seemingly dead with rigor mortis have been known to recover after several hours of treatment. Speed is essential as the brain is unlikely to survive circulatory arrest for more than an hour even at very low temperatures.

Hydrocortisone has been given in the field.

Hospital

(i) In the elderly gradual re-warming is essential: rapid re-warming may cause death.

The patient is placed between warm blankets in a warm ward and the aim is to raise the temperature at a rate of 0·55°C (1°F) per hour.

Dehydration should be corrected with parenteral fluids, such as 5 per cent glucose or low molecular weight dextran. Intestinal absorption has been shown to be diminished in rats, and the oral route should not be relied on.

In the presence of vasoconstriction, neither the intramuscular nor subcutaneous route is reliable.

A broad spectrum antibiotic should be given as a prophylactic against infection. Hydrocortisone should also be given as a routine to combat adrenocortical failure.

Oxygen at normal pressures, or hyperbaric oxygen if available, may be used to increase oxygen supply to the myocardium.

If the systolic blood pressure falls below 100, vasoconstrictor drugs may be necessary.

(ii) In young adults it is probably preferable to start active re-warming as soon as possible.

The trunk should be immersed in water, if necessary fully clothed, at 42°C or as hot as the hand can bear. The first effect is to accelerate the cooling of the deep tissues by causing vaso-dilatation of the skin. By this method, Niazi and Lewis (1958) revived a patient with a rectal temperature of 9°C, whose heart had stopped for 60 minutes. To minimise the 'after drop' in temperature the limbs may be left out of the water.

If cardiac arrest or atrial fibrillation has occurred external cardiac massage and mouth to mouth respiration should be started at half the normal rate if active re-warming does not restore heart beat or respiration. The lowered rate is preferable because of the low rate of metabolic production of carbon dioxide in hypothermia, and the fact that a drastic fall in $P\mathrm{CO_2}$ can cause ventricular fibrillation.

Once the patient has started to improve it is probably best to remove him from the bath and lie him flat in a temperature of 36–40°C either in blankets or air and allow him to re-warm slowly. His normal heat production will continue to re-warm him.

As intense peripheral vasoconstriction occurs in hypothermia, re-warming will cause peripheral vasodilatation, and the re-duced blood volume will fail to fill these dilated vessels. Some fall in arterial blood pressure will be inevitable. A boy of 15, whose rectal temperature had fallen to 32·5°C during the last five hours of a hill walk in the rain had a fall in blood pressure from 120/80 to 80/50 mmHg in ten minutes after the start of re-warming.

If the blood pressure of a patient in the bath does fall the patient should be removed and tipped head downwards.

It is important to monitor blood pressure, rectal temperature and the ECG. Blood pH, P_{CO_2}, glucose and potassium should be estimated on venous samples taken from the warmed arm.

The airway must be cleared, but endotracheal tubes should be used only when absolutely necessary since reflex bradycardia can precipitate ventricular fibrillation.

Artificial ventilation can also precipitate fibrillation by lowering P_{CO_2}. Although the respiration in hypothermia is slow it is proportionate to the tissue gas exchange in the body. If ventilation is necessary expired air is the safest.

In simple cases of hypothermia ventricular fibrillation is uncommon. If it occurs it should be treated on conventional lines by closed cardiac massage and electrical defibrillation. Antifibrillatory drugs are generally of no value in hypothermia and may be dangerous.

Falls in blood pH can occur as the body temperature returns to normal after hypothermia associated with surgical intervention, and lactate, with possibly potassium and glucose, may be required if the condition of the patient deteriorates. In simple hypothermia small falls only are usual. In any event correction of abnormal pH is not advisable until the body temperature is near normal, as the dangers of correcting supposed abnormalities is considerable in the cooled state, when body metabolism is ineffective. Warmed intravenous infusions should be used.

IPPV may be used to counteract hypoxaemia and to re-expand collapsed and oedematous alveoli. When used with a heated humidifier the central core temperature can be raised.

Steroids may be given as the prolonged stress of cold, exhaustion and other factors such as high altitude may result in some degree of adrenal exhaustion.

An Intensive Care Unit is the best place to treat severe cases of hypothermia, as the correction of complex blood electrolyte, pH, and other abnormalities is routine in these units. Arterial rather than venous blood too may give more accurate figures of blood electrolytes.

It should be stressed that death may be defined as a failure to revive—apparently dead individuals have recovered.

Acute Hypothermia

Immediate Treatment

The individual should be removed from the cold environment. He should not be massaged or rubbed but covered with blankets, or placed in a polythene bag. Oxygen should be given if available. If within about 30 minutes from a hospital he should be transferred; if not, curative treatment should be started.

Various complications may develop.

Cardiac Arrest

Ventricular fibrillation may occur as a result of efforts to revive the patient, as the myocardium is very sensitive to cold. Chilled re-circulating blood may also be a factor in the reviving patient.

External cardiac massage (at a slower rate than in the non-cooled individual) should be started.

If cardiac arrest has *not* occurred (i.e. bradycardia only is present) cardiac massage may induce ventricular fibrillation.

Hypotension

As the peripheral tissues re-warm, the peripheral vasoconstriction due to cold will be abolished, and hypotension occurs.

The patient should be transported head down. Alcohol and excess heating must be avoided.

Unconsciousness

This may be present at rescue, or develop some time later as the result of the continued fall of body temperature after rescue. Hypotension may also be the cause.

A clear airway should be maintained.

Respiratory Failure

Deep hypothermia is associated with respiratory depression and the diagnosis of respiratory arrest is correspondingly difficult. It may follow cardiac arrest.

Mouth to mouth respiration should be used but not too vigorously as hypocapnia may be produced (Keatinge 1969).

Curative

If the body temperature has been lowered rapidly and for a short period, there will have been insufficient time for major electrolyte disturbances to have occurred. Therefore the treatment of choice is rapid re-warming (Niazi and Lewis 1958) by immersion in a bath of water heated to 40–41°C if naked, or 44–46°C if clothed. Undressing a patient who may have some degree of muscular rigidity may precipitate ventricular fibrillation.

The patient should be left in the bath until he feels warm and then placed in a warm bed. Oxygen should be given if available.

Complications

(i) Cardiac arrest. At myocardial temperatures below 28°C ventricular fibrillation occurs. This is more likely when re-warming takes place and chilled acidotic blood returns to the 'central core'. In addition the blood is relatively hypoxic and hypoglycaemic.

Atrial fibrillation may also occur, but specific treatment does not appear to be required.

External cardiac massage should be carried out until DC fibrillation can restore sinus rhythm.

In severe acidosis defibrillation is unlikely to succeed and warmed I/V bicarbonate should be given.

Magnesium sulphate (0·1 g/kg body weight) has been given I/V in cases of ventricular fibrillation in by-pass surgery, and sinus rhythm restored at a body temperature of 30°C (Büky 1970).

In profound hypothermia when the individual appears dead, external cardiac massage with IPPV may be tried.

Defibrillation is only likely to succeed at core temperatures above 28°C (Linton and Ledingham 1966).

(ii) Respiratory depression. Shallow respiration (with sufficient oxygen consumption to supply the low metabolic needs) is not an indication for treatment. During resuscitation an increasing demand for oxygen will occur and a natural increase in respiration should provide this.

Insertion of an airway may cause bradycardia, and artificial ventilation may result in ventricular fibrillation. Over ventilation may cause hypocapnia.

However in partial drowning IPPV will expand collapsed alveoli, and may be used in conjunction with a heated humidifier (Ledingham and Mone 1972).

(iii) Hypotension. During re-warming sudden collapse due to hypotension may occur. The patient should be removed from the bath and tilted head down.

(iv) After drop in temperature. During re-warming, the after drop may be as much as 3°C (Alexander 1945). Survival chances are better with rapid than with slow re-warming in acute hypothermia.

If intravenous therapy is necessary all I/V fluid should be preheated to 38°C before transfusion (Freeman and Pugh 1969).

References

Alexander, L. (1945) Combined Intelligence Objective Subcommittee APO 413. No. 24.

Büky, B. (1970) *British Journal of Anaesthesia* **42**, 886.

Freeman, J. and Pugh, L. G. C. E. (1969) *International Anaesthesiology Clinic* **7**, 997.

Golden, F. St C. (1972) *Journal of the Royal Naval Medical Service* **58**, 199.

Keatinge, W. R. (1969) *Survival in cold water*. Blackwell Scientific publications: Oxford and Edinburgh.

Laufman, H. (1951) *Journal of the American Medical Association* **147**, 1201.

Ledingham, I. Mc A. and Mone, J. G. (1972) *Lancet* **1**, 534.

Linton, A. L. and Ledingham, I. Mc A. (1966) *Lancet* **1**, 25.

Niazi, S. A. and Lewis, F. J. (1958) *Annals of Surgery* **147**, 264.

Ward, M. P. (1961) Personal observation.

CHAPTER TWENTY-SIX

Frostbite and Immersion Injury

Frostbite

Frostbite occurs when the tissues freeze and ice cystals form. These may be intracellular, when cooling is extremely rapid or extracellular in environmental cold injury.

Pathophysiology

Tissues are damaged more easily by freezing than by non-freezing cold injury.

Experiments have shown that skin freezes when fingers were immersed in brine at $-1.9°C$. The true freezing point however was approximately $-0.53°C$.

Freezing at temperatures of $-1.9°C$ for seven minutes caused no lasting damage. The fingers were painful when thawed but became normal after a few minutes. After freezing for $11\frac{1}{2}$ minutes, the affected fingers were red and tender for several days. Blistering occurred after repeated exposure for 20 minutes or more (Keatinge and Cannon 1960).

However, the skin of the fingers can be cooled to temperatures below its true freezing point without freezing. This 'supercooling' is common if the skin is dry. On further cooling freezing

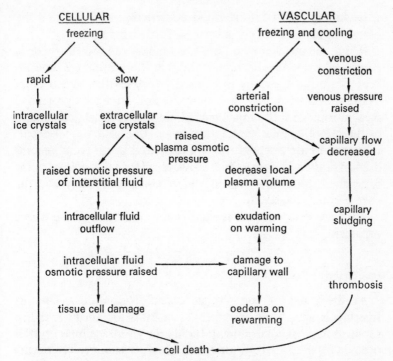

Fig. 21   Frostbite pathophysiology (Nelms 1972).

spreads rapidly in the supercooled tissues, with tissues hardening.

Two main reactions occur when tissues come in contact with a very cold object. These are a vascular reaction and ice crystal formation.

Vascular Reaction

The superficial tissues at the site of contact freeze to a depth which depends on the period of contact and the degree of cold.

Immediately below this zone damage occurs to the wall of the blood vessels, and plasma leaks into the tissues, forming blisters. The remaining intravascular blood becomes more viscous, with local haemo-concentration or 'sludging'. The small vessels may thus become blocked (Greene 1943).

If chilling continues arteriolar constriction remains, and the blood supply to the affected part is further reduced.

If due to the action of the precapillary sphincters there is complete stoppage of blood through the capillary, arterio-venous shunts open up and blood by-passes the frozen area. These shunts open and close in cycles and serve as a protective mechanism, for if too much chilled blood is recirculated cooling of the hypothalamic temperature-regulating centres will occur, the central core temperature will drop and death from genera-lised hypothermia is possible. However before this danger point is reached the arterio-venous shunts close completely and the part becomes avascular.

Thus the diseased part is sacrificed for survival of the whole organism.

Ice Crystal Formation

At the point of contact, ice crystal formation occurs. If freezing is very rapid intracellular crystals are formed; if less rapid, as in most environmental cold injury, extracellular crystals occur. Originating from interstitial fluid, crystal growth occurs at the expense of intracellular water. Intracellular osmotic pressure rises and enzyme mechanisms are disturbed with sub-sequent cell death.

Cellular death may thus result from vascular reaction, changes in osmotic pressure, or both causes.

Tissue death following frostbite is more likely to be due to interruption of the blood supply than the direct action of freez-ing. Skin from a severely frostbitten rabbit ear will survive if grafted onto a normal ear, whereas it will die if left *in situ*.

In immersion injury there is evidence that gangrene was more prevalent in tissues which had been subjected to trauma. Clinical observations suggest that the dry gangrene of frostbite appears thickest where pressure has been most marked, that is, on the heels, the plantar rather than the dorsal surface of the fingers and toes, at the tips of the toes, and over the distal part of the medial surface of the big toe, where contact with the boot is most pronounced.

Tissues vary in their resistance to frostbite. Skin appears to freeze at $-0.53°C$, whilst muscles, blood vessels and nerves are also highly susceptible. Connective tissue, tendons and bone are relatively resistant.

Thus the blackened extremities of a frostbitten hand or foot can be moved as the tendons under the gangrenous skin remain intact, and the muscles to which these tendons belong are far removed from the area of severe cold injury (Washburn 1962).

The incidence of frostbite at sea level will depend on the environmental factors which are responsible for the cooling of the atmosphere. These are ambient air temperature, the rate of air movement (wind), and length of time of exposure.

Certain modifying factors will also be involved—wetness of the skin surface due to sweat, immersion in water, or snow, and the amount of contact with cold objects.

Even under standard conditions there is no well defined value of wind-chill which causes freezing of the skin. This is because the skin tends to supercool, cold-induced vasodilatation occurs in the supercooled region, and this inhibits crystal formation.

Frostnip

The ambient air temperature seems to be the main factor in deciding the incidence of frostnip, since in acute cases the skin will very often not freeze at an ambient temperature above -10 to $-15°C$. The skin supercools to these levels and the heat loss is balanced by cold-induced vasodilatation.

For frostnip to occur on acute exposure the wind-chill index must exceed 1400, and the air temperature must be below the freezing point of skin. In an average person an ambient temperature of -10 to $-15°C$ is therefore necessary.

In chronic exposure the situation is different because of the ultimate reduction in cold-induced vasodilatation (Wilson and Goldman 1970).

Frostbite damages the tissues, whilst with frostnip the changes are reversible. The skin blanches and becomes numb with a sudden and complete cessation of the sensation of cold and discomfort in the affected part. A tingling may occur on rewarming. With immediate treatment frostnip will not progress to frostbite.

Superficial Frostbite

Only the skin and subcutaneous tissues immediately adjacent are involved in superficial frostbite.

The frozen part, though white and frozen on the surface, is soft and pliable when pressed gently before thawing. After rewarming, it becomes numb, mottled, blue or purple and it will then sting, burn, or swell for a period.

Blisters may occur within 24–48 hours, depending on the site of the injury. Thus blistering is more common on the dorsum of the fingers and hand, where tissues are lax, than on the palm. The blister fluid is slowly absorbed, the skin hardens and becomes black, producing a thick insensitive carapace of tissue. In certain sites the black carapace may occur without preceding blister formation. There is associated oedema, and within weeks a very marked line of demarcation occurs.

Throbbing or aching may persist for several weeks. If the contour of the blackened carapace corresponds to that of the original part, loss of tissue is unlikely. If, however, the contour of the pulp of the finger appears to be flattened and the carapace has a tendency to wrinkle, then loss of tissue is likely.

Unlike arteriosclerosis, gangrene following frostbite is essentially superficial, and the necrotic tissue may not extend more than a few millimetres in depth. The black carapace is fitted like a glove around the normal tissues and it peels off bit by bit over the months.

The nail may be lost but is likely to grow again either normally or with a wrinkled appearance.

After the carapace has been shed, the underlying shiny red 'babyskin' will be abnormally tender and unduly sensitive to heat and cold. Abnormal sweating may occur. In two to three months it will gradually take on the appearance of normal skin. The subcutaneous tissue generally feels rather wooden for the same period, but gradually becomes more pliable.

Deep Frostbite

Deep frostbite involves not only the skin and subcutaneous tissue but also the deeper structures, including muscle, bone and tendons.

Blistering may take weeks to develop but is not inevitable. The affected part becomes cold, mottled and blue or grey in colour, and may remain swollen for months.

Initially the part may be painless, but shooting and throbbing pain can occur and frequently abnormal sensations are encountered for up to two months.

As tendons are resistent to cold injury, the patient will be able to move his fingers and toes for long periods despite their gangrenous appearance. This is because the muscles responsible, although abnormally sensitive to cold injury, are situated a long distance from the affected area. This means that, even with severe frostbite, patients can walk and use their fingers and hands for crude movements such as gripping.

Eventually a carapace forms and sloughs off. Often a complete cast of the finger or toe with nail attached may separate.

Permanent loss of tissue is almost inevitable with deep frostbite, and this may be surmised from the shrivelled appearance of the affected finger-tip or toe. However, even with deep frostbite, a limb may return almost to normal over a period of months, and amputation should never be carried out until a considerable period, probably at least 6–9 months, has elapsed.

Prevention

An intelligent appreciation of the hazards of the environment and their effect on the individual, together with the knowledge that injury and illness may lead to frostbite, is the best protection.

It is extremely important to dress for the temperature with which the limbs will be in contact. In deep powder snow it is possible for the feet to be in snow many degrees below freezing-point, whilst at the same time the ambient temperature may be many degrees above freezing.

Even the ambient temperature may vary enormously, with a 50°C variation at sunset.

Curative Treatment

Frostnip

Frostnip is the only form of frostbite that should be treated immediately on the spot.

As this condition commonly occurs on the exposed portions of the body such as the cheek or nose, each person keeps a watch for the signs occurring in other members of the party, and as soon as whitening of the skin is observed it is treated immediately. A place sheltered from the wind is found, or the back is turned to the wind, and the affected part is warmed by the hand, or the glove. Once the normal colour and consistency of the area is obtained normal working is resumed.

Frostbite

For many years rubbing the affected part, either with snow or with the normal hand, has been advocated. This method neither melts the extracellular ice crystals by raising the temperature, nor increases the blood supply to the injured area. It also has the disadvantage of breaking the skin and allowing infection. Other forms of violent local therapy are open to the same objection, nor does the use of cold water fulfil either of the two criteria.

Anticoagulant treatment might prevent the sludged blood from coagulating permanently, but experimental results are equivocal.

Vasodilator agents (Schumacker *et al.* 1951) do not improve tissue survival; sympathectomy within 24 hours of thawing has sometimes been reported as reducing the amount of tissue necrosis but the results are not striking (Golding *et al.* 1964; Gildenbergh and Hardenbergh 1964).

Low molecular weight dextran either before or immediately after thawing might help to retain blood plasma in the vessels by osmotic action and so prevent sludging of the red cells, but, although dextran has been reported to reduce the amount of tissue loss in experimental frostbite in mice, it increased their death rate (Mundth *et al.* 1964; Anderson and Hardenbergh 1965). The sufficiently early use of dextran will rarely be practical and there does seem some possibility of danger in its use.

The use of hyperbaric oxygen at sea level and of supplementary oxygen at high altitude has been reported (Greene 1941; Ward *et al.* 1968). Over 17,500 ft (5334 m) oxygen appears to cause peripheral vasodilation, as an increased feeling of warmth has been reported when it has been used. At both sea level and high altitude an increased tissue tension of oxygen may just tip the balance in favour of a cell partially damaged by cold injury, and decrease tissue loss.

Warming seems to be the most effective treatment with rapid warming showing less loss of tissue than slow (Harkins and Harmon 1937; Finneran and Schumacker 1950; Fuhrman and Fuhrman 1957), possibly because the area of circulatory arrest is smaller after rapid warming (Crismon and Fuhrman 1947).

Rapid re-warming also decreases the damage to blood vessels, and may by the rapid restoration of a high blood flow result in little plasma being lost, and therefore no sludging (Aturson 1966).

It has the advantage that it may be undertaken with relative ease in the field, and therefore soon after the initial injury. This shortens the time that the blood vessels and cells are frozen and exposed to temperatures at which high electrolyte concentrations are dangerous. All other methods require admission to hospital.

The clinical experience obtained in Alaska (Mills *et al.* 1960). and elsewhere does suggest that rapid re-warming is a proven method of reducing tissue loss. Once active re-warming has been started it seems doubtful whether any other treatment is of benefit.

All cases diagnosed as frostbite should be treated either at a well-equipped camp from which evacuation by air or some other means is easy, or in a hospital. Attempts to treat frostbite at high camps or with inadequate facilities are ill-advised.

If the individual is uninjured or injured but able to move, he should be encouraged to make his own way, as walking on frostbitten feet does not appear to increase tissue loss.

In the case of a fracture the part should be splinted. The splint must be well padded as pressure will impede blood supply and increase the likelihood of frostbite. The part of the limb distal to the injury or fracture must be carefully examined at intervals to see that the blood supply is adequate.

No attempt should be made to treat the frostbitten part except under maximal conditions, as once re-warming has started, the tissues are liable to infection and loss of tissue will occur.

No patient should be allowed to walk on thawed or partly thawed feet.

Treatment should be directed at both the whole person and the affected part.

Care of the Person

The most important factor is to keep morale high.

Generalised re-warming may be necessary as some degree of hypothermia seems almost inevitable, especially at high altitude. This is best carried out by giving hot liquids, or even oxygen. The patient must be put in a sleeping bag and an extra source of heat may be provided by his companions lying alongside him in the same or another sleeping bag.

Food should be given as in itself it causes some peripheral vasodilation.

Alcohol can also be given, especially if some time is to be spent in shelter. This will cause vasodilation—but more important will boost morale and diminish any pain caused by the re-warming.

A broad-spectrum antibiotic must be started as a prophylactic against infection.

Mild analgesics such as aspirin may be used to alleviate pain.

The Affected Part

The affected part should be warmed, preferably using a container with water at 44°C. A thermometer should be available to measure the temperature accurately as water that is too hot will damage the limb. If a thermometer is not available the temperature should be tested with a normal, unfrostbitten finger. If it is too hot for comfort more cold water should be added. The temperature of the water should never be tested with a frostbitten finger, as partial anaesthesia due to nerve injury occurs. If no container is available, hot water poured over towels or a cloth wrapped around the part can be used.

Re-warming should last about 20 minutes at a time and the temperature of the water should be checked frequently to see that it does not fall below 42°C. Additional hot water should not be poured over the affected part.

If re-warming by fluid is impossible, the part should be placed against a warm abdomen, armpit or held in warm air. It should never be placed by an open fire.

After re-warming, the part should be cleaned very gently.

The tissues are extremely friable and liable to infection if broken, so dirt must be removed gradually and gently.

Blisters should be left, and should not be pricked or removed as they form a covering. However, some blisters may be broken and soft, dry, adsorbent dressing should be used as a cover. Similar dressings between the fingers or toes will prevent friction and prevent further damage to the skin. Even light pressure can cause pressure sores, infection and loss of tissue.

So long as the affected part is warm and does not get rubbed it may be kept exposed.

Swelling may occur, and this can be countered by elevation.

Local antibiotics in aerosol form can be used but it is unwise to rely on this method alone for combating infection.

No tissue should be removed surgically as (a) it is impossible to assess the depth of frostbitten tissue, (b) the black carapace acts as a protective covering for regenerating tissue, and (c) premature surgery appears to have been the most potent cause of the poor results of treatment.

Active movements should be carried out to prevent joint stiffening, and if these are not possible, passive movement should be employed.

Progress

It must be stressed that surgical intervention should be minimal.

The blackened carapace will gradually separate by itself without interference. Efforts to hasten separation are usually ill advised and are likely to lead to infection, loss of tissue and delay in healing.

Because of the disturbance of sensation that accompanies frostbite, pockets of infection may appear either under the nail or under the carapace, and abscesses may occur without causing pain. These are extremely difficult to diagnose in the early stages, but may necessitate removal of the nail or drainage.

Too few cases are seen by any individual and there is a tendency to try more than one treatment in the hope that more rapid healing will occur.

In general, however, provided no surgical intervention occurs the majority of cases of frostbite seem to heal in six months to a year.

Prognosis

This should be guarded but optimistic.

In one case the whole of the forepart of both feet extending to the ankle and including the heel became black six weeks after the initial injury. In three months the carapace had separated down to and including the fifth toe of each foot. After six months, the worst affected area, the plantar and medial surface of the left big toe, finally lost its carapace. In eight months the skin of the feet and all the toes appeared normal.

In another patient, both of whose legs were essentially blocks of frozen tissue to above the knees when first seen, conservative treatment for about a year resulted in recovery except for patches of persistent gangrene on the plantar surface of the heels. Bilateral amputation was carried out for this reason alone.

It is likely that too many unnecessary amputations have been carried out because of impatience at slow recovery. The black carapace may persist for months and the failure to appreciate that it is a 'superficial' rather than a 'deep' gangrene may lead to precipitate surgery.

After Effects

Once a part is frostbitten it is more liable to cold injury on subsequent occasions.

The skin may crack when dry, even at normal temperatures, causing painful fissures in the pulps of the thumb and fingers. The use of a hand cream at regular intervals will soften the skin.

It is important to differentiate the vasospastic and neuropathic sequelae of frostbite.

Sympathectomy produces good results in the former cases, while aggravating paraesthesia. In mixed cases a peripheral nerve block with procaine may differentiate the two. If the skin temperature rises, sympathectomy is useful (De Takats 1959).

Hyperhidrosis has also been reported in the affected area.

Decalcification of bone, possibly due to local ischaemic areas, the result of sludging of end arteries, has been observed.

Compensation neurosis has been reported. In these cases there is often diffuse hyperhidrosis and increased vaso-motor reactivity throughout the body and not only in the exposed part.

Immersion Injury

Immersion injury occurs with prolonged exposure to non-freezing temperatures below 15°C, which produces a characteristic pattern with lasting damage to muscle and nerve.

Clinical Features

At least six hours seems to be necessary to produce a fully developed case of immersion injury.

There is difficulty in walking and balancing and an apt description is that 'it feels like walking on cotton wool'.

After immersion at near 0°C limbs were red, numb and powerless—but with less extreme cooling they were whitish-yellow or mottled blue-black.

No pulsation could be felt in the arteries and there was complete sensory and motor paralysis with little blood flow.

After 2–5 hours in a warm environment a high blood flow

appeared with full arterial pulses. The limbs became hot, red, swollen and painful. Blistering may occur. There was a partial return of sensation and power, but a considerable degree of anaesthesia and weakness persisted.

After weeks or months blood flow returned to normal but the limb became very sensitive to temperature changes. Cooling caused intense vasoconstriction, and heating intense vasodilatation. Profuse sweating also occurred. Sensory loss was often persistent but the most serious disorder was loss of muscle power with resulting contraction.

In certain cases blood flow never returned to some areas, probably due to arterial thrombosis. These ischaemic areas became gangrenous (Ungley *et al.* 1945).

Pathophysiology

The sequence of events may be that initially cold-induced vasodilatation occurs to a varying degree. Body temperature falls, and stored heat is lost. The cold vasodilatation may then be completely replaced by vasoconstriction and blood flow is virtually nil. Some blood flow must occur as blistering is present but this could have taken place initially during vasodilatation.

Once vasodilatation is replaced by vasoconstriction the part cools to the temperature of the surroundings in an hour or two. Nerve conduction may cease at these temperatures, and some degree of ischaemia is inevitable.

In the early stages the direct effects of low temperature on nerve and muscle could account for sensory and motor paralysis (Bickford 1939). Evidence that local cooling blocked mammalian nerve directly and not through local ischaemia has been obtained experimentally (Paintal 1965). Biopsy of late cases of immersion injury in man showed extensive degeneration of nerves (Blackwood 1944).

Muscle damage in rats' tails can be demonstrated histologically within two days of immersion injury, while histological change in muscle due to denervation does not appear for four weeks (Blackwood and Russell 1943). Cooling must therefore damage by other means than interruption of its nerve supply, and it seems likely that prolonged cooling to temperatures above 0°C can damage nerve and muscle directly.

Arteries in limbs exposed to immersion injury were not normally thrombosed but there was some indication that arterial thrombosis and gangrene occurred in limbs exposed to trauma. Ischaemia due to thrombosis was not an important factor though the blood flow was diminished as a result of vasoconstriction.

If the circulation had been completely arrested during the period of cooling damage would have occurred, though evidence for this was lacking. A relative ischaemia could have occurred during warming if local warming increased oxygen requirements before adequate blood flow returned.

Fat necrosis and atrophy are also recorded (Friedman 1945).

Treatment

The trunk should be heated to 40–44°C while the limbs are allowed to warm spontaneously as blood flow returns. As the tissues are anaesthetic it is necessary strictly to supervise any 'local' application of heat.

When blood flow returns and the limbs become swollen, they should be raised.

Later, if excessive sweating and sensitivity to cold are troublesome, sympathectomy may be carried out (Schumacker and Abramson 1947).

References

Anderson, R. A. and Hardenbergh, E. (1965) *Journal of Surgical Research* 5, 256.

Aturson, G. (1966) *Acta chirurgica scandinavica* 131, 402.

Bickford, R. G. (1939) *Clinical Science* 4, 159.

Blackwood, W. (1944) *British Journal of Surgery* 31, 329.

Blackwood, W. and Russell, H. (1943) *Edinburgh Medical Journal* 50, 385.

Crismon, J. M. and Fuhrman, F. A. (1947) *Journal of Clinical Investigation* **26**, 468.

De Takats, G. (1959) *Vascular surgery*. W. B. Saunders Co: Philadelphia and London.

Finneran, J. C. and Schumacker, H. B. (1950) *Surgery, Gynecology and Obstetrics* **90**, 430.

Friedman, N. B. (1945) *American Journal of Pathology* **21**, 387.

Fuhrman, F. A. and Fuhrman, G. J. (1957) *Medicine* **36**, 465.

Gildenbergh, P. L. and Hardenbergh, S. D. (1964) *Annals of Surgery* **160**, 160.

Golding, M. R., Mendoza, M. F., Hennigar, G. R., Fries, C. C. and Wesolowski, S. A. (1964) *Surgery* **56**, 221.

Greene, R. (1941) *Lancet* **2**, 689.

Greene, R. (1943) *Journal of Pathology and Bacteriology* **55**, 259.

Harkins, H. N. and Harmon, P. H. (1937) *Journal of Clinical Investigation* **16**, 213.

Keatinge, W. R. and Cannon, P. (1960) *Lancet* **1**, 11.

Mills, W. J., Whaley, R. and Fish, W. (1960) *Alaska Medicine* **2**, 114.

Mundth, E. D., Long, D. M. and Brown, R. B. (1964) *Journal of Trauma* **4**, 246.

Nelms, J. D. (1972) *Journal of the Royal Naval Medical Service* **58**, 192.

Paintal, A. S. (1965) *Journal of Physiology* **180**, 1.

Schumacker, H. B. and Abramson, D. I. (1947) *Annals of Surgery* **125**, 203.

Schumacker, H. B., Radigan, L. R., Haskel, H., Ziperman, H. H. and Hughes, R. R. (1951) *Angiology* **2**, 100.

Ungley, G. G., Channell, G. D. and Richards, R. L. (1945) *British Journal of Surgery* **33**, 17.

Ward, M. P., Garnham, R., Simpson, B. R., Morley, G. H. and Winter, J. N. (1968) *Proceedings of the Royal Society of Medicine* **61**, 787.

Washburn, N. (1962) *New England Journal of Medicine* **266**, 974.

Wilson, O. and Goldman, R. F. (1970) *Journal of Applied Physiology* **29**, 658.

CHAPTER TWENTY-SEVEN

Accidents

Accurate figures for the incidence of accidents and their mortality and morbidity are extremely difficult to obtain.

Figures that are available—and it is only recently that attempts have been made to obtain accurate statistics—do indicate certain trends.

The two main occupations that are carried out in the mountain environment are mountain travel on foot, ski-mountaineering and downhill skiing.

The types of accident that affect individuals engaged in these two occupations differ so they will be considered separately.

Mountaineering

Essentially mountaineers are subjected to dangers either of their own making, such as a slip, or to dangers inherent in the en-

Table 36.   Mortality rate in the European Alps

Period	Deaths	Annual average
1859–1885	134	5
1886–1891	214	35
1911–1913	486	160

vironment such as an avalanche or rock fall. Judgement, which depends on experience, will play a large part in accidents of either category. Rough statistics dating back to 1859 are available for the European Alps.

In the Swiss Alps there were 58 deaths in 1956 and 113 in 1968 or the number of deaths had doubled in 12 years. Between 1964 and 1968 in the Swiss Alps there were 641 deaths or an average of 130 each year. In 1967, there were 210,000 overnight stays in Swiss Alpine Club huts and the death rate that year in the Swiss Alps was 136.

Statistics for the whole Alps are not available but 68 deaths were reported in the French Alps in 1971 and 35 deaths in the Bavarian Alps in 1968. If one adds the average Swiss figure of 130 and takes into account the Italian and Austrian Alps, it seems that the average number of deaths each year in the European Alps would be of the order of 300 to 350.

Some recent accident statistics have been published in Great Britian by the Mountain Rescue Committee of the British Mountaineering Council. Between 1959 and 1968, the total number of accidents was 1521. Of these, 304 or 20 per cent were fatal (Hartley 1970).

Table 37.   Analysis of British rescue statistics

Category	%	Contribution to total death rate %
Climbers	42	8
Hill walkers	53·4	10
Caves, miscellaneous	4·6	2
	100	20

Despite an increase in the number of accidents each year, which is probably explained by the increase in the number of people at risk (i.e. an increase in the numbers climbing and walking), the number of fatalities has remained much the same; in other words, the percentage of fatalities has fallen.

Table 38.   Climbing accidents in Great Britian, 1957–66 (Meldrum 1969)

Year	Number of accidents in summer and winter climbing	Number of climbers at risk (approx.)
1957	25	19,000
1958	49	25,000
1959	49	26,000
1960	54	28,000
1961	48	30,000
1962	58	33,000
1963	68	34,000
1964	59	37,000
1965	80	38,000
1966	64	40,000

This is probably due to better equipment, improved techniques and the use of safety devices, and a general improvement in knowledge.

Other factors undoubtedly are an increase in rescue facilities especially by helicopter and dog search, more rescue points, and more rescue teams.

However new techniques have more effect in raising climbing standards than in increasing safety.

Causes

The cause of each accident is compounded of many factors.

Generally it is possible, however, to subdivide them into three main categories: (a) individual, (b) equipment, and (c) environment.

Every cause has an immediate factor and a contributory factor.

Individual

The most frequent cause of an accident is a slip, and this is the immediate factor in about 60–70 per cent of cases.

Other immediate factors are loss of control while glissading, the rope sticking, faulty use of equipment, over-confidence, fatigue and poor judgement.

Contributory factors are inexperience, climbing alone, climbing unroped and poor equipment.

Equipment
Failure of equipment does occur but it is rare. In one American series it accounted for 5 per cent of accidents.

Environment
Falling rock, avalanches and lightning have caused accidents.

However the individual is the main factor, although the equipment and the environment may play roles of differing importance.

Age

Half the number of accidents in one American series occurred to those under 25 years old. Under 20, the percentage was 30 (*American Alpine Journal* 1966).

In the United Kingdom, about 44 per cent of accidents occur to those under 21 years of age.

Injury

The percentage of different types of injury in the United Kingdom series were, lower limbs, 31; head, 23; upper limbs, 11; and exposure, 10.

The comparatively high incidence of head injury has led to the increasing use of crash helmets and in the last few years this has resulted in the rate of head injuries showing a decline.

The relatively high incidence of exposure cases is due to the tardy recognition that hypothermia can occur in wet–cold conditions above 0°C in gale force winds.

Until recently it was not fully appreciated that the amount of heat lost in wet–cold conditions could be lethal. Cases of exposure also occur in dry–cold conditions but they seem less common, probably because it is more obviously 'cold'.

Injuries at High Altitude

At high altitude, above 17,500 ft (5334 m), the added factor of hypoxia becomes increasingly important (Ward 1968).

The Table gives the mortality on expeditions to the world's ten highest peaks up to the date of their first ascent.

It can be seen that the majority of deaths have been due to accidents and exhaustion. It is difficult to assess the part played by high altitude deterioration but it could be argued that errors in judgement due to chronic hypoxia played a particularly large part in a number of these disasters.

Diseases associated directly with high altitude, namely cerebrovascular accident and pulmonary oedema have accounted for five deaths and frostbite has been responsible for two.

In general it appears that environmental factors play a larger part in mortality at altitudes exceeding 17,500 ft (5334 m) than at lower level.

The incidence of slips and other individual causes of accident due to over-confidence and lack of experience is much reduced because personnel selected for this type of expedition are usually both very experienced and very expert.

The increase in physiological understanding of high altitude and cold does not appear to have reduced the overall accident rate. This is because individuals always tend to push themselves to the limits of their physiological capacity under these circumstances.

The overall mortality rates from these expeditions up to and including the successful assault on each mountain is 64 deaths. Of these 41 were Sherpa porters and 23 non-porters (usually Europeans).

The total number of porters at risk is unknown but the figure is probably two or three times the total number of non-porters who numbered about 300.

There was therefore a mortality rate of approximately 6–7 per cent amongst non-porters and probably a little lower for porters on these expeditions.

Table 39a. Mortality on world's ten highest peaks up to first ascent

Mountain	Year of first ascent	Number of expeditions	Year	Personnel	Mortality Cause
Everest 29,160 ft 8888 m	1953	9	1921	1 European 1 Porter	? Heart failure Enteric fever
			1922	7 Porters	Avalanche
			1924	2 Europeans	? Exhaustion
				1 Porter	Cerebral thrombosis
				1 Porter	Frostbite
			1934	1 European	Exhaustion
			1952	1 Porter	Chest injury following avalanche.
			Total 15 deaths		
K2 (Godwin-Austen) 28,253 ft 8611 m	1954	5	1939	1 European 3 Porters	Exhaustion Exhaustion
			1953	1 European	Avalanche (previous pulmonary embolus)
			1954	1 European	? Pneumonia ? Pulmonary oedema
			Total 6 deaths		
Kanchenjunga 28,168 ft 8585 m	1955	6	1905	1 European 4 Porters	Avalanche
			1929	1 European	Lost
			1930	1 Porter	Avalanche
			1931	3 Porters	? Cause
				1 European	Killed in accident
			1955	1 Porter	Cerebral haemorrhage
			Total 12 deaths		
Lhotse 28,028 ft 8545 m	1956	1	No deaths		
Makalu 27,790 ft 8470 m	1955	3	1955	1 Liaison Officer	? Cause
			Total 1 death		
Dhaulagiri 26,811 ft 8172 m	1960	7	1954 1959	1 European 1 Porter	Frostbite Accident
			Total 2 deaths		
Cho Oyu 26,904 ft 8200 m	1954	2	No deaths		
Manaslu 26,658 ft 8125 m	1956	3	No deaths		

Table 39a contd.

Mountain	Year of first ascent	Number of expeditions	Year	Personnel	Mortality Cause
Nanga Parbat 26,658 ft 8125 m	1953	6	1895	1 European 2 Porters	Avalanche Avalanche
			1934	1 European 3 Europeans 5 Porters	? Pulmonary oedema Exhaustion Frostbite Exhaustion Frostbite
			1937	7 Europeans 9 Porters Total 28 deaths	Avalanche Avalanche
Annapurna 26,504 ft 8078 m	1950	1	No deaths		

Total deaths = 64
Total expeditions = 43
Total non-porter deaths = 23
Total non-porters at risk = about 300.

Table 39b. Causes of death

Cause	
Cerebral vascular accident	2
Frostbite	2
Enteric fever	1
Heart failure (?) or pulmonary oedema (?)	3
Exhaustion and sequelae	15
Avalanche and accident	36
Unknown	5
Total	64

Downhill Skiing

The incidence of skiing injuries is also difficult to assess.

It has been suggested from American statistics that depending on conditions the accident rate is between 2·2 and 13 per 1000 skiers per day (McIntyre 1963).

In 1958 there were about 3·5 million skiers in the United

States and if each skied for 12 man-days a year this would mean about 42 million ski man-days. If the accident rate was 3 per 1000 ski man-days there would have been about 125,000 skiing accidents in the United States in 1958 (Erskine 1959).

This figure must be more than doubled by 1974.

The Swiss figures in 1972 suggested that more than 60,000 people are injured in skiing accidents in Switzerland each winter. About half are said to suffer serious injury (*The Guardian* 1972).

Age

About 80 per cent of injuries occurred in individuals under 30 years of age, but only 30 per cent of the ski population are over 30 years old (Howarth 1966).

Table 40. Age distribution of injuries

Age in years	Percentage of injuries
0–10	16
11–20	44
21–30	23
31–40	10
Over 40	7

In general women seemed more prone to accidents than men.

Skiing is predominantly a sport of the unmarried, there being more unmarried males than females taking part.

Occurrence

In one Scottish series 15 per cent of injuries occurred on the first day; 50 per cent occurred in those who have been skiing for one year or less (Waldie 1967).

About 60 per cent of injuries occurred in beginners, 35 per cent in competent skiers and 5 per cent in expert skiers.

Most accidents occurred after about three hours skiing either just before lunch or tea (Moritz 1959). Fatigue is one important factor but others can be implicated. The slopes are more crowded at these times, and touring skiers go downhill in the afternoon. Soft snow, which is commoner around midday, leads to more frequent falls as it is more difficult to ski and more dangerous when heavy. The sudden change from piste to soft snow is particularly dangerous as the tips of the skis dig in. Off-piste spring skiing is more dangerous as very sudden changes in snow consistency are common according to the degree and position of the slope. Skiing on steep bumpy ground is ten times more productive of accidents.

Velocity

If a normally built person weighing 150 lb moves at 30 mph (the average speed whilst skiing) he will develop a momentum (mass × velocity) of 6600 foot pounds/second.

If he stops in 2 feet his stopping force is 2250 pounds (Leidholt 1963).

In optimum conditions a man weighing 150 lb reaches about 24 mph on a 3° slope, 52 mph on a 10° slope and 120 mph on a 45° slope (Haddon *et al.* 1962).

Types of Injury

The mortality rate is negligible.

Over 90 per cent of injuries are to the lower limbs. About 40 per cent of patients lost a season's skiing and 5 per cent lost two seasons.

The average time in plaster of Paris was eight weeks.

The following figures give some indication of the type and distribution of injury.

An oblique fracture of the lateral malleolus and an associated tear of the medial ligament is not uncommon. Dislocation of the talus may occur.

A spiral fracture of the tibia occurring in the middle third of the shaft, and associated with a spiral fracture in the upper third of the shaft of the fibula was not uncommon.

Transverse (boot-top) fracture of the tibia is relatively uncommon. However in the last few years a 'higher' boot—i.e. one

Table 41a–c.   Types of injury

	Per cent
(a) All injuries (Erskine 1959)	
Sprains	46
Fractures	29
Laceration	13
Dislocations	8
Others	4
(b) Sprains (Ellison 1962)	
Lower limb	
Ankle	41
Knee	39
Foot	7·4
Upper limb	8
Others	4·6

There were more females in the beginners group and more men in the expert group. A combination of ipsilateral knee and ankle injury is common. About 25 per cent of knee strains are associated with a sprain or fracture of the ankle.

(c) Fractures (Ellison 1962)	
Lower limb	89
Lateral malleolus	33·8
Medial malleolus	8·4
Bimalleolar	5·1
Tibial shaft	15·2
Tibia and fibula	21·9
Fibula shaft	0·8
Foot	2·1
Femur	0·4
Others	1·3
Upper limb	7·7
Others	3·3

extending up the lower third of the lower leg—has resulted in a higher incidence of fracture of the tibial shaft in relation to fractures of the ankles.

In 1926 and 1936 Mock investigated 1200 skiing accidents and found that of leg fractures 45 per cent occurred at the ankle and 9 per cent in the lower leg.

In 1963, Gruenages showed in a similar number that ankle and tibial fractures occurred equally frequently.

As the incidence of transverse fractures of the tibia has increased over the years, it appears that the high boot protects the ankle at the expense of the tibia.

Some fractures appear to have been caused by the safety strap that keeps the skis attached to the boot after the release bindings have opened.

Few if any fractures occur under the age of 10 years, and age has an effect on the site. This was first recognised by Bruns in 1886 (Bruns 1886). With age, a progression occurs from fracture of the tibial shaft, tibia and fibula, to ankle.

Lacerations can be serious especially with steel tipped skis. Runaway skis may cause penetrating injuries of the chest and abdomen and a case of castration has been reported.

Causes

Causes may be divided into (a) individual (loss of control, and collision), (b) equipment (faulty or incorrectly applied bindings), and (c), environment (poor conditions and visibility).

The most important factor is the individual. Injury is caused by the differing forces between the body of the skier, and the skis. This force is transmitted through the legs when a fall occurs.

The main movements of the lower limbs in these circumstances are

Pitch, that is, up and down movement of the heel or flexion and extension of the ankle; Yaw, or rotation; and Roll, either inversion or eversion.

In an accident there is usually a combination of these forces with one predominating.

Release Bindings

The use of safety or release bindings has diminished the accident risk to the lower limbs, yet strains and fractures still occur.

In one series 37 per cent of casualties had release bindings; in another 50 per cent of those who had accidents did not know the purpose of the release bindings, and did not know the difference in function between the side release and forward release bindings.

Even with correct functioning serious injury can still occur. In one series of 36 oblique fractures of the fibula, six occurred despite correct functioning of the release bindings. Three out of 15 cases of rupture of the tendo Achilles, occurred despite correct release.

At the present time a factor in leg injury is the non-safety of safety bindings (Henry 1967).

To work properly safety bindings must be adjusted correctly. The force required to open the bindings is dependent on the individual setting. Their 'stiffness' must be below the breaking strain of bone or rupture of ligaments. They should be made in such a way as to be incapable of being tightened too much. Their functioning should not be impeded by freezing-up, self locking, catching or jamming in any way.

References

American Alpine Journal (1966) *Report on accidents in North American mountaineering.*

Bruns, P. (1886) *Deutsche Chirurgie* **27**, 8.

Ellison, A. E., Carroll, R. E., Haddon, W. and Wolf, M. (1962) *Public Health Reports* **77**, 985.

Erskine, L. A. (1959) *American Journal of Surgery* **97**, 667.

Hadden, W., Ellison, A. E. and Carroll, R. E. (1962) *Public Health Reports* **77**, 973.

Hartley, H. K. (1970) *Alpine Journal* **75**, 267.

Henry, P. H. (1967) *Report to Ski-club of Great Britain. On accident prevention.*

Howorth, B. (1966) *Clinical Orthopaedics* **43**, 171.

Leidholt, J. D. (1963) *Surgical Clinics of North America* **43**, 363.

McIntyre, J. M. (1963) *Canadian Medical Association Journal* **88**, 602.

Meldrum, K. I. (1969) *Alpine Journal* **74**, 308.

Moritz, J. R. (1959) *American Journal of Surgery* **98**, 493.

The Guardian (1972). Article, 5 January.

Waldie, W. (1967) *Report to Ski-club of Great Britain. On accident prevention.*

Ward, M. P. (1968) *Diseases occurring at altitudes exceeding 17,500 ft.* M.D. Thesis. University of Cambridge.

CHAPTER TWENTY-EIGHT

Mental Performance

Of all the tissues of the body those of the nervous system are the least capable of withstanding oxygen lack. The cortical region is the most sensitive whilst the respiratory and circulatory centres possess greater resistance. The cerebral cortex should function normally as long as its oxygen tension is well above 5 mmHg and it has a small reserve of dissolved oxygen.

The survival times of different nervous tissue when completely deprived of oxygen are given in Table 43.

Table 43. Survival times of oxygen-deprived nervous tissue (Drinker 1938)

Type of cell	Minutes
Small pyramidal cells of cerebrum	8
Purkinje cells of cerebellum	13
Medullary centres	20–30
Spinal cord	45–60
Sympathetic ganglia	60
Myenteric plexus	180

It has been suggested that changes occur in the cortical cells at partial pressures of oxygen equivalent to an altitude of 28,000 ft (8534 m) and that some of these changes may be irreversible (Van der Molen 1939).

The oxygen stores in the body are as follows:

Table 44. Oxygen stores in the body

Form	Site	ml (STPD)
Haemoglobin	Venous blood	600
	Arterial blood	280
Myoglobin	Muscles	240
Solution	Tissues	56
Gas	Lungs	370
	Total	1546

Rate of utilisation at rest is 250 ml/min.
At rest the total available stored oxygen needed to maintain metabolism will last approximately five minutes. (Rahn 1964).

The average unacclimatised individual cannot live much beyond an altitude of 25,000 ft (7620 m) and only the well acclimatised person can withstand an altitude of 28,000 ft (8534 m) without oxygen. There is no evidence of permanent brain damage in eight of 20 individuals who have been to this height without oxygen.

Like the heart, the brain has a metabolic requirement which is disproportionate to its blood supply—or in other words it is a relatively hypoxic organ. The resting human brain, which comprises about 2·0 per cent of the body weight accounts for 20 per cent of the total oxygen consumption of the body and 15 per cent of the total cardiac output. Its oxygen consumption therefore equals that of the liver which is twice its size (Schmidt 1964).

Impaired cerebral function is associated with a decreased oxygen consumption, though the converse is not true. The lower limit of the physiological range is about half the normal level.

In acute anoxia the brain tissue Po_2 may fall from 24 mmHg (normal in anaesthetised dogs) to 0·7 mmHg within three minutes (Cater 1964). Under hypothermic conditions it is possible to deprive the brain of oxygen for longer periods.

Blood Supply
Hypoxia produces cerebral vasodilatation and an increased

blood flow to the medulla oblongata, hypothalamus and pial vessels. Both oxygen lack and hypercapnia (increased carbon dioxide) increase cerebral blood flow, but the effect of hypoxia is greater.

Slight variations in oxygen tension do not effect cerebral blood flow but a moderate decrease does.

In acute hypoxia blood flow begins to increase when the arterial Po_2 falls below 50 mmHg, and at a Po_2 of 40 mmHg the flow increases rapidly (Lambertsen 1958).

In spite of vasodilatation, it is generally conceded that during the hypoxia of high altitude, the brain is one of the first organs to be affected.

Hyperventilation (hypocapnia) reduced the cerebral blood flow at a given arterial Po_2. Thus cerebral blood flow depends on both arterial Po_2 and Pco_2, the carbon dioxide acting against the oxygen.

This restriction of the rise of cerebral blood flow may be a factor in the aetiology of acute mountain sickness (Pugh 1965).

Cerebral glucose utilisation is also increased in men under hypoxic condition. The proportion of glucose converted to lactic acid is increased, and excess lactate appears in the venous cerebral blood (Cohen *et al.* 1964).

Hypoxia produces changes by a combination of direct action on nervous tissue and by indirect action on the cerebral circulation.

If severe and prolonged it causes an increase in capillary permeability which permits the passage of protein into the extravascular space with subsequent rise of extravascular osmotic pressure. Fluid is drawn out of the vessels and oedema is produced. This interferes with the oxygenation of the partially damaged brain cells. The cerebrospinal fluid pressure rises, venous obstruction is encouraged, and further hypoxia occurs.

The histological appearance confirms this picture. There is vascular dilatation, perivascular haemorrhage, and associated stasis. Perivascular and perineural oedema occurs.

The severest lesions are found in the cerebral and cerebellar cortex and in the hippocampus. If in acute hypoxia death is delayed for 30–36 hours, evidence of cerebral congestion will be minimal, but after 36 hours necrosis of the brain cells is often found.

In acute hypoxia a reduction of arterial blood saturation to 85 per cent (Po_2 = 50 mmHg) results in a decreased capacity for mental concentration and abolishes finer muscular co-ordination.

A reduction to 75 per cent (Po_2 = 40 mmHg) results in faulty judgement, emotional lability and impairment of muscular function, whilst below 60 per cent (Po_2 = 32 mmHg) the individual becomes unconscious and there is a progressive depression of the central nervous system. An arterial oxygen saturation of 75 per cent was the lowest safe limit for voluntary directed movement (Ivy 1946).

It is worth commenting that the normal average oxygen saturation of individuals on five Himalayan expeditions at be-tween 17,500–21,500 ft (5300–6500 m) was 65–70 per cent: during exercise this fell to 45 per cent.

All accounts of the effects of high altitude stress that mental performance diminishes with altitude. It should be emphasised that though hypoxia is usually the main factor, other conditions may make an important contribution to this deterioration. These include hypothermia, under-nutrition, and fatigue, each of which may be associated with severe mental symptoms.

Haldane (Haldane and Priestley 1935) drew attention to the effects of chronic hypoxia—a diminution of the acuteness of the senses and intellect, loss of memory and judgement, and a tendency to uncontrolled emotional outbursts.

The removal of higher cortical control appears to be the first effect of hypoxia (Greene 1957). Diminution in will power, lack of observation, poor memory and the necessity for recording each observation immediately are repeatedly noted. Sustained mental work is however possible, and the main effect of altitude is mental laziness which determination can overcome.

Dulling of the special sense was recognised rather from the recovery in appreciation of light and colour on descent, than from its loss during ascent.

The most compelling feature of life over 23,000 ft (7010 m) is mental lassitude, with an astonishing indifference to events.

Acute Hypoxia

Under certain conditions, for instance when a miner walks into a pocket of methane gas, acute hypoxia can result in instant loss of consciousness.

When initially exposed to low oxygen tensions the individual may be stimulated. As oxygen lack stimulates the nervous system a state of euphoria, associated with a feeling of self-satisfaction, may occur. This is usually followed by a period of depression. With depression, emotional outbursts of a different nature occur and the personality may change for the worse.

As hypoxia affects the higher centres more rapidly, there is a blunting of the finest susceptibilities and a loss of judgement and of initiative. This may be associated with inflexibility of purpose, and the individual may pursue his objective regardless of risk to his own life and the lives of others.

Level of Useful Consciousness

Useful consciousness may be defined as that state in which the individual remains attentive and is able to perform useful or purposeful acts. Alternatively it may be defined as a term expressing the period between the time when the subject's oxygen supply is totally deprived at various altitudes and the onset of physical and mental deterioration. This is influenced to a certain extent by the individual's degree of adaptation to hypoxia and also the type of test used to determine a 'useful or purposeful act'. The period of useful consciousness at 43,000 ft (13,106 m) while breathing air is 13–15 seconds (Holmstrom 1971).

Ivy (Ivy 1946) cut off the oxygen supply of subjects at different altitudes and observed how long they continued to write. He stated that at 26,000 ft (7925 m) none of his subjects was able to continue writing longer than 15 minutes. Ability to write persisted at an arterial oxygen saturation greater than 66 per cent. Ivy felt that an arterial oxygen saturation of 75 per cent was the lowest safe limit for voluntary directed movement. With a card-sorting test, the average arterial oxygen saturation was 64 per cent when the first error appeared (Hoffman *et al.* 1964).

It was observed by Riesin (Riesin *et al.* 1946) and his co-workers that loss of useful consciousness after 185·7 seconds occurred at about 27,000 ft (8200 m). Volunteers who had ingested glucose retained consciousness for an average of 261 seconds.

Acclimatisation also increased the period of useful consciousness (Mackenzie *et al.* 1945).

Mental Performance at Different Altitudes

Between 5000 and 8000 ft (1500 and 2500 m), two main reactions occur.

The majority are stimulated, with slight euphoria, increased motor drive and periods of stimulated thinking. Impatience and irritability are also recorded.

A few people become depressed, with drowsiness, emotional indifference, deterioration in physical fitness and mental fatigue.

Symptoms usually last from several hours to days.

Between 8000 and 18,000 ft (2500 and 5500 m), two main reactions are again recorded—depression and euphoria, with occasionally alternation between the two.

Depression is more common, with physical and mental fatigue, some degree of indifference to events, and aversion to physical exertion, lassitude, drowsiness and diminished sexual interests.

Euphoria was associated with increased physical activity, feelings of happiness, emotional tension, irritability and explosive behaviour.

Aggressive and anti-social behaviour has also been observed (Ryn 1971).

Some changes in psychological function seem inevitable over about 15,000 ft (4572 m) and become more marked at higher altitudes.

The most common alterations in behaviour seem to be as follow (McFarland 1937(a)).

(i) Greater effort in carrying out tasks.
(ii) A more critical attitude towards other people.
(iii) Mental laziness.
(iv) A heightened sensory irritability.

(v) Increased sensitivity on certain subjects.
(vi) A dislike of being told how to do things.
(vii) Difficulty in concentrating.
(viii) Slowness in reasoning.
(ix) Frequent recurrence of ideas.
(x) Difficulty in remembering.

Above 18,000 ft (5500 m), diminished physical activity, clumsiness, disorientation, labile moods and imperfect perceptions have been noted.

At 21,000 ft (6401 m) mental activity appeared to be little impaired. Crossword puzzles were solved in a comparable time and with no more difficulty than at sea level.

Gas analysis was carried out with relatively few errors (Pugh and Ward 1956).

Above 22,500 ft (6860 m) impairment of mental performance becomes more apparent, and mental disturbance is commoner if oxygen is not used.

Disorders of consciousness, lapses of memory, variations in mood, speech disturbances and disturbance of orientation in both space and time have all been recorded.

Many individuals have complained of poor memory, and periodic depression and decreased sexual potency for a fairly long period. Mental efficiency was often lower and outbreaks of irritability not uncommon.

Deterioration in character has been noted.

On one pre-war Everest expedition one man became withdrawn on the North Col 23,000 ft (7104 m) and as a result took little further part in the expedition. Delirious and paranoid psychoses have been recorded.

By contrast some men became more placid at high altitude.

Simple sensory and motor responses were not impaired until about 24,000 ft (7315 m). At this altitude too impairment of higher functions and memory were also noted.

Responses requiring the exercise of choice were impaired before those involving simple reactions. Routine tasks were undertaken without difficulty at 24,500 ft (7460 m), whereas unfamiliar situations requiring initiative took longer and were more difficult to begin.

Lack of critical judgement and foresight are all too familiar and vital items of food and equipment are forgotten. Poor decisions are common. This was probably a cause for pairing Irvine, a newcomer to altitude, rather than the experienced Odell, with Mallory on the summit attempt on Everest in 1924. Perhaps the 'fixity of purpose' induced by hypoxia was mainly responsible for the death of Mallory and Irvine on this occasion.

At 26,000 ft (7925 m) one member of the successful 1953 Everest Expedition collapsed on the ground. No sympathy was shown and the comment, 'Poor Tom, he's had it', summed up the feelings of the party.

Above 26,000 ft (7925 m) there is considerable retardation of thought and action associated with physical and mental depression.

Hallucinations have been recorded by one mountaineer climbing at 28,000 ft (8534 m) without oxygen (Smythe 1934).

Sleeping and Dreaming

It is common for sea-level visitors to high altitudes to complain of restless sleep and disturbing dreams. However these pass off as the individual becomes acclimatised.

Dreams tend to be fantastic and illusory in nature during the acclimatisation period but then become infrequent with little consciousness of sex or anxiety which occurred in dreams at sea level.

McFarland (McFarland 1937(a)) comments that the dreams which accompanied the greatest physiological disturbance were usually the most vivid and fantastic.

Nocturnal emission of semen has been reported during sleep at 27,400 ft (8350 m). Presumably this is a hypoxic effect.

Muscle Control

The more severe the hypoxia the greater the loss of the ability to exercise the muscular control required to write normally.

As hypoxia progresses the writing becomes less and less legible (McFarland 1932).

The type of paralysis produced by hypoxia is an ascending one.

Initially the legs lose their power, the arms then become affected, and the neck muscles are the last to become involved.

This was illustrated dramatically in acute hypoxia during a balloon ascent by Coxwell and Glaisher. Coxwell was paralysed apart from his neck muscles. He could still move his head and was able to grasp the rope release with his teeth. This enabled the balloon to descend and saved his own and his companion's life.

Accounts of mountaineering at high altitude are full of incidents indicating that control of the legs was poor and that walking, even downhill, demanded an infinite degree of concentration. Arm movements by contrast appear to be more normal.

Paraesthesia of the legs occurred in one mountaineer on the top of Everest after his oxygen set had been removed for a period.

Special Senses

Visual

The retina is closely related to the brain in its structure and it has a similar metabolism. It is therefore as sensitive to oxygen lack.

Balloonists were the first to comment that accommodation was affected by high altitude, and they experienced difficulty in making barometer readings.

Some visual disturbances were experienced by Barcroft's party at an altitude of 14,200 ft (4300 m) in the Andes, whilst at 28,000 ft (8534 m) on Everest one mountaineer described a pulsating object in the sky.

There appears to be a diminution in sensitivity to light above 7400 ft (2300 m). At a simulated altitude of 15,000 ft (4570 m) a light intensity 2·5 times greater than normal was required in order for it to be seen (McFarland and Evans 1939).

Visual acuity is also reduced at high altitude.

While the central field of vision appears to be unaffected there does appear to be evidence that peripheral vision is slightly constricted (Evans and McFarland 1938).

The diameter of the retinal vessels increases at high altitude, the veins dilating more than the arteries (Cusick *et al.* 1940). It is interesting that patients with disease due to high altitude have been noted to suffer dilation of the retinal capillaries.

Some fatigue of accommodation and convergence has been reported. This seems to start at about 15,000 ft (4572 m). At 18,000 ft (5486 m), there is a general tendency towards diminished precision in ocular fixation and certain latent defects in normal ocular muscle balance were shown up.

Aural

In progressively increasing hypoxia at simulated altitudes, the sense of hearing is the last to disappear.

A decrease in auditory sensitivity has been noted at about 14,000–15,000 ft (4267–4572 m) and above, both in simulated conditions and in the field.

In general, acclimatisation to altitude seems to increase the auditory threshold (McFarland 1937).

All sensation is damped at high altitude. This is almost impossible to detect subjectively. It is only on descent to lower levels that the individual is aware of heightened perception and the appreciation of sensations which he had not realised were impaired.

References

Cater, D. B. (1964) *Cerebral blood supply and cerebral oxidative metabolism. In*, General discussion to, *Oxygen in the animal organism. Ed.* Dickens, F. and Neil, E. Pergamon Press: Oxford.

Cohen, P. J., Wollman, M., Alexander, S. C., Chase, P. E., Smith, T. C., Melman, E., Behar, M. G. and Price, H. L.

(1964) *Federation Proceedings. Federation of American Societies for Experimental Biology* **23**, 521.

Cusick, P. L., Benson, O. O. and Boothby, W. M. (1940) *Proceedings. Mayo Clinic* **15**, 500.

Drinker, C. K. (1938) *Carbon monoxide asphyxia.* Oxford University Press: New York.

Evans, J. N. and McFarland, R. A. (1938) *American Journal of Ophthalmology* **21**, 968.

Greene, R. (1957) *British Medical Journal* **1**, 1028.

Haldane, J. S. and Priestley, R. (1935) *Respiration.* Oxford.

Hoffman, C. E., Clark, R. T. and Brown, E. B. (1946) *American Journal of Physiology* **145**, 685.

Holmstrom, F. M. G. (1971) Hypoxia. In, *Aerospace medicine. Ed.* Randell, H. W. Williams Wilkins: Baltimore.

Ivy, A. C. (1946) *Federation Proceedings. Federation of American Societies for Experimental Biology* **5**, 319.

Lambertsen, C. J. (1958) In, *Man's dependence on his earthly atmosphere. Ed.* Schafer, K. E. Macmillan: New York.

McFarland, R. A. (1932) *Archives of Psychology* **145**, 110.

McFarland, R. A. (1937(a)) *Journal of Comparative Psychology* **24**, 147.

McFarland, R. A. (1937(b)) *Journal of Comparative Psychology* **23**, 191.

McFarland, R. A. and Evans, J. N. (1939) *American Journal of Physiology* **127**, 37.

Mackenzie, C. G., Riesen, A. H., Bailey, J. R., Tahmisian, T. N. and Crocker, P. L. (1945) *Journal of Aviation Medicine* **16**, 156.

Pugh, L. G. C. E. (1965) *High Altitude.* In, *Physiology of human survival. Ed.* Edholm, O. and Bacharach, A. L. Academic Press: New York and London.

Pugh, L. G. C. E. and Ward, M. P. (1956) *Lancet* **271**, 1115.

Rahn, H. (1964) *Oxygen stores in man.* In, *Oxygen in the animal organism. Ed.* Dickens, F. and Neil, E. Pergamon Press: Oxford.

Riesin, A. M., Tahmisian, T. N. and Mackenzie, C. G. (1946) *Proceedings of the Society for Experimental Biology and Medicine* **63**, 250.

Ryn, Z. (1971) *Acta medica polonica* **12**, 3.
Schmidt, C. F. (1964) *Cerebral blood supply and cerebral oxidative metabolism.* In, *Oxygen in the animal organism.* Ed. Dickens, F. and Neil, E. Pergamon Press: Oxford.
Smythe, F. S. (1934) In, *Everest 1933.* Ed. Ruttledge, H. Hodder and Stoughton.
Van der Molen, H. R. (1938) *Nederlands tijdschrift voor geneeskunde* **83**, 4921.

CHAPTER TWENTY-NINE

Psychological Survey of Mountaineers

The mountaineer, through a long and patient study of his craft and as a result of a variety of experiences gained in many different kinds of mountain country, can learn to move safely in situations which, but for his skill, would be unacceptably dangerous. Once he makes climbing a substitute for living a normal life he takes the danger inherent to the mountain environment as a stimulant and becomes a danger to himself and others.

Investigations were carried out at the Leeds Institute of Education into four separate groups of British mountaineers and a control of nonclimbers (those with no further interest or who had never climbed and had no desire to do so) using the Cattell and Eban 16 Personality Factor Questionnaire (Gray 1968).

The groups were classified as:

(i) Top climbers. (28 subjects)

All were members of the Alpine Climbing Group. This contains a high proportion of outstanding mountaineers and rock climbers, many with considerable expedition experience. The standard for entry is high and with few exceptions disqualification is automatic at the age of 40 or if climbs of a high enough standard are not continued.

(ii) Rock-climbing instructors. (28 subjects)
(iii) Average rock climber. (39 subjects)
(iv) General interest in mountain activities. (45 subjects)
(v) Nonclimbers. (11 subjects)

The main findings could be summarised as follows.

The top climbers were more reserved, detached, critical and cool than the average rock climber, the nonclimber and the mountain activities group. The rock climbing instructors were also more aloof than the others.

There was no significant difference in emotional stability between the groups.

All those who were interested in mountain activities and rock climbing were more aggressive, asserted themselves more, and were more stubborn than the non-rock climbers.

The top climbers were prone to act from expediency, evaded rules more and felt fewer obligations than the others.

The top climbers and instructors were more self sufficient, preferred their own decisions and were more resourceful than those interested in general mountain activities. The nonclimbers were also more self sufficient than the mountain activities group.

Both the top climbers and nonclimbers were more intelligent and abstract thinking than the mountain activities group and average rock climbers.

The instructors and nonclimbers were more trusting, adaptable, free of jealousy and easier to get on with than the mountain activities group and rock climbers.

The instructors were more placid, self assured and confident than the average rock climber.

The instructors were more experimental, critical, liberal, analytical and free thinking than the mountain activities group and the average rock climber.

The top climbers appeared to be more intelligent, abstract thinking, socially reserved, detached and cool than the other groups. They tended to be withdrawn and cautious, and preferred one or two close friends to large groups. In addition they were very self sufficient, liked to make their own decisions, were highly competitive and aggressive and resourceful in their chosen sphere of activity.

The mountain instructors were more closely aligned to the nonclimbers than to other climbing groups. With the non-climbers they were more adaptable, less competitive, more concerned with other people and easier to get along with than the other groups. They were also placid, confident and serene, whilst in thought they were liberal and analytic.

As far as emotional stability and sociability were concerned climbers and nonclimbers were about equal.

Personality characteristics of members of the 1963 American Everest team were investigated by the California Personality Inventory Scales (Lester 1969).

The Everest teams average scores were highest and definitely above normal on the following scales.

Scale	High scorers tend to be
Psychologically-mindedness	Observant, spontaneous, changeable, rebellious against rules, restrictions and constraints.
Achievement via independence	Mature, forceful, strong, demanding, dominant, foresightful.
Dominance	Aggressive, confident, persistent, self reliant and independent (having leadership potential and initiative).
Flexibility	Adventurous, confident, humorous, rebellious, idealistic, egoistic, sarcastic and cynical, highly concerned with personal pleasure and diversion.

| Self-acceptance | Intelligent, outspoken, sharpwitted, demanding, aggressive and self-centred. |
| Intellectual efficiency | Efficient, capable, progressive, planful, thorough, alert, well informed. Placing a high value on cognitive and intellectual matters. |

The Everest teams average scores were lowest on the following:

Scale	Low scores tend to be
Socialisation	Defensive, demanding, stubborn, opinionated, headstrong, rebellious and undependable.
Good impression	Inhibited, cautious, shrewd, wary, aloof. Cool and distant in relationships with others. Self centred.

Studies by Ryn (Ryn 1971) on twenty Polish men and ten women mountaineers revealed that two main types of personality could be distinguished—the schizoid–psychasthenic and the asthenio–neurotic.

The schizoid–psychasthenic personality was commonest, characterised by features such as secretiveness, reserve and the avoidance of contact with other people. They were distinguished by great emotional sensitivity but had difficulty in revealing this. Not at all sure of themselves they had a feeling of inferiority associated with a high level of aspiration. As a rule they were extremely active, self-reliant, and tended towards eccentric and unconventional behaviour.

They had marked difficulty in submitting to social and collective discipline. Emotionally they were unstable, obstinate, over-sensitive and often aggressive. All were in good physical condition and had a high degree of tolerance to frustration.

Within this group a few individuals had a tendency to isolate themselves and to seek to be alone; they showed outward emotional coolness and mistrust and suspicion of contacts with others.

The other type of personality—the asthenic–neurotic—was especially characterised by timidity, shyness, a feeling of inferiority and many neurotic symptoms. These individuals felt a great need to be conspicuous among their contemporaries and had high ambitions and aspirations. For many, childhood illness and other factors in early life had led to a feeling of inferiority in personal worth and physical efficiency, and had resulted in them avoiding people of their own age and a desire to test themselves so that they sought difficulties and danger.

Often the feeling of inferiority, and especially of general muscular weakness, resulted either from their physical build or from susceptibility to disease in childhood, or prolonged childhood illness leading to impaired physical development. The feeling of restricted physical movement and inability to take part in games or gymnastics was often very marked and resulted, when the person was able to take part in physical activities such as mountaineering, in his driving himself to become exceptionally fit physically.

In both groups most showed outstanding intelligence.

Women seemed less well adjusted and had more neurotic symptoms, were more sensitive and less able to resist frustration.

Men were well adjusted, had a strong need to dominate and to stress their own ego, had a great tolerance of frustration and a feeling of security and self-sufficiency.

All these studies were characterised by weak sexuality and little interest in their occupations.

In most mountaineers the first encounter with mountains brought an experience of fascination and wonder—an emotional revelation of something new and unknown. Many chose occupations and places to work so that they could be near mountains. Often the experience brought back from the mountains gave inspiration for creative work.

The most attractive aspect was the opportunity of experiencing emotion mingled in their nature. For many it became impossible to replace the desire to climb mountains by any other form of activity.

Other motives mentioned were the taking of independent decisions, absence of social restrictions, freedom of movement, the chance to take risks and expose oneself to danger, and the need for freedom from conventional daily life which was often unattractive and emotionally monotonous.

The aesthetic interest in landscape played a secondary role.

By comparison with other sports which involve extreme conditions, the elements of heroism, combating loneliness, the overcoming of natural difficulties and the feelings of fear and other weakness played an important part.

These mountaineers fully realised the dangers inherent in their sport and in fact one outstanding factor of the modern climber is that he makes every effort to be as safe as possible. Essentially the psychological satisfaction gained is stronger than their fear.

It appears therefore that there is a good deal of overlap in the type of person chosen for an American Everest team and the top British climbers. This is not surprising as Everest teams tend to be chosen from the best mountaineers. The Polish group also tended to have similar personality traits.

References

Gray, D. (1968) *Alpine Journal* **73**, 167.
Lester, J. T. (1969) *Alpine Journal* **74**, 101.
Ryn, Z. (1971) *Acta medica polonica* **12**, 3.

Index